AF556808

The Biology of Echinococcus

and Hydatid Disease

The Biology of Echinococcus and Hydatid Disease

Edited by R. C. A. Thompson

School of Veterinary Studies,

Murdoch University, Western Australia

London
GEORGE ALLEN & UNWIN
Boston Sydney

**George Allen & Unwin (Publishers) Ltd,
40 Museum Street, London WC1A 1LU, UK**

George Allen & Unwin (Publishers) Ltd,
Park Lane, Hemel Hempstead, Herts HP2 4TE, UK

Allen & Unwin Inc.,
Fifty Cross Street, Winchester, Mass 01890 USA

George Allen & Unwin Australia Pty Ltd,
8 Napier Street, North Sydney, NSW 2060, Australia

First published in 1986

British Library Cataloguing in Publication Data

The Biology of Echinococcus and hydatid disease.
1. Echinococcosis 2. Veterinary parasitology
I. Thompson, R. C. A.
616.9′64 RC184.T6
ISBN 0-04-591020-0

Library of Congress Cataloging-in-Publication Data
Main entry under title:
The Biology of Echinococcus and hydatid disease.
Includes bibliographies and index.
1. Echinococcosis. 2. Echinococcus. I. Thompson, R. C. A.
[DNLM: 1. Echinococcosis. 2 Echinococcus.
WC 840 B615]
RC184.T6B56 1985 616.9′64 85-9066
ISBN 0-04-591020-0 (alk. paper)

Set in 10 on 11½ point Bembo by Columns of Reading
and printed in Great Britain by Butler & Tanner Ltd,
Frome and London

Preface

Although the need for a volume restricted entirely to *Echinococcus* and hydatid disease has been evident for some time, it was the recent retirement of James Desmond Smyth which acted as the stimulus for this book.

In 1964, Desmond Smyth commented – 'considering the status of hydatid disease as a disease of world importance, surprisingly little is known regarding the general biology of the causative organism'. Today, 20 years later, the medical, veterinary and economic significance of hydatid disease has not diminished, in fact there is evidence that the causative agent, *Echinococcus*, is spreading into areas previously free of infection. However, the nine chapters assembled in this volume are striking evidence of the major advances which have been made in our understanding of *Echinococcus* and hydatid disease. Since the early 1960s, biological, epidemiological and immunological research on *Echinococcus* has expanded rapidly and there is now much fresh knowledge of life-cycle patterns, host–parasite relationships and the speciation of the organism. Similarly, marked progress has been achieved in the surveillance, control, treatment and diagnosis of hydatid disease.

It is perhaps surprising that such a volume devoted to a parasite that has been recognised as a serious pathogen since the time of Hippocrates (see Ch. 3) has not appeared before now. My aim has therefore been to embrace all aspects of *Echinococcus* and hydatid disease, the only area consciously avoided concerns surgical treatment of the disease in man, which probably warrants a volume in itself. This book thus provides a comprehensive and authoritative account of the present state of knowledge of one of the world's major zoonoses. As such, it is hoped that students and research workers in parasitology and human and veterinary medicine will find this book of value, as well as personnel directly involved with the surveillance, treatment and control of hydatid disease. However, I do not wish to suggest a limited readership, quite the contrary. Research on this fascinating and intriguing tapeworm has contributed enormously to the broad field of cestode biology, and in particular to host–parasite relationships, immunobiology, biochemistry, physiology and speciation. These contributions are abundantly evident throughout this book.

It is clear from Professor Rogers' Appreciation that Desmond Smyth's contribution to the field of tapeworm biology, and in particular his inspiring and varied research on *Echinococcus*, has been enormous. His name appears frequently throughout the pages of this book, thus demonstrating his broad influence in this field of parasitological endeavour.

I am honoured to have had the enjoyable task of editing this volume. The high quality of the contributions by Desmond Smyth's colleagues and their wide-ranging and up-to-date coverage makes this *Festschrift* a most appropriate tribute to the stimulating force of Desmond Smyth's work and the extent of his influence on *Echinococcus* and hydatid disease research.

Finally, I should like to acknowledge the thoughtfulness of Professor Roy Anderson who initially conceived this volume.

Murdoch, Western Australia R. C. A. THOMPSON
July 1984

Cover illustration A glazed pottery ceramic of the scolex of adult *Echinococcus* showing hooks and suckers. It was sculpted by Dr Sheila White, Lecturer in Anatomy in the School of Veterinary Studies, Murdoch University, who was inspired by a scanning electron micrograph of the scolex. Mr Geoff Griffiths, of the same department, took the photograph.

Contents

Contributors

C. Bryant, Professor of Zoology, Department of Zoology, Australian National University, Canberra, ACT 2601, Australia

J. Eckert, Professor of Parasitology and Director, Institute of Parasitology, University of Zurich, Winterthurestrasse 266, Switzerland

M. A. Gemmell, Director, Hydatid Research Unit, Ministry of Agriculture and Fisheries, University of Otago Medical School, Dunedin, New Zealand

D. D. Heath, Section Leader, Hydatid Research, Research Division, Ministry of Agriculture and Fisheries, Wallaceville Animal Research Centre, Private Bag, Upper Hutt, New Zealand

M. J. Howell, Reader in Zoology, Department of Zoology, Australian National University, Canberra, ACT 2601, Australia

J. R. Lawson, Scientist, Hydatid Research Unit, Ministry of Agriculture and Fisheries, University of Otago Medical School, Dunedin, New Zealand

M. W. Lightowlers, National Health and Medical Research Council Senior Research Officer, Veterinary Clinical Centre, University of Melbourne, Princes Highway, Werribee, Victoria 3030, Australia

D. P. McManus, Lecturer in Parasitology, Department of Pure and Applied Biology, Imperial College of Science and Technology, London, England

R. L. Rausch, Professor of Animal Medicine and Professor of Pathobiology, Division of Animal Medicine and Department of Pathobiology, University of Washington, Seattle, Washington 98195, USA

M. D. Rickard, Reader in Veterinary Parasitology, Veterinary Clinical Centre, University of Melbourne, Princes Highway, Werribee, Victoria 3030, Australia

W. P. Rogers, Emeritus Professor, Department of Plant Physiology, Waite Agricultural Research Institute, University of Adelaide, Glen Osmond, South Australia 5064, Australia

C. W. Schwabe, Professor of Epidemiology, Department of Epidemiology and Preventive Medicine, University of California, Davis, California 95616, USA

R. C. A. Thompson, Senior Lecturer in Parasitology and Head, World Health Organisation Collaborating Centre for Echinococcosis/Hydatidosis, Division of Veterinary Biology, School of Veterinary Studies, Murdoch University, Western Australia 6150, Australia

Professor J. D. Smyth – an appreciation on his retirement

James Desmond Smyth is a distinguished academic and scientist. As a teacher, author of books, guide and mentor of postgraduate students, he is regarded with respect and – for many who worked more closely with him – affection. As a research worker he has achieved distinction for his study of parasites and especially for his work on *Echinococcus granulosus*. The study of parasites is apt to invite the uncritical collection of data: Smyth was not of that school. His research, from the earliest to his latest papers, has been directed towards the solution of problems largely concerned with the fundamental features of parasitism.

Smyth was born in Dublin, Ireland, in 1917. At Trinity College of the University of Dublin he obtained the degrees of BA and BSc in 1940, his PhD in 1942 and his DSc in 1958. After serving as Lecturer in Zoology at the University of Leicester (1942–5) and the University of Leeds (1945–7) he returned to Trinity College where he became Professor of Experimental Biology in 1955.

I got to know him well when he came to Australia in 1959 as Foundation Professor of Zoology in the School of General Studies at the Australian National University, Canberra. To the regret of his colleagues and friends in Australia he left in 1970 to become Professor of Parasitology at Imperial College of Science and Technology, London, where he remained until he retired in 1982. He is now Emeritus Professor of Parasitology, University of London and Senior Research Fellow of the College. Just recently he was awarded a Leverhulme Trust Emeritus Fellowship at the London School of Hygiene and Tropical Medicine where he will prepare a new edition of his monograph, *The physiology of cestodes*.

That is the bare outline of a successful academic career. It was the outcome of a wide knowledge of biology, intellectual ability, experience and hardwork. But to this must be added the man's personal charm – his rather withdrawn depreciating manner, his gentle Irish sense of humour, humanity and generosity. His personal charm and an underlying determination to achieve the goals he set himself are important factors in Smyth's success as an academic. This was especially notable in the setting-up of his new department at the Australian National University in competition with other newly established departments in the Faculty of Science. As a result the Department of Zoology had a good start: indeed it has been said that Smyth's skill in pursuing the needs of his own department led to a general lift in the standards of the whole new faculty. But it also led, as might be expected in the fiercely competitive arena of academia, to criticism and outright opposition – especially among members of the Faculty of Science outside his own department.

Smyth came to Australia with an established reputation and at the Australian National University he flourished. In a decade he not only built up an excellent department from scratch, but he also published a fine textbook and two monographs which, in my opinion, are still the best in the field. And he continued his personal research work with vigour and even greater success.

At Imperial College Smyth followed Professor B. G. Peters, a nematologist, in a long-established and distinguished department. The contrast with the Australian National University must have been considerable. In the one, life in what was then a small town in the bush, building up a new department with great scope for individual initiative in selecting courses, staff, and even in the design of laboratories. In the other, a member, with several other professors, in a department long-established materially and intellectually, in central London. It says much for the man that he was able to accommodate himself to the change and to continue successfully in his own chosen field of research.

It is as a research worker in parasitology rather than as an academic zoologist on which Desmond Smyth's international reputation is based. Parasitology is a branch of science for which a specifically unique intellectual content cannot be claimed; with the notable exception of some early papers, much of the advance in our knowledge of parasitology has been based on previous advances in other branches of biology, chemistry and, more rarely, in physics. Indeed, in the past, research in parasitology has seldom – again with the exception of some early papers – illustrated other areas of science. In recent years, however, this has become more common: a change which Smyth, in his general approach to the study of parasites has accelerated.

J. D. Smyth was one of that small group of research workers who directed the emphasis in parasitological research from the pragmatic investigation of parasites as pests of economic importance to the investigation of parasitism as a biological phenomenon. And he used a wide range of scientific expertise: from biochemistry and physiology to experimental biology and morphology. The breadth of his knowledge of biology is shown in his imaginative article on 'Parasites as biological models' (Smyth 1969). In this paper he discussed the use of parasites for research in a broad range of disciplines from immunology to cytodifferentiation. Of particular interest to me was his proposal that development in complex life cycles might involve a series of gene sets controlled by mechanisms based on the Jacob–Monod model of gene action.

During his career as a research worker Smyth frequently returned to a basic problem of parasitism: the nature of the factors which govern host specificity. He has been primarily concerned with the properties of the gut and its secretions which favour or prevent infection, especially with *Echinococcus*. The major outcome of this work, I believe, is the recognition that the nature of the hosts' bile is, in some species, an important factor in determining specificity (see, for example, Smyth 1962a, Smyth & Haslewood 1963). These studies culminated, fittingly enough, in results which indicated the potential infectivity to man of various strains of *Echinococcus granulosus*.

I think that Smyth's major contribution to biological science stems from his work with whole organisms in artificial environments which are complex in their physical structure as well as in their chemistry. Most notable in this respect was the discovery of the cultural conditions which controlled the differentiation of protoscoleces of *Echinococcus granulosus* in either the cystic form or the adult strobilated tapeworm (Smyth 1967, and see Ch. 5 for further details). Initially Smyth (1962b) was successful, by manipulating the biochemical and biophysical character of a liquid medium, in cultivating individual protoscoleces to the formation of small hydatid cysts, thus duplicating, to a considerable degree, the differentiation and development which takes place when a hydatid cyst is ruptured and protoscoleces are freed in the tissues of the intermediate host. Next, Smyth developed a 'diphasic medium' – a liquid phase overlying a solid serum base – for the development of the strobilar stage. This was the outcome of a series of papers in which the nutritional features of the liquid and solid phases necessary for growth were examined. It was also inspired by Smyth's observations on the physiology of the rostellum (Smyth 1964) and of the process of evagination of protoscoleces.

In recent years 'The insemination–fertilisation problem in cestodes cultured *in vitro*' (reviewed under this title by Smyth 1982) has been in the forefront of Smyth's research interests. This problem was tackled, with considerable success, in early work with *Schistocephalus solidus* (see, for example, Smyth 1954). And at the time of his retirement Smyth was engaged in similar but more difficult studies with *Echinococcus granulosus*.

Two of Professor Smyth's textbooks, an *Introduction to animal parasitology* (1962c, and a second edition, 1976) and *Frogs as host–parasite systems* (1980, with Mildred Smyth) have been widely used for the teaching of parasitology to undergraduates which became a special interest of his later years. But, as might be expected, the postgraduate students from many countries who studied in Smyth's laboratories at Trinity College, the Australian National University and Imperial College were mostly responsible for broadening his influence in parasitology.

In recognition of his contribution to knowledge J. D. Smyth has been honoured by scientific societies: in UK, where he is an Honorary Member and past President of the British Society for Parasitology; in USA an Honorary Member of the American Society of Parasitologists; and in Australia, past President and Honorary Fellow of the Australian Society for Parasitology. He is also a Fellow of the Linnean Society of London and a Fellow of the Royal Society of Tropical Medicine and Hygiene.

Smyth has been a member of the editorial boards of *Experimental Parasitology*, and at present serves on the board of *Zeitschrift für*

Parasitenkunde, he was also foundation editor of the *International Journal for Parasitology*. During 1963–1964 he was Visiting Overseas Fellow, Churchill College, Cambridge.

It would be remiss of me to end this article without mentioning Mrs Mildred Smyth, 'Mim' to her friends, who worked and published with research worker Desmond Smyth, and who so ably supported the Professor J. D. Smyth socially, and in the handling of his academic problems.

Adelaide, South Australia W. P. ROGERS

REFERENCES

Smyth, J. D. 1954. Studies in tapeworm physiology. VII. Fertilization of *Schistocephalus solidus in vitro*. *Exp. Parasitol.* **3**, 64–71.

Smyth, J. D. 1962a. Lysis of *Echinococcus granulosus* by surface active agents in bile and the role of this phenomenon in determining host specificity in helminths. *Proc. R. Soc. B* **156**, 553–72.

Smyth, J. D. 1962b. Studies in tapeworm physiology. X. Axenic cultivation of the hydatid organism, *Echinococcus granulosus*; establishment of a basic technique. *Parasitology* **52**, 441–57.

Smyth, J. D. 1962c. *Introduction to animal parisitology*. London: Hodder & Stoughton.

Smyth, J. D. 1964. Observations on the scolex of *Echinococcus granulosus* with special reference to the occurrence and cytochemistry of secretory cells in the rostellum. *Parasitology* **54**, 515–26.

Smyth, J. D. 1967. Studies in tapeworm physiology. XI. Axenic cultivation of the protoscoleces of *Echinococcus granulosus* to the strobilate stage. *Parasitology* **57**, 111–33.

Smyth, J. D. 1969. Parasites as biological models. *Parasitology* **59**, 73–91.

Smyth, J. D. 1976. *Introduction to animal parasitology*, 2nd edn. London: Hodder & Stoughton.

Smyth, J. D. 1982. The insemination–fertilization problem in cestodes cultured *in vitro*. In *Aspects of parasitology. A* Festschrift *dedicated to the fiftieth anniversary of the Institute of Parasitology of McGill University 1932–1982*, E. Meerovitch (ed.), 393–406. Montreal: McGill University.

Smyth, J. D. and G. A. D. Haslewood 1963. The biochemistry of bile as a factor in determining host specificity in intestinal parasites, with particular reference to *Echinococcus granulosus*. *Ann. N.Y. Acad. Sci.* **113**, 234–60.

Smyth, J. D. and M. M. Smyth, 1980. *Frogs as host–parasite systems*. London: Macmillan.

1 Biology and systematics of *Echinococcus*

R. C. A. Thompson

INTRODUCTION

Echinococcus Rudolphi, 1801 is a small endoparasitic flatworm belonging to Class Cestoda. It is a 'true tapeworm' (Subclass Eucestoda) and as such exhibits the features which characterise this group (Table 1.1). It has no gut and all metabolic interchange takes place across the syncytial outer covering, the tegument. Anteriorly, the adult possesses a specialised attachment organ (scolex) bearing two rows of hooks and four muscular suckers (Figs 1.2 & 1.3). The body, or strobila, is segmented and consists of a number of reproductive units (proglottids) (Fig. 1.3). *Echinococcus* has an indirect life-cycle in which the adult is hermaphroditic and the larva, the hydatid cyst, proliferates asexually. For general accounts of cestode biology the reader is referred to Smyth (1969a, 1976), Schmidt and Roberts (1981) and Arme and Pappas (1983).

Classification

The classification given in Table 1.1 is practical and universally recognised. Proposals have been put forward which employ different names for both class and subclass (e.g. Cestoidea: Cestoda) and in 1974, Wardle *et al.* suggested that the family Taeniidae be promoted to ordinal status. However, the justification for this is not apparent and their revised classification has not so far been widely accepted.

Basic life-cycle

Echinococcus exhibits certain unique characteristics that set it apart from the other major genus in the family, *Taenia*. An adult *Echinococcus* is only a few millimetres long and rarely possesses more than five proglottids, whereas species of *Taenia* can grow to several metres in length and consist of several thousand proglottids. Unlike *Taenia*, the larval stage (metacestode) of *Echinococcus* exhibits a low degree of host specificity and has a much greater reproductive potential. As with all members of the family Taeniidae, *Echinococcus* requires two mammalian hosts for completion of its life-cycle. A definitive (final) host in which the adult, strobilar stage develops in the small intestine, and an intermediate host in which the cystic metacestode usually develops in the viscera (Fig. 1.1). The definitive

Table 1.1 Classification of *Echinococcus*.

Phylum Platyhelminthes
: soft-bodied, triploblastic and acoelomate; dorsoventrally flattened with cellular outer body covering; excretory system protonephridial

Class Cestoda
: endoparasites; gut absent; outer body covering a living syncytial tegument with microtriches

Subclass Eucestoda
: true tapeworms; adults characteristically with elongated body (strobila) consisting of linear sets of reproductive organs (proglottids); specialised anterior attachment organ a scolex; hermaphrodite with indirect life-cycles

Order Cyclophyllidea
: scolex with four muscular suckers and a rostellum usually armed with hooks; strobila consisting of proglottids in various stages of development and each proglottid clearly demarcated by external segmentation; eggs round, not operculate, containing non-ciliated six-hooked oncosphere

Family Taeniidae
: adults in small intestine of carnivores and man; intermediate hosts all mammalian; scolex with rostellum usually armed with double row of hooks; genitalia unpaired in each proglottid with marginal genital pore irregularly alternating; eggs with radially striated hardened 'shell' (embryophore); metacestode a cysticercus, coenurus, hydatid or strobilocercus

Genera
: genera include *Taenia, Echinococcus, Anoplotaenia, Dasyurotaenia*

host is always a carnivore. It becomes infected by ingesting protoscoleces which are produced by asexual multiplication of the metacestode. There may be several thousand protoscoleces within a single cyst, and each one is capable of developing into a sexually mature adult worm. Adult worms produce eggs, each containing a single embryo (oncosphere), which are voided in the faeces of the definitive host. The eggs, which are capable of surviving in the environment for varying periods, are infective to numerous species of herbivorous or omnivorous intermediate hosts upon ingestion. In this chapter, the biology of *Echinococcus* will be discussed in detail by examining the development of each life-cycle stage; the adult, egg and metacestode.

Hydatid disease

Infection with *Echinococcus* may be naturally transmitted between man and other animals. It thus claims membership of the most significant group of communicable diseases, the zoonoses. The clinical and economic significance of the parasite are almost completely confined to infection with the

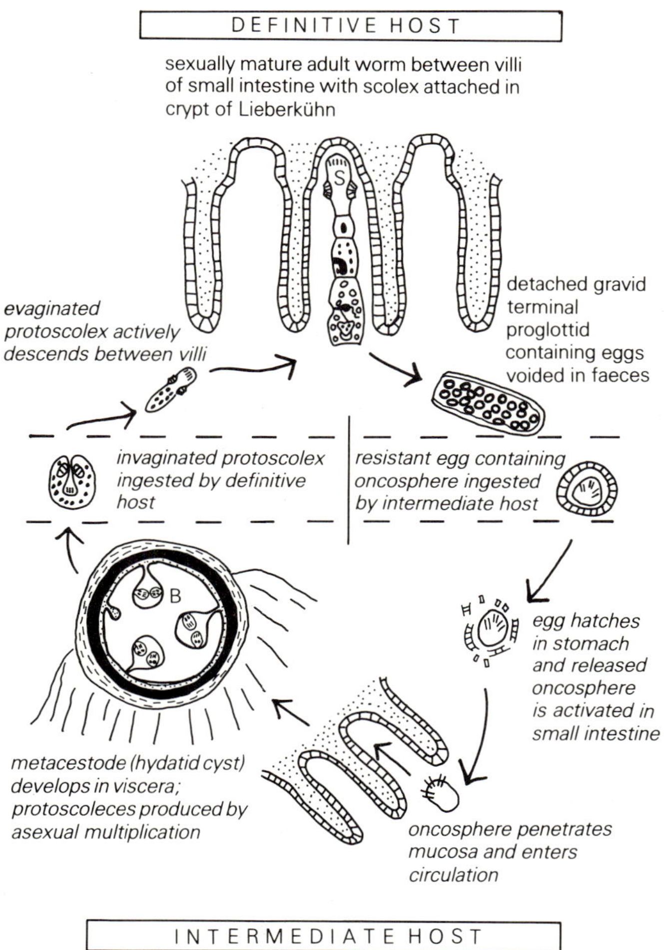

Figure 1.1 Basic life-cycle of *Echinococcus*. S, scolex; B, brood capsule containing protoscoleces.

metacestode. Hydatid disease, hydatidosis and echinococcosis are all terms used to refer to infection with the metacestode. Strictly speaking, the terms hydatid disease and hydatidosis should be restricted to infection with the metacestode, and echinococcosis to infection with the adult stage. This is the convention with *Taenia* infections in which the terms cysticercosis and taeniasis apply to infection with the metacestode (cysticercus) and adult respectively. However, since recent monographs dealing with the control of *Echinococcus* infections use the three terms interchangeably, no attempt will be made to restrict their usage here.

Taxonomy

At the present time four species, *Echinococcus granulosus, E. multilocularis, E. oligarthrus* and *E. vogeli* are considered to be valid taxonomically and their characteristics are summarised in Table 1.2. The status of a fifth species, *E. cruzi*, has been in doubt (Rausch *et al.* 1978, Kumaratilake & Thompson 1982). However, a recent study in which paratype material of *E. cruzi* was compared with the two species, *E. vogeli* and *E. oligarthrus*, found that *E. cruzi* was synonymous with *E. oligarthrus* (Rausch *et al.* 1984), thus confirming the earlier conclusions of Cameron (1926).

In the past, the taxonomy of the genus *Echinococcus* at both specific and subspecific levels has been a matter of controversy and some confusion. The current situation has been comprehensively reviewed (Kumaratilake & Thompson 1982) and some historical aspects are discussed in Chapter 2. The apparent variability of *Echinococcus* which has given rise to much of the taxonomic uncertainty within the genus will be considered further in the section on strain variation at the end of this chapter.

ADULT

Host specificity and susceptibility

The definitive host of *Echinococcus* is always a carnivore (Table 1.2) and the degree of host specificity expressed is far greater than at the intermediate host level. For example, apart from a strain which utilises the lion (Graber & Thal 1980), felids appear to be refractory to infection with *E. granulosus*. Extensive laboratory and field studies in different parts of the world have demonstrated that the domestic cat plays no role as a definitive host for *E. granulosus* (see Thompson 1977a for a review). The red fox (*Vulpes vulpes*) is a suitable definitive host for only certain strains of *E. granulosus* (see Thompson 1977a, 1983 for reviews). However, *E. multilocularis* has the fox as its major definitive host and may also utilise the domestic cat (Schantz 1982, Thompson & Eckert 1983, and see Ch. 2). Of the four species of *Echinococcus*, only *E. oligarthrus* does not appear to mature in dogs and characteristically uses wild felids as definitive hosts (see Schantz 1982, and Ch. 2).

The factors responsible for such differences in host specificity are not completely understood. The microtopography of the small intestine (e.g. crypt and villous size) between species of definitive host may be more suited to certain species, or strains, of *Echinococcus* than others (Smyth & Smyth 1968, Smyth 1968). Such physical factors may play an important role in the initial establishment of the parasite but do not explain why in certain hosts, such as *E. granulosus* in cats, the parasite may initially establish but fails to complete its development. In this respect, differences in the composition of bile between definitive host species may influence host specificity (reviewed by Smyth 1968, 1969a). A particular type or concentration of bile constituent may be necessary for evagination, establishment or development of certain species or strains of *Echinococcus*, or, alternatively, may act as a toxic or lytic agent in unfavourable hosts. Apart from bile there are likely to be many biochemical and nutritive factors, as well as physiochemical and immunological characteristics, that could play an important role in specificity. Such factors may also influence susceptibility. For example, although a particular strain of *Echinococcus* may develop normally in a range of definitive hosts, the number of worms which initially establish and the rate of development may vary markedly between host species. In Australia two closely related canids, the dingo (*Canis familiaris dingo*) and the domestic dog (*C. f. familiaris*) both act as suitable definitive hosts for the sylvatic strain of *E. granulosus* (Kumaratilake & Thompson 1984a). However, considerably more worms initially establish and develop more quickly in dingoes than in dogs (Thompson & Kumaratilake 1985). Presumably the metabolic or physiological requirements of this strain of *E. granulosus* are better catered for in the dingo. A similar situation was reported in the United Kingdom where sheep-dogs were more susceptible to experimental infection with the UK sheep strain of *E. granulosus* than beagles (Walters & Clarkson 1980).

Establishment in the definitive host

The definitive host acquires infection by ingesting viable protoscoleces. These may be ingested still within the hydatid cyst and thus the masticatory actions of the host will assist in tearing open the cyst and freeing the brood capsules. The process of excystment – removal of brood capsule and other cystic tissue – is further assisted by the action of pepsin in the stomach (Smyth 1969a). Prior to ingestion, the apical region of the protoscolex (suckers, rostellum and hooks) is invaginated within the mucopolysaccharide-coated basal region of the protoscolex tegument (Marchiondo & Andersen 1983). This protects the scolex until it is stimulated to evaginate. In dogs experimentally infected with evaginated protoscoleces of *E. granulosus*, far fewer worms establish than in dogs infected with invaginated protoscoleces (L. M. Kumaratilake & R. C. A. Thompson unpublished).

The precise nature of the stimulus for evagination is not known. Protoscoleces are sensitive to environmental changes and evaginate in response to variations in temperature and osmotic pressure, and to agitation (De Rycke 1968, R. C. A. Thompson unpublished). In an intact hydatid cyst removed from the intermediate host and maintained between 10 and 20 °C, the protoscoleces will invariably begin to evaginate after a few days although temperatures below 10 °C appear to inhibit evagination (R. C. A. Thompson unpublished). Specific enzymes or bile are not essential but the rate of evagination is increased in the presence of bile (Smyth 1967). However, aerobic conditions appear to be essential for evagination (Smyth 1969a).

The time required for evagination in the definitive host is variable.

Table 1.2 Species which have been taxonomically recognised within the genus *Echinococcus*★.

	Echinococcus granulosus (Batsch, 1786)	*Echinococcus multilocularis* Leuckart, 1863	*Echinococcus oligarthrus* (Diesing, 1863)	*Echinococcus vogeli* Rausch and Bernstein, 1972
Geographical distribution (see Ch. 2 for details)	cosmopolitan	holarctic	central and South America	central and South America
Host range (see Ch. 2 for details)				
definitive host	primarily dogs and other canids	primarily foxes but also other canids and cats	wild felids	bush dog (*Speothos venaticus*)
intermediate host	primarily ungulates but also primates and marsupials; MAN	primarily arvicolid rodents; MAN	agoutis (*Dasyprocta* spp.), paca (*Cuniculus paca*) and spiny rats (*Proechimys* spp.)	agoutis (*Dasyprocta* spp.), paca (*Cuniculus paca*) and spiny rats (*Proechimys* spp.); MAN
Metacestode				
type	unilocular (cystic)	multivesicular (alveolar)	polycystic	polycystic
location	visceral, primarily liver and lungs	visceral, primarily liver	peripheral, primarily muscles, occasionally visceral	visceral, primarily liver
protoscolex hooks				
mean length (μm) of large hooks (range)	25.9–35.0 (19.4–44.0)	26.7–28.5 (25.0–29.7)	30.5–33.4 (29.1–37.9)	39.3–41.6 (38.2–45.6)
mean length (μm) of small hooks (range)	22.6–27.8 (17.0–31.0)	23.1–25.4 (21.8–27.0)	25.4–27.3 (22.6–29.2)	32.5–34.0 (30.4–36.9)

Adult				
mean length (μm) of large hooks (range)	32.0–42.0 (25.0–49.0)	31.0 (24.9–34.0)	52.0 (43.0–60.0)	53.0 (49.0–57.0)
mean length (μm) of small hooks (range)	22.6–27.8 (17.0–31.0)	27.0 (20.4–31.0)	39.0 (28.0–45.0)	42.6 (30.0–47.0)
mean number of segments (range)	3 (2–7)	5 (2–6)	3	3
total length of strobila (mm)	2.0–11.0	1.2–4.5	2.2–2.9	3.9–5.5
position of the genital pore				
mature segment	near (usually posterior) to middle	anterior to middle	anterior to middle	posterior to middle
gravid segment	posterior to middle	anterior to middle	approximately at middle	posterior to middle
mean number of testes (range)	32–68 (25–80)	18–26 (16–35)	29 (15–46)	56 (50–67)
distribution of testes (in relation to genital pore)	equal or majority posterior	majority posterior	majority posterior	majority posterior
position of mature segment	penultimate or antepenultimate	antepenultimate	antepenultimate	antepenultimate
form of the uterus	lateral sacculations	sac-like	sac-like	long, tubular and sac-like
ratio of anterior part of strobila:gravid segment	1:0.86–1.30	1:0.31–0.80	1:0.96–1.10	1:1.90–3.00

⋆*Sources of information:* Vogel 1957, Sweatman and Williams 1963, Williams and Sweatman 1963, Verster 1965, Thatcher and Sousa 1966, Sousa and Thatcher 1969, Rausch and Bernstein 1972, Rausch *et al.* 1978, D'Alessandro *et al.* 1979.

Although up to 86.5 per cent of ingested protoscoleces may have evaginated after 6 h, complete evagination can take up to 3 d (Thompson 1977b). Following evagination, protoscoleces are initially very active. They are rich in glycogen which acts as an energy reserve, although *in vitro* studies have shown that these reserves are rapidly used up, usually within 3 h (Smyth 1967). Activity then declines during the first 8 d of cultivation but increases thereafter, presumably as energy reserves are replenished. These observations have been confirmed *in vivo* with the demonstration of a lag phase in growth during the first 3 d of infection in dogs (Thompson 1975). The initial activity of the newly evaginated protoscolex or juvenile adult is an obvious prerequisite to establishment in the small intestine of the definitive host. Studies in dogs have shown that juvenile adult worms of *E. granulosus*, still in the process of evaginating, are already deep between the villi with some actually within the crypts of Lieberkühn by 6 h after infection (Thompson 1977b). If young worms fail to do this they will presumably be swept out of the small intestine. Developing worms attach mainly by grasping substantial plugs of tissue with their suckers (Smyth *et al.* 1969a, Thompson *et al.* 1979, Thompson & Eckert 1983) (Fig. 1.2). The hooks only superficially penetrate the mucosal epithelium but their shape ensures that they act as anchors to assist in preventing the worm being dislodged. As in all cestodes, the tegument of *Echinococcus* is covered with numerous minute 'microvilli-like' projections termed microtriches (Jha & Smyth 1969, 1971, Thompson *et al.* 1979, Thompson 1982). One possible function ascribed to microtriches is that they assist in attachment by interdigitating with host microvilli (Mettrick & Podesta 1974). However, ultrastructural studies on the host–parasite interface of adult *E. granulosus in situ* in the dog found no evidence of interdigitation (Thompson *et al.* 1979).

Featherston (1969) presented evidence that developing *Taenia hydatigena* undergo migration in the intestine of dogs and it has been suggested that developing *T. ovis* and *T. pisiformis* may also migrate (Coman & Rickard 1975). It is not known to what extent the developing adult of *Echinococcus* migrates within the small intestine, although it does move between adjacent villi. However, once the adult worm reaches maturity it appears to be confined to a particular region of the small intestine (Thompson *et al.* 1979). Mature *E. granulosus* is found in the anterior quarter of the small intestine whereas *E. multilocularis* occurs in the posterior region (Thompson & Eckert 1983). This variation in distribution between *E. granulosus* and *E. multilocularis* is probably related to differences in their metabolic requirements which are provided by the different physiological environments of the anterior and posterior small intestine. *In vitro* studies strongly suggest that *E. granulosus* and *E. multilocularis* are physiologically distinct (Smyth 1979).

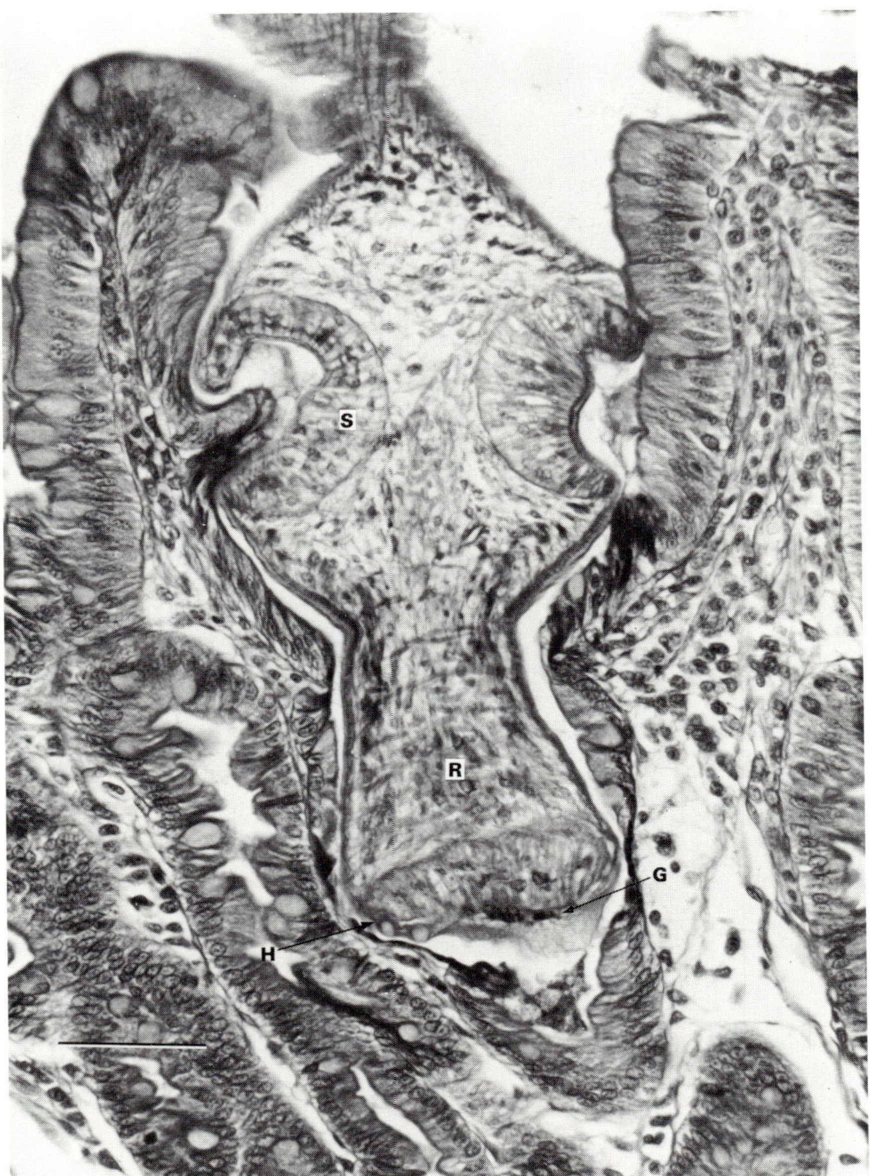

Figure 1.2 Section of mucosal wall of an experimentally infected dingo (*Canis familiaris dingo*) showing 35 d old *Echinococcus granulosus in situ*. Rostellum (R) is extended into a crypt of Lieberkühn and the suckers (S) are grasping the epithelium at the base of the villi. G, 'rostellar gland'; H, hooks. Section stained with Martius Scarlet Blue. Scale bar, 50 μm.

Activities at the interface

Although an adult *Echinococcus* may alter its position and move up and down and between adjacent villi during development, this may not occur once the worm reaches maturity. From 20 and 35 d after infection respectively, *E. multilocularis* and *E. granulosus* are found in a position characteristic of the mature worm. The rostellum is deeply inserted into a crypt of Lieberkühn with the mobile apical rostellar region usually fully extended, the hooks superficially penetrating the mucosal epithelium and the suckers grasping the epithelium at the base of the villi (Smyth *et al.* 1969a, Thompson *et al.* 1979, Thompson & Eckert 1983; Fig. 1.2).

Invasion of the crypts of Lieberkühn by the mature worm may be of particular physiological significance to *Echinococcus*. It is a characteristic not shared by other taeniids, which achieve only a relatively superficial attachment to the mucosa of the definitive host (Beveridge & Rickard 1975, Featherston 1971), presumably because of their greater size. *Echinococcus* has a very mobile and extensible apical rostellar region. Extension of this region into the crypts coincides with the commencement of secretory activity of a modified group of tegumental cells ('rostellar gland') situated in the apical rostellum (Fig. 1.2) and the release of secretory material into the interface between parasite and host (Smyth 1964a, b, Smyth *et al.* 1969b, Thompson *et al.* 1979, Thompson & Eckert 1983). The mechanism for release of secretory material is analogous to holocrine secretory processes. The nature of the secretion is unclear. It is a protein or polypeptide containing a relatively large amount of cystine and possibly a lipid component. The origin and site of synthesis of the secretion has not been determined, although large amounts occur in both the perinuclear and distal cytoplasm of the tegument as well as in the tegumental nuclei (Thompson *et al.* 1979).

The crypts of Lieberkühn may represent a site of particular nutritional significance for mature *Echinococcus*. Nutrients could be derived from the lysis of host cells but there is no evidence that the secretion is histolytic or has any enzymatic activity. An important factor to be considered is the timing of secretory activity, which coincides with a levelling off in growth of the worm at around 30 d after infection and the commencement of egg production (Thompson *et al.* 1979). The secretion may therefore be associated with the maturation of ova and/or subsequent release of the gravid proglottid (apolysis). Gland activity could be recurrent with a cycle of activity associated with the maturation and release of each proglottid. Modified glandular parts of the scolex tegument have been described in other cestodes (Öhman-James 1973, Sawada 1973, Hayunga 1979, Richards & Arme 1981, Specian & Lumsden 1981). In these cases the most favoured role for the secretion is one of attachment. In *Echinococcus*, perhaps firm attachment is a prerequisite for apolysis, since unattached gravid worms *in vitro* do not shed their terminal proglottids (Thompson & Eckert 1982). An adhesive function to assist in retention of the worms most adequately accounts for the special location of the rostellar secretory cells, site of release, and timing if apolysis necessitates particularly firm positioning. Mature *E. granulosus* possesses two morphologically distinct types of microthrix (Thompson *et al.* 1982). On the strobila, they are blade-like and rigid for most of their length and probably serve to keep the absorptive surface of the parasite and host apart, thus maintaining a free flow of nutrients at the interface between the two absorptive surfaces. On the apical rostellum and scolex the microtriches are long, slender filamentous types apparently flexible for most of their length, thus allowing the scolex and rostellum to achieve close contact with the host, perhaps to enhance adhesion.

One other possible function for the rostellar secretion that can not be dismissed at this stage, is that of protection. It is feasible that the secretion may protect the worm either by inhibiting or inactivating host digestive enzymes or by interfering with the host's immune effector mechanisms (see also Ch. 6). However, it would be reasonable to expect such a protective mechanism to operate throughout the life of the adult worm, unless, as seems to be the case, it is only after maturity that a permanent and very intimate association is achieved between parasite and host.

An interesting feature of this host–parasite relationship is that the presence of the adult parasite appears to go virtually unnoticed by the host. Like the majority of adult tapeworms (Rees 1967), *Echinococcus* seldom engenders a morphologically apparent host response. Occasionally in heavy infections, there may be an excessive production of mucus. The host tissue that is grasped by the suckers is usually necrotic, but the hooks cause little damage (Thompson *et al.* 1979) (Fig. 1.2). Observations at the ultrastructural level have shown hook damage is restricted to columnar cells with an associated loss of some host microvilli (Thompson *et al.* 1979). The epithelium of parasitised crypts is commonly flattened and there may be occasional rupture of a crypt wall with release of host cells into the crypt (Smyth *et al.* 1969a). Adult worms have been observed to invade the lamina propria, but this appears to be a rare event. No substantial pathology or evidence of a host cellular reaction has been observed in infections with adult *E. granulosus* or *E. multilocularis* (Thompson *et al.* 1979, Thompson & Eckert 1983).

Development

DIFFERENTIATION

The development of the adult parasite involves germinal and somatic differentiation and can be divided into the following processes: proglottisation; maturation; growth; segmentation. Germinal differentiation comprises proglottisation, which refers to the sequential formation of new reproductive units (proglottids), and the maturation of the proglottids. Somatic differentiation consists of growth, i.e. increase in size, and the somatic delineation of each proglottid by segmentation (strobilisation). Segmentation in cestodes is not to be confused with true mesodermal segmentation (metamerism) which occurs by distal growth not proximally as in cestodes (Freeman 1973). In some cestodes, including *Echinococcus* (see below), proglottisation may occur without segmentation. Thus both terms are necessary for a full comprehension of the process of development (Freeman 1973), but should not be referred to interchangeably. Segmentation in cestodes, including *Echinococcus*, does not involve the formation of any separatory structure or 'inter-proglottid' membrane between adjoining proglottids (Mehlhorn *et al.* 1981). The demarcation of each proglottid is purely an external phenomenon caused by an infolding of the tegument which gives rise to the characteristic constricted appearance. It also appears that the microtriches in the infolded regions of the tegument may be linked together thus stabilising the infoldings (Mehlhorn *et al.* 1981).

The four developmental processes described above take place independently. This has been demonstrated by studies on *E. granulosus* and *E. multilocularis in vitro* (Smyth 1971, Smyth & Davies 1975, Smyth & Barrett 1979), and *E. granulosus in vivo* (Thompson 1977b). This suggests a very complicated process of cytodifferentiation and the possible existence of several primitive cell lines as in *Hymenolepis diminuta* (Sulgostowska 1972, 1974). However, preliminary studies on cytodifferentiation in adult *E. granulosus* suggest that only one primitive cell type exists (Gustafsson 1976). These 'germinative cells' make up approximately 24 per cent of the total number of cells in the neck region, most of them occurring in the inner parenchyma and in the vicinity of the nerve cords. This germinative cell is obviously extremely sensitive to environmental and/or nutritive conditions, as demonstrated by the results of *in vitro* studies on *Echinococcus* (Smyth & Barrett 1979 and see Ch. 5). In some cultures mainly genital cells are produced, leading to proglottisation and maturation but no segmentation, whereas in other cultures more somatic cells are produced leading to growth without sexual maturation. Obviously a fine balance exists that can easily be upset if environmental factors are not correct.

INDUCTION OF DEVELOPMENT

The factor, or factors, which induce the evaginated protoscolex to develop into an adult worm are not understood. Studies on *E. granulosus in vitro* suggested that contact of the scolex with a solid nutritive substrate is necessary to initiate adult differentiation (Smyth 1967 and see Ch. 5). The contact stimulus was thought to be nutritional by a form of membrane digestion (Smyth 1972). However, recent studies have found that *E. multilocularis* will differentiate sexually in monophasic media (without a solid serum base) (Smyth & Davies 1975, Smyth 1979). Since it is unlikely that the factors which initiate adult differentiation will differ between the two species, the stimulus must be more complex than previously thought.

SEQUENTIAL DEVELOPMENT

The newly evaginated protoscolex contains an abundance of calcareous corpuscles (Fig. 1.3), which consist of an organic base and inorganic material (Smyth 1969a). Their function is not clear but may be that of a buffering system (Smyth 1969a). Alternatively they could be a source of inorganic ions, CO_2 and phosphates. The latter function seems quite likely because such a reserve of potential energy would be required during initial establishment (Smyth 1969a). The rapid disappearance of calcareous corpuscles, usually within 7–8 d, supports this hypothesis (Smyth & Davies 1974a). Within 3–4 d after infection, the lateral excretory canals of the young worm are clearly evident and by the end of the first week a posterior excretory bladder is seen (Smyth & Davies 1974a). The excretory system of *Echinococcus*, like all other cestodes, is based on the platyhelminth protonephridial system with the lateral excretory canals (Fig. 1.3) acting as collecting ducts for numerous flame cells distributed throughout the parenchyma. However, the physiology of excretion has not been investigated. Recent evidence that the excretory ducts of some pseudophyllideans are capable of absorption (Lindroos & Gardberg 1982) raises the possibility that the excretory system of *Echinococcus* could also function as a distributive system.

The sequence of development described below and illustrated in Figure 1.3 refers to *E. granulosus* (Smyth *et al.* 1967, Smyth & Davies 1974a). Although it is essentially the same in other species, the rate of development varies, particularly in relation to growth, onset of egg production and number of proglottids produced. The first sign of proglottisation is the appearance of a genital rudiment or anlagen which may appear as early as 11 d after infection, separated from the scolex by a clear band. By 14 d the first proglottid is clearly evident as a darkly staining body demarcated from the scolex by the transverse infolding of the tegument which delineates the first segment. Within 1–2 d a lateral branch forms from the genital rudiment which will eventually open to the exterior via the genital pore. Subsequent stages of maturation follow the general cestode pattern and are summarised in Figure 1.3. Growth, as determined by total worm length, exhibits a steady log–linear increase throughout the first 35 d of infection apart from a lag period during the first 3 d (Thompson 1975). Growth also levels off prior to egg production (Thompson 1975, 1977b).

SEXUAL REPRODUCTION

Mature *Echinococcus* is hermaphroditic (Fig. 1.3) and capable of self-insemination (Smyth & Smyth 1969). It is not known whether cross-insemination between two individuals takes place. Hermaphroditism combined with self-insemination is obviously an advantage to a small worm such as *Echinococcus*, which might find it difficult to find another worm, particularly in light infections. Further, such a reproductive mechanism has a significant evolutionary potential as will be detailed below. The requirements for self-insemination in *Echinococcus* appear to be extremely complex as suggested by the repeated failure to achieve fertilisation *in vitro* (see Smyth & Davies 1974a, Smyth 1979 and Ch. 5). It has been suggested that there may be specific or non-specific factors in the

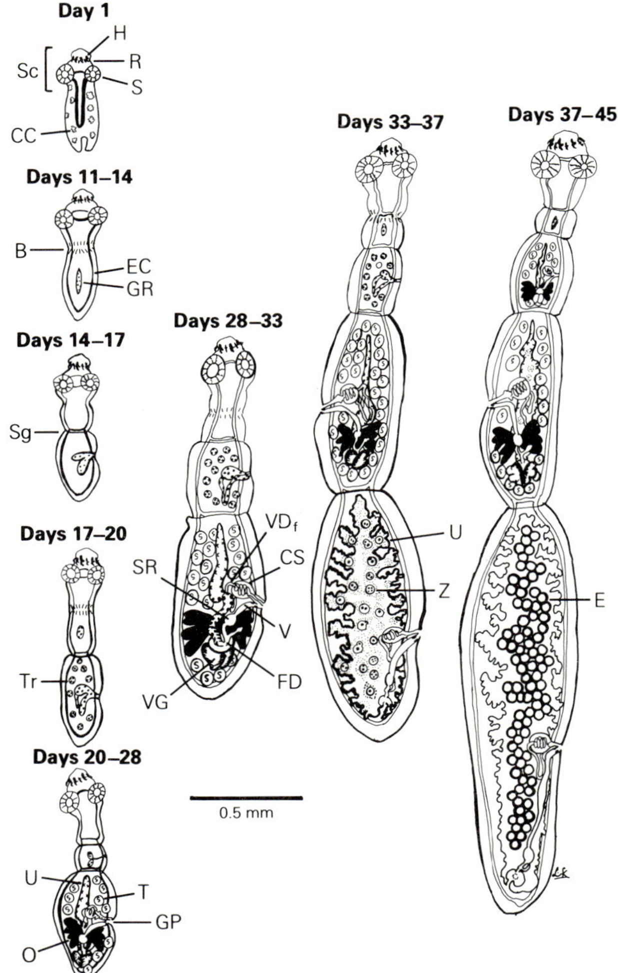

Figure 1.3 Stages of development of adult *Echinococcus granulosus* in the definitive host. (The periods at which various stages appear may vary and are dependent on strain of parasite and various host factors.) Day 1: Protoscolex has evaginated and elongated; contains numerous calcareous corpuscles. Days 11–14: calcareous corpuscles have disappeared; lateral excretory canals are conspicuous; genital rudiment present denoting formation of first proglottid; constriction and clear area below the neck ('banding') marks the site of the first segment. Days 14–17: genital rudiment has divided into two and extends unilaterally; first segment fully formed. Days 17–20: rudimentary testes appear in first proglottid; initial stages in formation of second proglottid. Days 20–28: two-segmented worm; male genitalia – testes, cirrus and vas deferens – have developed; female genitalia – ovary, Mehlis' gland and vitelline gland – still developing; uterus appears as a streak; both cirrus and vagina open to exterior via lateral genital pore. Days 28–33: male and female genitalia in terminal proglottid fully mature; uterus still dilating; penultimate proglottid has developing genitalia; either a band or third segment appears. Days 33–37: ovulation and fertilisation in terminal proglottid; fully dilated uterus

intestinal secretions of the definitive host which activate the cirrus to commence its copulatory movements and that without such stimulation self-insemination may not occur (Smyth 1982a).

EGG PRODUCTION AND SUBSEQUENT DEVELOPMENT

The initial onset of egg production varies between species and even between strains. In *E. granulosus* it ranges from 34 to 58 d, whereas *E. multilocularis* has a far more rapid rate of maturation with egg production commencing between 28 and 35 d after infection (see Thompson & Eckert 1982, Thompson *et al.* 1984). In *E. oligarthrus*, available evidence suggests that adults do not become gravid until 80 d after infection (Sousa & Thatcher 1969).

Although development up to the initial onset of egg production has been extensively studied, little is known of subsequent development. The lack of detailed sequential studies is directly related to the dangers of maintaining definitive hosts harbouring gravid infections. Consequently, there are several aspects of development which have still to be clarified. The number of eggs produced is uncertain, with reports varying between 100 and 1000 per proglottid (Rausch 1975, Arundel 1972). A recent study demonstrated that the numbers may be higher than this in *E. granulosus*, with approximately 1500 eggs per proglottid, whereas *E. multilocularis* rarely produces more than 200 eggs per proglottid (Thompson & Eckert 1982). Similarly, it is not known how often species of *Echinococcus* produce gravid proglottids. Based on the rate of development during the first 40 d of infection, it has been estimated that gravid proglottids are produced and detach every 7–14 d (Smyth 1964a, Schantz 1982). However, Yasmashita *et al.* (1956) monitored the faeces of dogs infected with *E. granulosus* and found that there was a delay of between 4 and 6 weeks between the first and second appearance of eggs in the faeces. Observations by Kumazawa and Suzuki (1983) on *Hymenolepis nana* demonstrated a drastic decrease in maturation rate after the onset of apolysis. Without further investigation it is impossible to conclude whether the rate of proglottisation after apolysis in *Echinococcus* is constant or declines. It is also not known how long the adult parasite may survive in the definitive host. It has been reported that

---

contains dividing zygotes; male and female genitalia degenerating in terminal proglottid; mature genitalia in penultimate proglottid and developing genitalia in ante-penultimate proglottid; strobila divided by three or four segments. Days 37–45: gravid with embryonated eggs in uterus of terminal proglottid – eggs have fully formed embryophore ('thick-shelled') and contain embryo (oncosphere); zygotes in uterus of penultimate proglottid and maturing genitalia in ante-penultimate proglottid; strobila divided by three, four or five segments. *Abbreviations*: B, band; CC, calcareous corpuscles; CS, cirrus sac; E, embryonated eggs; EC, excretory canal; FD, female reproductive ducts; GP, genital pore; GR, genital rudiment; H, hooks; O, ovary; R, rostellum; S, sucker; Sc, scolex; Sg, segment; SR, seminal receptacle; Tr, rudimentary testes; T, testes; U, uterus; V, vagina; VD_f, vas deferens; VG, vitelline gland; Z, zygotes. Scale bar, 0.5 mm. (Original drawing by L. M. Kumaratilake.)

adult worms become senescent after 6–20 months, although worms may live for 2 years or longer (Schantz 1982). In the absence of accurate information on the rate of production and release of gravid proglottids and the life-span of the adult parasite, it is impossible to determine the reproductive potential of *Echinococcus* in the definitive host. Such information is obviously essential for an understanding of the epidemiology of hydatid disease (see Ch. 7).

Another assumption that has not been adequately confirmed is whether gravid proglottids pass out of the definitive host containing their full complement of eggs. Observations suggest that some eggs of *E. granulosus* are liberated from the proglottid prior to exit from the definitive host (Yamashita *et al.* 1956). This is similar to the situation for *Taenia hydatigena, T. pisiformis* and *T. multiceps*, in which the majority of eggs are released within the intestinal tract (Featherston 1969, Coman & Rickard 1975, Willis *et al.* 1981).

EGG

Infectivity

When released from the definitive host, the egg of *Echinococcus* is presumed to be fully embryonated and infective to a suitable intermediate host. However, as discussed in Chapter 7, taeniid eggs at the time of expulsion are probably at different stages of maturation and immature eggs may mature in the environment under appropriate conditions. A recent study on *T. multiceps* suggests that freshly shed eggs require a short period of maturation before being infective (Willis *et al.* 1981).

Morphology

Taeniid eggs are spherical to ellipsoid in shape and usually range in size from 30 to 50 μm and from 22 to 44 μm in their two diameters. They are morphologically indistinguishable at the light microscope level and ultrastructural studies of the eggs of *E. granulosus*, *E. multilocularis* and various *Taenia* species have shown that they possess similar structures consisting of several layers and membranes (Fig. 1.4) (Morseth 1965, Sakamoto 1981, Swiderski 1982). The embryophore is the principal layer affording physical protection to the embryo, or oncosphere, since the vitelline layer ('egg shell' or outer envelope) is stripped from the egg before it is liberated. The embryophore is relatively thick and impermeable, consisting of polygonal blocks composed of an inert keratin-like protein, which are held together by a cementing substance (Morseth 1966, Nieland 1968, Sakamoto 1981). *Echinococcus* eggs are extremely resistant, enabling them to withstand a wide range of environmental temperatures (see Ch. 7).

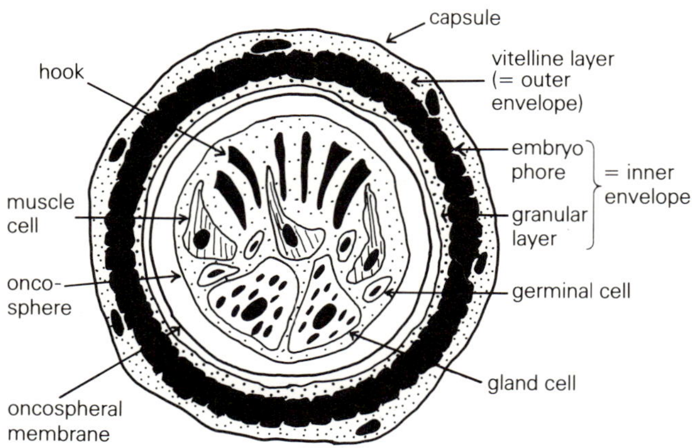

Figure 1.4 Diagram of the egg of *Echinococcus*. [For details of cytology and musculature see Lethbridge (1980), Sakamoto (1981), Swiderski (1983).]

Hatching and activation

When ingested by a suitable intermediate host, viable eggs of *Echinococcus* hatch in the stomach and small intestine. Hatching is a two-stage process involving (1) the passive disaggregation of the embryophoric blocks in the stomach and intestine and (2) the activation of the oncosphere and its liberation from the oncospheral membrane (reviewed by Lethbridge 1980). Disaggregation of the embryophoric blocks appears to require the action of proteolytic enzymes, including pepsin and pancreatin, in the stomach and/or intestine but does not depend on any one specific enzyme. The oncosphere plays no part in disaggregation of the embryophore and remains essentially dormant until activated. Evidence suggests the oncosphere may be stimulated to free itself from the oncospheral membrane following changes in membrane permeability brought about by the surface active properties of bile salts. This has led to the proposal that bile may play a part in determining intermediate host specificity, since its composition varies between different species of vertebrate (Smyth 1969a). However, the situation is certainly not as straightforward since eggs hatch in extra-intestinal sites. Borrie *et al.* (1965) demonstrated that eggs of *E. granulosus* administered to sheep by tracheostomy developed into hydatid cysts in the lungs, indicating that the eggs hatched, and that the oncospheres were activated and penetrated the lung tissues in an extra-intestinal site devoid of both digestive enzymes and bile salts. Similarly, hydatid cysts of *E. granulosus* have been shown to develop in the liver, pleural cavity, lungs and peritoneal cavity of rodents following inoculation of eggs by intraperitoneal injection or laparotomy (Blood & Lelijveld 1969, Williams & Colli 1970, Colli & Williams 1972, Kumaratilake & Thompson 1981, R. C. A. Thompson in preparation). In the last-mentioned study, eggs inoculated into the peritoneal cavity were rapidly surrounded by adhering neutrophils and macrophages which probably released hydrolytic enzymes causing dissolution of the embryophore. More circumstantial data has been provided for *E. multilocularis* eggs which apparently hatched when injected into the liver of mice (Sakamoto *et al.* 1982). Thus hatching requirements do not depend on the physiological characteristics of the gut and are not specific. The latter view has been emphasised by Coman and Rickard (1975), who found that eggs of *Taenia pisiformis, T. ovis* and *T. hydatigena* hatched and activated in the small intestine of the canine definitive host. Consequently, factors which regulate whether eggs of a particular taeniid species will or will not develop in a particular intermediate host must operate on the oncosphere either during the invasive or establishment phases.

Penetration and tissue localisation

The liberated, activated oncosphere exhibits intricate rhythmic movements involving the body and hooks, the co-ordinated movement of the latter effected by a complex muscular system (Swiderski 1983). The so-called 'penetration glands' are also prominent at this stage. Studies in sheep and rabbits have shown that the oncospheres of *E. granulosus* penetrate the tips of the villi in the jejunal and upper ileal region of the small intestine (Heath 1971). The oncospheres initially attach to the microvillous border of the villi, presumably using their hooks as anchors. Studies on several taeniid species, including *E. granulosus*, have shown that oncospheres rapidly migrate through the epithelial border of the villi, reaching the lamina propria within 30–120 min after hatching (reviewed by Lethbridge 1980). Penetration appears to involve hook and body movements presumably assisted by the penetration gland secretions. Stainable material in the penetration glands is totally extruded from between the hooks at the time, and in the place where the oncosphere is actively engaged in penetration (reviewed by Fairweather & Threadgold 1981). Degeneration of host tissue also occurs in the vicinity of the invading oncosphere (Heath 1971). It is therefore assumed that penetration gland secretions must aid the penetration process by causing lysis of host tissue. However, the putative enzymatic nature of the secretion has yet to be established. Alternatively, penetration may be purely mechanical, involving hook and body movements. The secretion may have other functions such as to assist adhesion, act as a lubricant or afford protection against host digestive enzymes or immunological factors (Lethbridge 1980, Fairweather & Threadgold 1981). Recent ultrastructural studies (Swiderski 1983) have shown that the oncosphere of *E. granulosus* has three types of gland cells (Fig. 1.4). Thus several secretions with different functions may be produced during penetration.

The factors that determine the final localisation of the metacestode of *Echinococcus* in a given host are not clear but probably include anatomical and physiological characteristics of the host as well as the species and strain of parasite. Heath (1971) provided strong circumstantial evidence that oncospheres of *E. granulosus* are capable of completing a lymphatic or venous migration. He further postulated that since the lymphatic lacteals of the villus differed in size between different hosts, the size of the oncosphere in relation to the venules and lacteals in various animals may determine the distribution of cysts between the liver and lungs.

Post-oncospheral development

Once the oncosphere attains a site of predilection (Table 1.2), post-oncospheral development proceeds leading to the formation of the metacestode. Studies *in vivo* (Rausch 1954, Sakamoto & Sugimura 1970) and *in vitro* (Heath & Lawrence 1976) demonstrated that the oncosphere of *Echinococcus* very rapidly undergoes a series of reorganisational events during the first 10–14 d, involving cellular proliferation, degeneration of oncospheral hooks, muscular atrophy, vesicularisation and central cavity formation, and development of both germinal and laminated layers. Post-oncospheral development is initiated by the growth and division of primary germinal cells (Slais 1973), five pairs of which have been described in the posterior pole of the oncosphere (Swiderski 1983) (Fig. 1.4).

METACESTODE

Metacestodes of the four species of *Echinococcus* have certain basic features in common which can be illustrated by a detailed examination of *E. granulosus*. Differences exhibited by the other three species will then be discussed.

Structure

ECHINOCOCCUS GRANULOSUS

The fully developed metacestode of *E. granulosus* is typically unilocular, subspherical in shape, fluid-filled and exhibits the least complex structure of the four species (Cameron & Webster 1969, Rausch *et al.* 1981, Schantz 1982). The cyst consists of an inner germinal or nucleated layer supported externally by a tough, elastic, acellular laminated layer of variable thickness, surrounded by a host-produced fibrous adventitial layer (Fig. 1.5). Typically *E. granulosus* produces a single-chambered unilocular cyst in which growth is expansive by concentric enlargement. Asexual proliferation of the germinal layer and brood capsule formation takes place entirely endogenously. Pouching of the cyst walls may occur giving rise to secondary chambers communicating with the central cavity (Vanek 1980). Sometimes the central cavity may be partly separated from the secondary chambers by incomplete septa. Occasionally cysts may abut and coalesce, forming groups or clusters of small cysts of different size. In some hosts,

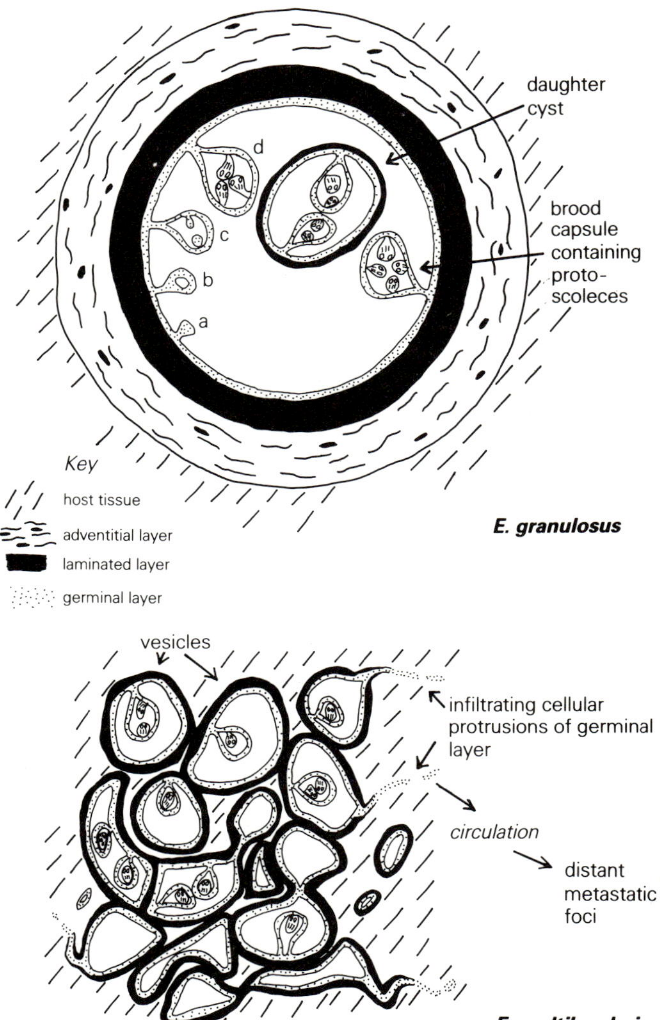

Figure 1.5 Diagrammatic representation of the metacestodes of *Echinococcus granulosus* and *E. multilocularis*. a, b, c, d are stages in the development of the brood capsule in *E. granulosus*.

particularly man, where unusually large cysts may develop, daughter cysts may form within the primary cyst (Fig. 1.5).

The germinal layer is similar in structure to the tegument of the adult worm, consisting of a distal cytoplasmic syncytium from which microtriches project into the overlaying laminated layer (Morseth 1967, Lascano *et al.* 1975, Bortoletti & Ferretti 1973, 1978). The cell bodies and nuclei comprise the perinuclear, or proliferative cell layer, which contains several cell types including tegumental, muscle, glycogen-storing and undifferentiated cells. Cytoplasmic connections between the two layers maintain continuity. The undifferentiated cells of the perinuclear layer are proliferative and are responsible for the formation of brood capsules which originate as small nuclear masses, or buds, which proliferate towards the cystic cavity (Fig. 1.5; Slais 1973, Thompson 1976). Brood capsules enlarge, vacuolate and become stalked. Within their lumen, a repetition of the asexual budding process takes place, leading to the production of numerous protoscoleces.

The delicate germinal layer is supported externally by the laminated layer. All species of *Echinococcus* are characterised by the possession of a laminated layer which, because it is periodic acid–Schiff (PAS) positive (Kilejian *et al.* 1961), provides a useful diagnostic marker. It is a polysaccharide protein complex with a predominance of galactosamine over glucosamine (Kilejian & Schwabe 1971). Ultrastructurally it consists of a microfibrillate matrix in which aggregates of electron-dense material occur (Richards *et al.* 1983). Electron microscopy (Bortoletti & Ferretti 1973, Lascano *et al.* 1975, Verheyen 1982, Richards *et al.* 1983) and *in vitro* studies (Smyth 1962, Heath & Osborn 1976) support the theory that the laminated layer is of parasite origin and is secreted by the germinal layer, although the precise site of synthesis has still to be convincingly demonstrated. The finding of common parasite antigens in the laminated layer, germinal layer and protoscoleces also suggests that the germinal layer gives rise to the laminated layer (Varela-Diaz & Torres 1977). Ultrastructural studies of larval *E. multilocularis* have led to the suggestion that the degeneration of cells of the host's defence system along the surface of the tegument contribute to the formation of the laminated layer (Mehlhorn *et al.* 1983). However, this does not explain the presence of a laminated layer around daughter cysts (Fig. 1.5) of *E. granulosus* which may develop within a primary cyst to which host cells have been denied access. That the origin of the laminated layer is different in *E. multilocularis* and *E. granulosus* seems unlikely. It has recently been proposed that the laminated layer is an exaggerated glycocalyx (Richards *et al.* 1983), i.e. a much thicker version of the ubiquitous outer carbohydrate coat of tapeworms which is produced by the tegument (Whitfield 1979). The laminated layer undoubtedly assists in supporting the cyst and allows an often considerable intracystic tension to develop (Cameron & Webster 1969, Slais 1973). It may also protect the cyst from immunological attack by offering an immunogenically inert barrier which can deny access to host defence cells (Coltorti & Varela-Diaz 1974). Immunoglobulin, however, can pass through the laminated layer and the capacity to regulate penetration of macromolecules into the cyst appears to be a function of the germinal rather than the laminated layer (Coltorti & Varela-Diaz 1974).

The host fibrous capsule (adventitial layer) which typically surrounds fully developed, viable cysts of *E. granulosus*, is the product of a three-layered host cellular inflammatory reaction initiated in the early stages of post-oncospheral development (Cameron & Webster 1969, Smyth & Heath 1970, Slais & Vanek 1980). The initial intensity of this reaction varies between hosts and governs the fate of the developing metacestode.

If too intense it will cause the degeneration and eventual death of the parasite, whereas in suitable intermediate hosts the initial reaction resolves, leaving a fibrous capsule. The latter situation is common where a stable host–parasite relationship has evolved, as appears to be the case, for example, between the British horse strain of *E. granulosus* and the horse (Thompson 1977a, Ronéus *et al.* 1982).

ECHINOCOCCUS MULTILOCULARIS

The metacestode of *E. multilocularis* is the most complex and develops quite differently to that of *E. granulosus* (Ohbayashi *et al.* 1971, D'Alessandro *et al.* 1979, Wilson & Rausch 1980, FAO 1982, Braithwaite *et al.* 1985). It is a multivesicular, infiltrating structure with no limiting host-tissue barrier (adventitial layer), consisting of numerous small vesicles embedded in a dense stroma of connective tissue (Fig. 1.5). The larval mass usually contains a semisolid matrix rather than fluid. Proliferation occurs both endogenously and exogenously and is attributable to the undifferentiated cells of the germinal layer (Sakamoto & Sugimura 1970). The metacestode consists of a network of filamentous solid cellular protrusions of the germinal layer which are responsible for infiltrating growth (Fig. 1.5) transforming into tube-like and cystic structures (Vogel 1978, Eckert *et al.* 1983, Mehlhorn *et al.* 1983). Furthermore, the detachment of germinal cells from infiltrating cellular protrusions and their subsequent distribution via the lymph or blood can give rise to the distant metastatic foci characteristic of *E. multilocularis* (Ali-Khan *et al.* 1983, Eckert *et al.* 1983, Mehlhorn *et al.* 1983).

ECHINOCOCCUS VOGELI AND *ECHINOCOCCUS OLIGARTHRUS*

The metacestodes of *E. vogeli* and *E. oligarthrus* have been less studied but exhibit developmental and structural characteristics considered intermediate to those of *E. granulosus* and *E. multilocularis* (Rausch *et al.* 1981). The metacestodes of both species are termed polycystic since they are characterised by the internal division of fluid-filled cysts to form multichambered growths (D'Alessandro *et al.* 1979, Morales *et al.* 1979, Rausch *et al.* 1981). *E. vogeli* produces cysts varying greatly in size from 2 to 80 mm, which may occur singly, in small groups, or occasionally in dense aggregations in which each cyst is enclosed by its separate adventitia. In *E. vogeli*, endogenous proliferation and convolution of both germinal and laminated layers leads to the formation of secondary subdivisions of the primary vesicle with production of brood capsules and protoscoleces in the resultant chambers, which are often interconnected. In *E. oligarthrus*, there is less subdivision into secondary chambers and the laminated layer is much thinner than that of *E. vogeli* (Sousa & Thatcher 1969, Rausch *et al.* 1981). Exogenous proliferation has been reported in both species but, at least in *E. vogeli*, it appears to be abnormal and does not occur in the natural intermediate host.

Rate of development

Although in both *E. granulosus* and *E. multilocularis*, initial reorganisation of the oncosphere and formation of the germinal and laminated layers occurs rapidly, usually within the first 14 d (see above), the rate of subsequent development differs markedly. In *E. granulosus*, it is slow and variable and dependent on a number of factors including the strain of parasite, the species and strain of host and the degree of infection. Heath (1973) concluded that *E. granulosus* cysts increase in diameter by between 1 and 5 cm per year depending on factors yet unresolved. The time taken for brood capsule formation is also extremely variable. The earliest recorded is 195 d in mice following oral infection with eggs (Colli & Schantz 1974). In pigs, 10–12 months has been reported (Slais 1980), whereas in sheep reports range from 10 months to 4 years (Heath 1973, and see Ch. 7). The production of brood capsules and protoscoleces does not seem to depend on cyst size and in mice it has been found that it is not always the largest cysts which develop protoscoleces (Colli & Schantz 1974). In horses, fertile cysts as small as 2 mm in diameter have been reported (Edwards 1981). The life-span of hydatid cysts of *E. granulosus* can be as long as 16 years in horses (Ronéus *et al.* 1982) and 53 years in man (Spruance 1974).

In contrast to *E. granulosus, E. multilocularis* develops rapidly in its natural intermediate host, producing protoscoleces in only 2–4 months, an adaptation to the short-lived arvicoline rodents it utilises (Rausch 1975). Thereafter, proliferation of vesicles is curtailed and there is little if any further increase in size (Rausch & Wilson 1973). In man, growth is very different. Proliferation continues indefinitely although there are few if any protoscoleces produced (Rausch & Wilson 1973). The larval mass proliferates peripherally and at the same time regressive changes occur centrally. Thus a progressively enlarging mass of necrotic tissue with a relatively thin zone of viable proliferating parasite is produced. The term 'alveolar hydatid' is used to describe this form of growth, which is not a feature of the development in natural intermediate host species.

Asexual reproduction and differentiation

The asexual reproduction exhibited by species of *Echinococcus* has a potential unsurpassed by other tapeworms and is of particular evolutionary significance (see below). The metacestode has a potentially unlimited sequential generative capacity (reviewed by Whitfield & Evans 1983). Although some germinal cells initiate the production of new brood capsules and protoscoleces, a pool of uncommitted, undifferentiated, germinal cells remain. This fact makes possible the indefinite perpetuation of larval *Echinococcus* in rodents by repeated intraperitoneal passage of protoscoleces or germinal layer material (secondary hydatidosis), and the development in man and other animals of secondary cysts following the rupture of a primary cyst. Thus undifferentiated cells retained in the germinal layer and protoscolex are capable of initiating new cycles of asexual multiplication. Apart from being able to initiate the production of new protoscoleces, a protoscolex has a dual capability since if ingested by a suitable definitive host it will develop into an adult worm. However, even the adult worm must retain some undifferentiated multipotential germinal cells, since adult worms can de-differentiate in a cystic direction under unfavourable conditions (Smyth 1969b). Unfortunately, as with adult *Echinococcus*, there is a pronounced lack of ultrastructural and developmental information relating to germinal cells in the metacestode, and very little is known of the origin and cytodifferentiation of such cells.

STRAIN VARIATION

Taxonomy and terminology

A total of 16 species and 13 subspecies have been described in the genus *Echinococcus* but only the four species *E. granulosus, E. multilocularis, E. oligarthrus* and *E. vogeli* are now recognised as valid taxonomically (Table 1.2). The reasons for dismissing the remainder as taxonomic entities have been discussed in depth (Rausch 1967, Krotov 1979, Kumaratilake & Thompson 1982) and rest largely on evaluation of the morphological descriptions and, in the case of subspecies, lack of evidence for geographical or ecological segregation.

In the past, the extent and significance of the inherent variability exhibited by *Echinococcus* was neglected. As a result certain features that characterised a particular population were overlooked because of uncertainty regarding its taxonomic status. It is now clear that many of the populations previously given taxonomic status exhibit strongly defined and distinct characteristics. Indeed, the possibility that some invalidated subspecies could be reproductively isolated and represent sibling species has been proposed (Rausch, cited by Schantz 1982). However, until more information is available such populations are referred to as strains. It is now firmly established that numerous strains which are of uncertain taxonomic status exist in different parts of the world (Kumaratilake & Thompson 1982). Furthermore, much emphasis is now being given to the importance of strain variation in the epidemiology and control of hydatidosis (Thompson 1982, FAO 1982).

Speciation

The complexity of speciation within *Echinococcus* was discussed over 20 years ago when it was emphasised that the systematic categorisation of *Echinococcus* into well defined species or subspecies may be an oversimplification of a complicated speciation problem. Smyth and Smyth (1964) pointed out that *Echinococcus* has a mode of reproduction which favours the expression of mutants, with the result that new variants can readily arise. In the sexual phase of the life-cycle, the hermaphroditic adult is capable of self-insemination. Thus, if a mutation occurs it will appear in both ova and sperm, resulting in the formation of a homozygote. Because the metacestode reproduces asexually, a large population of genetically identical individuals could arise from a single mutation. *Echinococcus* therefore has the potential to speciate instantaneously and sympatrically without any geographical or ecological isolation. For example, if embryos carrying a mutant gene proved to be infective to a suitable intermediate host, which may represent a new or unusual host, subsequent asexual development would give rise to a clone of genetically identical individuals (protoscoleces). A population of this new variant running into millions could therefore be rapidly established.

Extent of strain variation

ECHINOCOCCUS GRANULOSUS

United Kingdom The turning point in our understanding of strain variation came in the early 1970s with the first demonstration of physiological differences between populations of *E. granulosus*. Smyth and Davies (1974b) compared the *in vitro* development of *E. granulosus* from British sheep and horses and found that in identical culture media the parasite of sheep origin developed to sexual maturity whereas that from horses failed to do so (see Ch. 5 for details). This demonstrated that the two populations, now informally referred to as the British sheep and horse strains, had quite different metabolic requirements. Interestingly, these two populations were initially described as two subspecies, *E. g. granulosus* and *E. g. equinus* (Williams & Sweatman 1963). Comprehensive studies carried out over the last decade have shown that the two populations differ in a range of characteristics and to such an extent that perhaps consideration should be given in the future to proposing that the horse strain is a separate species (*E. equinus*?!). Apart from well documented morphological differences between the two strains, they also differ in host specificity, developmental biology of the adult and metacestode stages, physiology, biochemical characteristics and epidemiology (Thompson & Smyth 1975, Thompson 1978, 1979, Smyth 1977, 1982b, Thompson & Kumaratilake 1982).

Australia Similar studies have been applied to populations of *E. granulosus* in Australia where geographical separation may be a major factor in the selection of strains, since hydatid endemic areas are separated by vast distances of desert or sea (Thompson & Kumaratilake 1982). A variety of criteria have been simultaneously applied to populations of *E. granulosus* from both domestic and wild host assemblages in different geographical areas. It has been possible to differentiate and characterise three distinct strains which differ in the morphology of the adult and metacestode stages (Kumaratilake & Thompson 1984a), the developmental characteristics of both adult and metacestode *in vivo* and *in vitro* (Kumaratilake *et al.* 1983, Kumaratilake & Thompson 1983), and the nature of the protein profiles obtained for each strain by isoelectric focusing (Kumaratilake & Thompson 1984a). Two strains are confined to the Australian mainland; one is maintained principally in a typical sheep–dog cycle and the other in a sylvatic cycle involving dingoes and macropod marsupials (wallabies and kangaroos) (Thompson & Kumaratilake 1982). The third strain is restricted to the Australian island state of Tasmania and is perpetuated in a sheep–dog cycle. The mainland domestic strain is identical to that occurring in sheep in the United Kingdom and New Zealand and was probably introduced with early settlers from Europe, as was probably the case also in New Zealand. The sylvatic strain is quite distinct and shows little in common with forms of *E. granulosus* described in other countries. It seems logical to assume that it was brought into Australia with the dingo accompanying migrating aboriginals many thousands of years ago and has since become well adapted to a cycle between the dingo and macropod marsupials. This is supported by the fact that the sylvatic strain develops normally in dingoes whereas development is retarded in the domestic dog (Thompson & Kumaratilake 1985). The origin of the Tasmanian domestic strain is more difficult to explain. It was presumably introduced into Tasmania with European settlers at about the same time as the domestic strain of *E. granulosus* on the mainland. However, one of the characteristic features of the Tasmanian strain of *E. granulosus* is its more rapid rate of maturation in dogs compared to that of the mainland domestic strain. In particular, the onset of egg production of the Tasmanian strain occurs nearly 1 week earlier than that of its mainland counterpart. It is possible that the intensive control programme adopted in Tasmania over the last 20 years against hydatidosis, involving regular drug treatment of dogs, may have selected for a new strain. A reduced prepatent period would have obvious advantages for a parasite subjected to regular anthelmintic treatment. Similar control measures to those in Tasmania have not been instituted on the Australian mainland and thus *E. granulosus* has not been exposed to the same selection pressure. If this is the case, it demonstrates the rapid evolutionary potential of *Echinococcus*.

Africa An important aspect emphasised by the Australian studies is that a particular strain of *E. granulosus* can occur in more than one intermediate host species and, furthermore, that a particular host species may be susceptible to more than one strain of *E. granulosus*. A similar situation has been described in Kenya, where an unusually complex strain picture apparently exists. Extensive biochemical studies suggest the occurrence of at least three strains, one which occurs in man, sheep and goats, another which occurs in camels and goats, and a third which may be peculiar to cattle, although the status of the cattle form has still to be resolved (McManus 1981, Macpherson & McManus 1982). However, further comparative studies on Kenyan isolates are required since investigations on morphology and development *in vitro* indicate that isolates of *E. granulosus* from different intermediate hosts may be more closely related than the biochemical data suggests (Macpherson 1981, Macpherson & Smyth 1985). Biochemical evidence has also been presented which indicates that the Kenyan sheep strain of *E. granulosus* is different from that occurring in sheep in the United Kingdom (McManus 1981). The Kenyan sheep strain appears to be the major source of infection in man (Macpherson 1983) and it has been suggested that the parasite affecting man may represent a particularly virulent strain, thus accounting for the high level of infection in certain tribes (Thompson 1979, French *et al.* 1982).

In other parts of Africa, a distinct strain of *E. granulosus* apparently occurs in lions. Sylvatic cycles involving the lion and a number of intermediate host species have been reported from several African countries (reviewed by Nelson 1982, 1983, Macpherson *et al.* 1983). The most significant evidence for the existence of a distinct lion strain has been reported by Graber and Thal (1980) in the Central African Republic; they suggest that a sylvatic cycle between the lion and wart-hog occurs and have experimental evidence to show that the local parasite is not only distinct morphologically but also not infective to dogs.

North America A population of *E. granulosus* occurs in northern North America perpetuated in a sylvatic cycle between wolves, moose and reindeer. This parasite, which is considered to represent the original form of the cestode (see Ch. 2), does not readily infect domestic ungulates and, in contrast with domestic strains of *E. granulosus*, is virtually asymptomatic in man (Cameron 1960, Cameron & Webster 1961, Wilson *et al.* 1968). It also differs serologically from domestic strains of the parasite (Cameron 1960) and exhibits characteristic differences in the type of infection produced in laboratory mice (Webster & Cameron 1961).

Switzerland In Switzerland, a cattle–dog cycle is the most important for the maintenance of *E. granulosus* and hydatid cysts in cattle are usually fertile (Eckert 1970, 1981). In the majority of countries from which hydatidosis in cattle has been reported, cysts are rarely fertile and cattle are presumed to be accidental hosts for the parasite maintained in other cycles (reviewed by Thompson *et al.* 1984). For example, in both Australia and the United Kingdom, experimental studies have shown that sheep and cattle isolates are similar. However, the developmental, morphological and biochemical characteristics of *E. granulosus* from Swiss cattle are quite different to those of *E. granulosus* of domestic animal origin from other European countries and Australia (Thompson *et al.* 1984). In particular, adult *E. granulosus* of Swiss cattle origin has a remarkably rapid rate of maturation, producing eggs as early as 34 d after infection! Furthermore, *E. granulosus* of Swiss cattle origin was found to be identical to that occurring in cattle in South Africa, where high fertility rates have also been reported in bovine cysts (Thompson *et al.* 1984). It is of interest that this South African bovine form was initially described as the species *E. ortleppi* by Lopez-Neyra and Soler Planas in 1943.

Russia and Bulgaria Extensive studies have been undertaken in Russia and Bulgaria on different populations of *E. granulosus* (reviewed by Kumaratilake & Thompson 1982). On the basis of a variety of differential criteria, including cross-infection experiments, it appears that in each country a pig strain of the parasite exists which is quite distinct from that occurring in other domestic animals.

Asia There is also evidence of different strains of *E. granulosus* in parts of Asia. The possible existence of a sylvatic strain involving deer and jackals in Sri Lanka has been reported (Paramananthan & Dissanaike 1961) and hydatid cysts with a high fertility rate and unusually large numbers of protoscoleces have been observed in cattle and buffaloes in Sri Lanka (Dissanaike 1957, 1962, Paramananthan 1961). In India, morphological and developmental studies have led to the suggestions that separate buffalo and goat strains occur (Gill & Rao 1967, Rao 1968, Pandey 1972).

ECHINOCOCCUS MULTILOCULARIS

Of the other three species of *Echinococcus*, evidence of strain variation has so far only been reported in *E. multilocularis*. Populations of *E. multilocularis* from Europe, Alaska and central North America differ in a variety of characteristics, including morphology, degree of pathogenicity, developmental characteristics in definitive and intermediate hosts and host specificity (Vogel 1957, Rausch & Richards 1971, Ohbayashi *et al.* 1971, Thompson & Eckert 1983).

Significance of strain variation

From what has been discussed above, it is evident that knowledge of the existence and extent of strain variation is essential if hydatidosis is to be controlled (see Ch. 7). Strain characteristics may influence local patterns of transmission. In Australia, for example, and also other countries where sylvatic and domestic cycles operate, control may be difficult if not impossible if strains of *Echinococcus* perpetuated in wild host assemblages are found to be infective to domestic animals. Control programmes incorporating the regular drug treatment of dogs must also take into account that strains of *E. granulosus* differ in their onset of egg production, as in Switzerland and Australia (Thompson *et al.* 1984, Kumaratilake *et al.* 1983). Evidence of differences in clinical manifestations, pathogenicity and susceptibility to man must also be considered. In Britain the horse strain of *E. granulosus* appears not to be infective to man whereas man is highly susceptible to infection with the sheep strain (Thompson & Smyth 1976, Thompson 1977a). In northern North America the sylvatic strain of *E. granulosus* causes a benign infection in man (Wilson *et al.* 1968), in contrast to the situation in parts of Kenya and Libya, where it has been suggested that virulent strains of *E. granulosus* may exist locally (French *et al.* 1982, Gebreel *et al.* 1983). Differences in the antigenic characteristics between strains of *E. granulosus* will have a bearing on the development of immunodiagnostic procedures in different countries (Cameron 1960, Huldt *et al.* 1973, Gottstein *et al.* 1983, Lightowlers *et al.* 1984, see also Ch. 8). An obvious corollary to this must be the assumption that a vaccine developed against one particular strain of *Echinococcus* may not protect against infection with another strain.

Finally, it has been suggested that strains of *Echinococcus* may differ in their response to particular chemotherapeutic regimes (Saimot *et al.* 1981, Schantz *et al.* 1982, Kammerer & Schantz 1984). This is supported by the detailed information being obtained on the biochemical differences between strains. For example, variation in the activity of individual enzymes has been demonstrated and it has been emphasised that such information is vital if new chemotherapeutic agents are to be developed in the future which may act by inhibiting one or several of the enzymes catalysing energy-synthesising reactions (McManus & Smyth 1982). Furthermore, the fact that strains of *Echinococcus* exhibit variations in their energy metabolisms raises the important question of what advantages do these differences confer on the strains that possess them? (see Bryant 1983).

CONCLUDING REMARKS

Since the early 1960s there has been a flood of new information concerning the developmental biology and host–parasite relationships of *Echinococcus*. The application of *in vitro* cultivation procedures and ultrastructural techniques have probably contributed more than anything else to this new knowledge. However, the story obviously does not end here. The preceding discussion shows that as one question has been answered several more have been uncovered.

We still know very little about cytodifferentiation in both the adult and the metacestode, and can only hypothesise as to the functional significance of tegumental secretions and microtrichial polymorphism in the adult. Much has been deduced about the ontogeny of the adult worm, but several significant aspects have still to be resolved particularly relating to egg production. The factors responsible for stimulating larval–adult differentiation and fertilisation are also not understood. Although *in vitro* culture and ultrastructural studies have revealed a great deal of information on post-oncospheral development and subsequent morphogenesis of the metacestode, we still do not know with certainty the origin of the laminated layer. Furthermore, many areas such as the physiology of excretion and osmoregulation, and the function of calcareous corpuscles, have been completely neglected.

Our understanding and appreciation of the taxonomy and speciation of *Echinococcus* has changed dramatically over the last 25 years. The situation is now much less complex and controversial, and a more rational approach has been taken in designation of species and subspecies. As with many other organisms, biochemical, developmental and behavioural criteria are being used to complement morphology in studies on the differentiation and characterisation of *Echinococcus* populations. A direct result has been the realisation that *Echinococcus* is extremely variable and exists, at least in some species, as a series of strains. The recognition of these strains as species or subspecies by some workers in the past undoubtedly led to previous confusion regarding the taxonomy of the genus. However, the extent and practical significance of strain variation are now widely recognised and new variants are being described and characterised with increasing frequency – an essential prerequisite if adequate control measures are to be defined. As the number of strains which have been identified increase and the characteristics by which they differ become more diverse, an obvious question to be resolved is what advantages these various characteristics bestow on particular strains.

The biology and speciation of this unique and fascinating tapeworm will undoubtedly provide areas for much fruitful research in the future.

REFERENCES

Ali-Khan, Z., R. Siboo, M. Gomersall and M. Faucher 1983. Cystolytic events and the possible role of germinal cells in metastasis in chronic alveolar hydatidosis. *Ann. Trop. Med. Parasitol.* **77**, 497–512.

Arme, C. and P. W. Pappas (eds) 1983. *The biology of the eucestoda.* London: Academic Press.

Arundel, J. H. 1972. A review of cysticercoses of sheep and cattle in Australia. *Aust. Vet. J.* **48**, 140–53.

Beveridge, I. and M. D. Rickard 1975. The development of *Taenia pisiformis* in various definitive host species. *Int. J. Parasitol.* **5**, 633–9.

Blood, B. D. and J. L. Lelijveld 1969. Studies on sylvatic echinococcosis in southern South America. *Z. Tropenmed. Parasitol.* **20**, 475–82.

Borrie, J., M. A. Gemmell and B. W. Manktelow 1965. An experimental approach to evaluate the potential risk of hydatid disease from inhalation of *Echinococcus* ova. *Br. J. Surg.* **52**, 876–8.

Bortoletti, G. and G. Ferretti 1973. Investigation on larval forms of *Echinococcus granulosus* with electron microscope. *Riv. Parassitologia* **34**, 89–110.

Bortoletti, G. and G. Ferretti 1978. Ultrastructural aspects of fertile and sterile cysts of *Echinococcus granulosus* developed in hosts of different species. *Int. J. Parasitol.* **8**, 421–31.

Braithwaite, P. A., R. J. S. Thomas and R. C. A. Thompson 1985. Hydatid disease: the alveolar variety in Australia. A case report with comment on the toxicity of mebendazole. *Aust. N.Z. J. Surg.* (in press).

Bryant, C. 1983. Intraspecies variations of energy metabolism in parasitic helminths. *Int. J. Parasitol.* **13**, 327–32.

Cameron, T. W. M. 1926. Observations on the genus *Echinococcus* Rudolphi, 1801. *J. Helminthol.* **4**, 13–22.

Cameron, T. W. M. 1960. The incidence and diagnosis of hydatid cyst in Canada. *Echinococcus granulosus* var. *canadensis*. *Parassitologia* **2**, 381–90.

Cameron, T. W. M. and G. A. Webster 1961. The ecology of hydatidosis. In *Studies in disease ecology* **2**, 141–60. Washington, D.C.: American Geographical Society.

Cameron, T. W. M. and G. A. Webster 1969. The histogenesis of the hydatid cyst (*Echinococcus* spp.). Part 1. Liver cysts in large mammals. *Can. J. Zool.* **47**, 1405–10.

Colli, C. W. and P. M. Schantz 1974. Growth and development of *Echinococcus granulosus* from embryophores in an abnormal host (*Mus musculus*). *J. Parasitol.* **60**, 53–8.

Colli, C. W. and J. F. Williams 1972. Influence of temperature on the infectivity of eggs of *Echinococcus granulosus* in laboratory rodents. *J. Parasitol.* **58**, 422–6.

Coltorti, E. A. and V. M. Varela-Diaz 1974. *Echinococcus granulosus*: penetration of macromolecules and their localization on the parasite membranes of cysts. *Exp. Parasitol.* **35**, 225–31.

Coman, B. J. and M. D. Rickard 1975. The location of *Taenia pisiformis*, *Taenia ovis* and *Taenia hydatigena* in the gut of the dog and its effect on net environmental contamination with ova. *Z. ParasitKde* **47**, 237–48.

D'Alessandro, A., R. L. Rausch, C. Cuello and N. Aristizabal 1979. *Echinococcus vogeli* in man, with a review of polycystic hydatid disease in Colombia and neighboring countries. *Am. J. Trop. Med. Hyg.* **28**, 303–17.

De Rycke, P. H. 1968. The evagination of *Echinococcus granulosus* in media with different osmotic pressures. *Z. ParasitKde* **30**, 192–8.

Dissanaike, A. S. 1957. Some preliminary observations on *Echinococcus* infection in local cattle and dogs. *Ceylon Med. J.* **4**, 69–75.

Dissanaike, A. S. 1962. Observations on *Echinococcus* infection in Ceylon. In *First regional symposium on scientific knowledge of tropical parasites*, 223–40. Singapore: University of Singapore.

Eckert, J. 1970. Echinokokkose bei Mensch und Tier. *Schweiz. Arch. Tierheilk.* **112**, 443–57.

Eckert, J. 1981. Echinokokkose. *Berl. Münch. Tierärztl. Wscht* **94**, 369–78.

Eckert, J., R. C. A. Thompson and H. Mehlhorn 1983. Proliferation and metastases formation of larval *Echinococcus multilocularis*. I. Animal model, macroscopical and histological findings. *Z. ParasitKde* **69**, 737–48.

Edwards, G. T. 1981. Small fertile hydatid cysts in British horses. *Vet. Rec.* **108**, 460–1.

Fairweather, I. and L. T. Threadgold 1981. *Hymenolepis nana*: the fine structure of the 'penetration gland' and nerve cells within the oncosphere. *Parasitology* **82**, 445–58.

FAO 1982. *Echinococcosis/hydatidosis surveillance, prevention and control: FAO/UNEP/WHO guidelines*, FAO Animal Production and Health Paper No. 29. Rome: Food and Agriculture Organisation of the United Nations.

Featherston, D. W. 1969. *Taenia hydatigena*. I. Growth and development of adult stage in the dog. *Exp. Parasitol.* **25**, 329–38.

Featherston, D. W. 1971. *Taenia hydatigena*. II. Evagination of cysticerci and establishment in dogs. *Exp. Parasitol.* **29**, 242–9.

Freeman, R. S. 1973. Ontogeny of cestodes and its bearing on their phylogeny and systematics. *Adv. Parasitol.* **11**, 481–557.

French, C. M., G. S. Nelson and M. Wood 1982. Hydatid disease in the Turkana district of Kenya. I. The background to the problem with hypotheses to account for the remarkably high prevalence of the disease in man. *Ann. Trop. Med. Parasitol.* **76**, 425–37.

Gill, H. S. and B. V. Rao 1967. On the biology and morphology of *Echinococcus granulosus* (Batsch, 1786) of buffalo-dog origin. *Parasitology* **57**, 695–704.

Gebreel, A. O., H. M. Gilles and J. E. Prescott 1983. Studies on the sero-epidemiology of endemic diseases in Libya. *Ann. Trop. Med. Parasitol.* **77**, 391–7.

Gottstein, B., J. Eckert and H. Fey 1983. Serological differentiation between *Echinococcus granulosus* and *E. multilocularis* infections in man. *Z. ParasitKde* **69**, 347–56.

Graber, M. and J. Thal 1980. L'échinococcose des artiodactyles sauvages de la République Centrafricaine: existence probable d'un cycle lion-phacochère. *Rev. Elev. Méd. Vét. Pays Trop.* **33**, 51–9.

Gustafsson, M. K. S. 1976. Basic cell types in *Echinococcus granulosus* (Cestoda, Cyclophyllidea). *Acta Zool. Fenn.* **146**, 1–16.

Hayunga, E. G. 1979. The structure and function of the scolex glands of three caryophyllid tapeworms. *Proc. Helminthol. Soc. Wash.* **46**, 171–9.

Heath, D. D. 1971. The migration of oncospheres of *Taenia pisiformis, T. serialis* and *Echinococcus granulosus* within the intermediate host. *Int. J. Parasitol.* **1**, 145–52.

Heath, D. D. 1973. The life cycle of *Echinococcus granulosus.* In *Recent advances in hydatid disease*, R. W. Brown, J. R. Salisbury, W. E. White (eds), 7–18. Victoria, Australia: Hamilton Medical and Veterinary Association.

Heath, D. D. and S. B. Lawrence 1976. *Echinococcus granulosus*: development *in vitro* from oncosphere to immature hydatid cyst. *Parasitology* **73**, 417–23.

Heath, D. D. and P. J. Osborn 1976. Formation of *Echinococcus granulosus* laminated membrane in a defined medium. *Int. J. Parasitol.* **6**, 467–71.

Huldt, G., G. S. O. Johansson and S. Lantto 1973. Echinococcosis in northern Scandinavia. *Archs. Environ. Health* **26**, 35–40.

Jha, R. K. and J. D. Smyth 1969. *Echinococcus granulosus*: ultrastructure of microtriches. *Exp. Parasitol.* **25**, 232–44.

Jha, R. K. and J. D. Smyth 1971. Ultrastructure of the rostellar tegument of *Echinococcus granulosus* with special reference to biogenesis of mitochondria. *Int. J. Parasitol.* **1**, 169–77.

Kammerer, W. S. and P. M. Schantz 1984. Long term follow-up of human hydatid disease (*Echinococcus granulosus*) treated with a high-dose mebendazole regimen. *Am. J. Trop. Med. Hyg.* **33**, 132–7.

Kilejian, A. and C. W. Schwabe 1971. Studies on the polysaccharides of the *Echinococcus granulosus* cyst, with observations on a possible mechanism for laminated membrane formation. *Comp. Biochem. Physiol.* **40B**, 25–36.

Kilejian, A., L. A. Schinazi and C. W. Schwabe 1961. Host–parasite relationships in echinococcosis. V. Histochemical observations on *Echinococcus granulosus. J. Parasitol.* **47**, 181–8.

Krotov, A. I. 1979. [The question of the subspecies and strains of representatives of *Echinococcus* Rudolphi, 1801.] *Meditsinskaya Parazitologiya i Parazitarnye Bolezni* **48**, 22–6 [in Russian].

Kumaratilake, L. M. and R. C. A. Thompson 1981. Maintenance of the life cycle of *Echinococcus granulosus* in the laboratory following *in vivo* and *in vitro* development. *Z. ParasitKde* **65**, 103–6.

Kumaratilake, L. M. and R. C. A. Thompson 1982. A review of the taxonomy and speciation of the genus *Echinococcus* Rudolphi 1801. *Z. ParasitKde* **68**, 121–46.

Kumaratilake, L. M. and R. C. A. Thompson 1983. A comparison of *Echinococcus granulosus* from different geographical areas of Australia using secondary cyst development in mice. *Int. J. Parasitol.* **13**, 509–15.

Kumaratilake, L. M. and R. C. A. Thompson 1984a. Morphological characterisation of Australian strains of *Echinococcus granulosus. Int. J. Parasitol.* 14, 467–11.

Kumaratilake, L. M. and R. C. A. Thompson 1984a. Biochemical characterisation of Australian strains of *Echinococcus granulosus* by isoelectric focusing of soluble proteins. *Int. J. Parasitol.* 14, 581–6.

Kumaratilake, L. M., R. C. A. Thompson and J. D. Dunsmore 1983. Comparative strobilar development of *Echinococcus granulosus* of sheep origin from different geographical areas of Australia *in vivo* and *in vitro*. *Int. J. Parasitol.* **13**, 151–6.

Kumazawa, H. and N. Suzuki 1983. Kinetics of proglottid formation, maturation and shedding during development of *Hymenolepis nana*. *Parasitology* **86**, 275–89.

Lascano, E. F., E. A. Coltorti and V. M. Varela-Diaz 1975. Fine structure of the germinal membrane of *Echinococcus granulosus* cysts. *J. Parasitol.* **61**, 853–60.

Lethbridge, R. C. 1980. The biology of the oncosphere of cyclophyllidean cestodes. *Helminthol. Abstr. A* **49**, 59–72.

Lightowlers, M. W., M. D. Rickard, R. D. Honey, D. L. Obendorf and G. F. Mitchell 1984. Serological diagnosis of *Echinococcus granulosus* infection in sheep using cyst fluid antigen processed by antibody affinity chromatography. *Aust. Vet. J.* **61**, 101–8.

Lindroos, P. and T. Gardberg 1982. The excretory system of *Diphyllobothrium dendriticum* (Nitzsch 1824) plerocercoids as revealed by an injection technique. *Z. ParasitKde* **67**, 289–97.

Lopez-Neyra, C. R. and M. Soler Planas 1943. Revisión del género *Echinococcus* Rud. y descripción de una especie nuéva parasita intestinal del perro en Almería. *Rev. Ibér. Parasitologia* **3**, 169–94.

McManus, D. P. 1981. A biochemical study of adult and cystic stages of *Echinococcus granulosus* of human and animal origin from Kenya. *J. Helminthol.* **55**, 21–7.

McManus, D. P. and J. D. Smyth 1982. Intermediary carbohydrate metabolism in protoscoleces of *Echinococcus granulosus* (horse and sheep strains) and *E. multilocularis*. *Parasitology* **84**, 351–66.

Macpherson, C. N. L. 1981. *Epidemiology and strain differentiation of* Echinococcus granulosus *in Kenya*. PhD thesis, University of London.

Macpherson, C. N. L. 1983. An active intermediate host role for man in the life cycle of *Echinococcus granulosus* in Turkana, Kenya. *Am. J. Trop. Med. Hyg.* **32**, 397–404.

Macpherson, C. N. L. and D. P. McManus 1982. A comparative study of *Echinococcus granulosus* from human and animal hosts in Kenya using isoelectric focusing and isoenzyme analysis. *Int. J. Parasitol.* **12**, 515–21.

Macpherson, C. N. L. and J. D. Smyth 1985. *In vitro* culture of the strobilar stage of *Echinococcus granulosus* from protoscoleces of human, camel, sheep and goat origin from Kenya and buffalo origin from India. *Int. J. Parasitol.* 15, 137–40.

Macpherson, C. N. L., L. Karstad, P. Stevenson and J. H. Arundel 1983. Hydatid disease in the Turkana district of Kenya. III. The significance of wild animals in the transmission of *Echinococcus granulosus*, with particular reference to Turkana and Masailand in Kenya. *Ann. Trop. Med. Parasitol.* **77**, 61–73.

Marchiondo, A. A. and F. L. Andersen 1983. Fine structure and freeze-etch study of the protoscolex tegument of *Echinococcus multilocularis* (Cestoda). *J. Parasitol.* **69**, 709–18.

Mehlhorn, H., B. Becker, P. Andrews and H. Thomas 1981. On the nature of the proglottids of cestodes: a light and electron microscopic study on *Taenia, Hymenolepis* and *Echinococcus*. *Z. ParasitKde* **65**, 243–59.

Mehlhorn, H., J. Eckert and R. C. A. Thompson 1983. Proliferation and metastases formation of larval *Echinococcus multilocularis*. II. Ultrastructural investigations. *Z. ParasitKde* **69**, 749–63.

Mettrick, D. F. and R. B. Podesta 1974. Ecological and physiological aspects of helminth–host interactions in the mammalian gastrointestinal canal. *Adv. Parasitol.* **12**, 183–277.

Morales, G. A., V. H. Guzman, E. A. Wells and D. Angel 1979. Polycystic echinococcosis in Columbia: the larval cestodes in infected rodents. *J. Wilde. Dis.* **15**, 421–8.

Morseth, D. J. 1965. Ultrastructure of developing taeniid embryophores and associated structures. *Exp. Parasitol.* **16**, 207–16.

Morseth, D. J. 1966. Chemical composition of embryophoric blocks of *Taenia hydatigena, Taenia ovis* and *Taenia pisiformis* eggs. *Exp. Parasitol.* **18**, 347–54.

Morseth, D. J. 1967. Fine structure of the hydatid cyst and protoscolex of *Echinococcus granulosus. J. Parasitol.* **53**, 312–25.

Nelson, G. S. 1982. Carrion-feeding cannibalistic carnivores and human disease in Africa with special reference to trichinosis and hydatid disease in Kenya. *Symp. Zool. Soc. Lond.* **50**, 181–98.

Nelson, G. S. 1983. Wild animals as reservoir hosts of parasitic diseases of man in Kenya. In *Tropical parasitoses and parasitic zoonoses*, J. D. Dunsmore (ed), 59–72. 10th Meeting of the World Association for the Advancement of Veterinary Parasitology, Australia.

Nieland, M. L. 1968. Electron microscope observations on the egg of *Taenia taeniaeformis. J. Parasitol.* **54**, 957–69.

Ohbayashi, M., R. L. Rausch and F. H. Fay 1971. On the ecology and distribution of *Echinococcus* spp. (Cestoda: Taeniidae), and characteristics of their development in the intermediate host. II. Comparative studies on the larval *E. multilocularis* Leuckart, 1863, in the intermediate host. *Jap. J. Vet. Res.* **19**, Suppl. 3, 1–53.

Öhman-James, C. 1973. Cytology and cytochemistry of the scolex gland cells in *Diphyllobothrium ditremum* (Creplin, 1825). *Z. ParasitKde* **42**, 77–86.

Pandey, V. S. 1972. Observations on the morphology and biology of *Echinococcus granulosus* (Batsch, 1786) of goat–dog origin. *J. Helminthol.* **46**, 219–33.

Paramananthan, D. C. 1961. Some observations on brood capsules of hydatid cysts from local animals. *Ceylon J. Med. Sci.* **10**, 57–9.

Paramananthan, D. C. and A. S. Dissanaike 1961. Sylvatic hydatid infection in Ceylon. *Trans. R. Soc. Trop. Med. Hyg.* **55**, 483.

Rao, B. V. 1968. Experimental transmission of *Echinococcus* of buffalo origin to foxes (*Vulpes bengalensis*). *Vet. Rec.* **83**, 56–7.

Rausch, R. L. 1954. Studies on the helminth fauna of Alaska. XX. The histogenesis of the alveolar larva of *Echinococcus* species. *J. Infect. Dis.* **94**, 178–86.

Rausch, R. L. 1967. A consideration of intraspecific categories in the genus *Echinococcus* Rudolphi, 1801 (Cestoda: Taeniidae). *J. Parasitol.* **53**, 484–91.

Rausch, R. L. 1975. Taeniidae. In *Diseases transmitted from animals to man*, W. T. Hubbert, W. F. McCulloch and P. R. Schurrenberger (eds), 678–707. Springfield, Ill.: Thomas.

Rausch, R. L. and J. J. Bernstein 1972. *Echinococcus vogeli* sp. n. (Cestoda: Taeniidae) from the bush dog, *Speothos venaticus* (Lund). *Z. Tropenmed. Parasit.* **23**, 25–34.

Rausch, R. L. and S. H. Richards 1971. Observations on parasite–host relationships of *Echinococcus multilocularis* Leuckart, 1863, in North Dakota. *Can. J. Zool.* 1317–30.

Rausch, R. L. and J. F. Wilson 1973. Rearing of the adult *Echinococcus multilocularis*

Leuckart, 1863, from sterile larvae from man. *Am. J. Trop. Med. Hyg.* **22**, 357–60.

Rausch, R. L., A. D'Alessandro and M. Ohbayashi 1984. The taxonomic status of *Echinococcus cruzi* Brumpt and Joyeux, 1924 (Cestoda: Taeniidae) from an agouti (Rodentia: Dasyproctidae) in Brazil. *J. Parasitol.* **70**, 295–302.

Rausch, R. L., A. D'Alessandro and V. R. Rausch 1981. Characteristics of the larval *Echinococcus vogeli* Rausch and Bernstein, 1972 in the natural intermediate host, the paca, *Cuniculus paca* L. (Rodentia: Dasyproctidae). *Am. J. Trop. Med. Hyg.* **30**, 1043–52.

Rausch, R. L., V. R. Rausch and A. D'Alessandro 1978. Discrimination of the larval stages of *Echinococcus oligarthrus* (Diesing, 1863) and *E. vogeli* Rausch and Bernstein, 1972 (Cestoda: Taeniidae). *Am. J. Trop. Med. Hyg.* **29**, 1195–202.

Rees, G. R. 1967. Pathogenesis of adult cestodes. *Helminthol. Abstr. A* **36**, 1–23.

Richards, K. S. and C. Arme 1981. The ultrastructure of the scolex–neck syncytium, neck cells and frontal gland cells of *Caryophyllaeus laticeps* (Caryophyllidea: Cestoda). *Parasitology* **83**, 477–87.

Richards, K. S., C. Arme and J. F. Bridges 1983. *Echinococcus granulosus equinus*: an ultrastructural study of the laminated layer, including changes on incubating cysts in various media. *Parasitology* **86**, 399–405.

Ronéus, O., D. Christensson and N.-G. Nilsson 1982. The longevity of hydatid cysts in horses. *Vet. Parasitol.* **11**, 149–54.

Saimot, A. G., A. Meulemans, J. M. Hay, J. Mohler, C. Manuel and J. P. Coulaud 1981. Etude pharmacocinétique du flubendazole au cours de l'hydatidose humaine á *E. granulosus*. Résultats préliminaies. *Nouv. Presse Med.* **10**, 3121–24.

Sakamoto, T. 1981. Electron microscopical observations on the egg of *Echinococcus multilocularis*. *Mem. Fac. Agr. Kagoshima Univ.* **17**, 165–74.

Sakamoto, T. and M. Sugimura 1970. Studies on echinococcosis. XXIII. Electron microscopical observations on histogenesis of larval *Echinococcus multilocularis*. *Jap. J. Vet. Res.* **18**, 131–44.

Sakamoto, T., I. Kono and N. Yasuda 1982. Experimental infection of mice by intrahepatic inoculation of oncospheres and eggs of *Echinococcus granulosus*. *Mem. Fac. Agr. Kagoshima Univ.* **18**, 141–7.

Sawada, I. 1973. The mode of attachment of the larval tapeworm to the mucosa of the chicken intestine. *Jap. J. Zool.* **17**, 1–9.

Schantz, P. M. 1982. Echinococcosis. In *CRC handbook series in zoonoses, Section C: Parasitic zoonoses*, J. Steele (ed.), **1**, 231–77. Boca Raton, Fla: CRC Press.

Schantz, P. M., H. Van den Bossche and J. Eckert 1982. Chemotherapy for larval echinococcosis in animals and humans: report of a workshop. *Z. ParasitKde* **67**, 5–26.

Schmidt, G. D. and L. S. Roberts 1981. *Foundations of parasitology*. St Louis: Mosby.

Slais, J. 1973. Functional morphology of cestode larvae. *Adv. Parasitol.* **11**, 395–480.

Slais, J. 1980. Experimental infection on sheep and pigs with *Echinococcus granulosus* (Batsch, 1786), and the origin of pouching in hydatid cysts. *Acta Vet. Acad. Sci. Hung.* **28**, 375–87.

Slais, J. and M. Vanek 1980. Tissue reactions to spherical and lobular hydatid cysts of *Echinococcus granulosus* (Batsch, 1786). *Folia Parasitol.* **27**, 135–43.

Smyth, J. D. 1962. Studies on tapeworm physiology. X. Axenic cultivation of the hydatid organism, *Echinococcus granulosus*; establishment of a basic technique. *Parasitology* **52**, 441–57.

Smyth, J. D. 1964a. The biology of the hydatid organism. *Adv. Parasitol.* **2**, 169–219.

Smyth, J. D. 1964b. Observations on the scolex of *Echinococcus granulosus*, with special reference to the occurrence and cytochemistry of secretory cells in the rostellum. *Parasitology* **54**, 515–26.

Smyth, J. D. 1967. Studies on tapeworm physiology. XI. *In vitro* cultivation of *Echinococcus granulosus* from the protoscolex to the strobilate stage. *Parasitology* **57**, 111–33.

Smyth, J. D. 1968. *In vitro* studies and host-specificity in *Echinococcus. Bull. Wld Hlth Org.* **39**, 5–12.

Smyth, J. D. 1969a. *The physiology of cestodes.* Edinburgh: Oliver & Boyd.

Smyth, J. D. 1969b. Parasites as biological models. *Parasitology* **59**, 73–91.

Smyth, J. D. 1971. Development of monozoic forms of *Echinococcus granulosus* during *in vitro* culture. *Int. J. Parasitol.* **1**, 121–4.

Smyth, J. D. 1972. Changes in the digestive surface of cestodes during larval/adult differentiation. In *Functional aspects of parasite surfaces*, A. E. R. Taylor and R. Muller (eds), *Symp. Br. Soc. Parasitol.* **10**, 41–70. Oxford: Blackwell Scientific.

Smyth, J. D., 1976. *Introduction to animal parasitology.* London: Hodder and Stoughton.

Smyth, J. D. 1977. Strain differences in *Echinococcus granulosus*, with special reference to the status of equine hydatidosis in the United Kingdom. *Trans. R. Soc. Trop. Med. Hyg.* **71**, 93–100.

Smyth, J. D. 1979. *Echinococcus granulosus* and *E. multilocularis: in vitro* culture of the strobilar stages from protoscoleces. *Angew. Parasitol.* **20**, 137–47.

Smyth, J. D. 1982a. The insemination–fertilization problem in cestodes cultured *in vitro*. In *Aspects of parasitology. A* Festschrift *dedicated to the fiftieth anniversary of the Institute of Parasitology of McGill University* 1932–1982, E. Meerovitch (ed.), 393–406. Montreal: McGill University.

Smyth, J. D. 1982b. Speciation in *Echinococcus*: biological and biochemical criteria. *Revta Ibér. Parasitol.* Vol. Extra, 25–34.

Smyth, J. D. and N. J. Barrett 1979. *Echinococcus multilocularis*: further observations on strobilar differentiation *in vitro*. *Revta Ibér. Parasitol.* **39**, 39–53.

Smyth, J. D. and Z. Davies 1974a. *In vitro* culture of the strobilar stage of *Echinococcus granulosus* (sheep strain): a review of basic problems and results. *Int. J. Parasitol.* **4**, 631–44.

Smyth, J. D. and Z. Davies 1974b. Occurrence of physiological strains of *Echinococcus granulosus* demonstrated by *in vitro* culture of protoscoleces from sheep and horse hydatid cysts. *Int. J. Parasitol.* **4**, 443–5.

Smyth, J. D. and Z. Davies 1975. *In vitro* suppression of segmentation in *Echinococcus multilocularis* with morphological transformation of protoscoleces into monozoic adults. *Parasitology* **71**, 125–35.

Smyth, J. D. and D. D. Heath 1970. Pathogenesis of larval cestodes in mammals. *Helminthol. Abstr. A* **39**, 1–23.

Smyth, J. D. and M. M. Smyth 1964. Natural and experimental hosts of *Echinococcus granulosus* and *E. multilocularis*, with comments on the genetics of speciation in the genus *Echinococcus*. *Parasitology* **54**, 493–514.

Smyth, J. D. and M. M. Smyth 1968. Some aspects of host specificity in *Echinococcus granulosus*. *Helminthologia* **9**, 519–27.

Smyth, J. D. and M. M. Smyth 1969. Self insemination in *Echinococcus granulosus in vivo*. *J. Helminthol.* **43**, 383–8.

Smyth, J. D., M. Gemmell and M. M. Smyth 1969a. Establishment of *Echinococcus granulosus* in the intestine of normal and vaccinated dogs. *Ind. J. Helminthol.* Srivastava Commemorative Volume, 167–78.

Smyth, J. D., H. J. Miller and A. B. Howkins 1967. Further analysis of the factors controlling strobilization, differentiation, and maturation of *Echinococcus granulosus in vitro*. *Exp. Parasitol.* **21**, 31–41.

Smyth, J. D., D. J. Morseth and M. M. Smyth 1969b. Observations on nuclear secretions in the rostellar gland cells of *Echinococcus granulosus* (Cestoda). *The Nucleus* **12**, 47–56.

Sousa, O. E. and V. E. Thatcher 1969. Observations on the life-cycle of *Echinococcus oligarthrus* (Diesing, 1863) in the Republic of Panama. *Ann. Trop. Med. Parasitol.* **63**, 165–75.

Specian, R. D. and R. D. Lumsden 1981. Histochemical, cytochemical and autoradiographic studies on the rostellum of *Hymenolepsis diminuta*. *Z. ParasitKde* **64**, 335–45.

Spruance, S. L. 1974. Latent period of 53 years in a case of hydatid cyst disease. *Archs. Int. Med.* **134**, 741–2.

Sulgostowska, T. 1972. The development of organ systems in cestodes. I. A study of histology of *Hymenolepsis diminuta* (Rudolphi, 1819) Hymenolepididae. *Acta Parasitol. Pol.* **20**, 449–62.

Sulgostowska, T. 1974. The development of organ systems in cestodes. II. Histogenesis of the reproductive system in *Hymenolepis diminuta* (Rudolphi, 1819) (Hymenolepididae). *Acta Parasitol. Pol.* **22**, 179–90.

Sweatman, G. K. and R. J. Williams 1963. Comparative studies on the biology and morphology of *Echinococcus granulosus* from domestic livestock, moose and reindeer. *Parasitology* **53**, 339–90.

Swiderski, Z. 1982, *Echinococcus granulosus*: embryonic envelope formation. *Proc. 10th Int. Cong. Electron Microsc.* **3**, 513.

Swiderski, Z. 1983. *Echinococcus granulosus*: hook-muscle systems and cellular organisation of infective oncospheres. *Int. J. Parasitol.* **13**, 289–99.

Thatcher, V. E. and O. E. Sousa 1966. *Echinococcus oligarthrus* Diesing, 1863, in Panama and a comparison with recent human hydatid. *Ann. Trop. Med. Parasitol.* **60**, 405–16.

Thompson, R. C. A. 1975. *Studies on equine hydatidosis in Great Britain*. PhD thesis, University of London.

Thompson, R. C. A. 1976. The development of brood capsules and protoscolices in secondary hydatid cysts of *Echinococcus granulosus*. *Z. ParasitKde* **51**, 31–6.

Thompson, R. C. A. 1977a. Hydatidosis in Great Britain. *Helminthol. Abstr. A* **46**, 837–61.

Thompson, R. C. A. 1977b. Growth, segmentation and maturation of the British horse and sheep strains of *Echinococcus granulosus* in dogs. *Int. J. Parasitol.* **7**, 281–5.

Thompson, R. C. A. 1978. Equine hydatidosis (echinococcosis) in Great Britain. *Proc. 2nd Eur. Multicoll. Parasitol, Trogir, 1975*, 301–9. Belgrade: Association of Yugoslav Parasitologists.

Thompson, R. C. A. 1979. Biology and speciation of *Echinococcus granulosus*. *Aust. Vet. J.* **55**, 93–8.

Thompson, R. C. A. 1982. Intraspecific variation and parasite epidemiology. In *Parasites: their world and ours*, D. F. Mettrick and S. S. Desser (eds), 369–78. Amsterdam: Elsevier Biomedical Press.

Thompson, R. C. A. 1983. The susceptibility of the European red fox (*Vulpes vulpes*) to infection with *Echinococcus granulosus* of Australian sheep origin. *Ann. Trop. Med. Parasitol.* **77**, 75–82.

Thompson, R. C. A. and J. Eckert 1982. The production of eggs by *Echinococcus multilocularis* in the laboratory following *in vivo* and *in vitro* development. *Z. ParasitKde* **68**, 227–34.

Thompson, R. C. A. and J. Eckert 1983. Observations on *Echinococcus multilocularis* in the definitive host. *Z. ParasitKde* **69**, 335–45.

Thompson, R. C. A. and L. M. Kumaratilake 1982. Intraspecific variation in

Echinococcus granulosus: the Australian situation and perspectives for the future. *Trans. R. Soc. Trop. Med. Hyg.* **76**, 13–6.

Thompson, R. C. A. and L. M. Kumaratilake 1985. Comparative development of Australian strains of *Echinococcus granulosus* in dingoes (*Canis familiaris dingo*) and domestic dogs (*C. f. familiaris*) with further evidence for the origin of the sylvatic strain. (in press).

Thompson, R. C. A. and J. D. Smyth 1975. Equine hydatidosis: a review of the current status in Great Britain and the results of an epidemiological survey. *Vet. Parasitol.* **1**, 107–27.

Thompson, R. C. A. and J. D. Smyth 1976. Attempted infection of the rhesus monkey (*Macaca mulatta*) with the British horse strain of *Echinococcus granulosus*. *J. Helminthol.* **50**, 175–7.

Thompson, R. C. A., J. D. Dunsmore and A. R. Hayton 1979. *Echinococcus granulosus*: secretory activity of the rostellum of the adult cestode *in situ* in the dog. *Exp. Parasitol.* **48**, 144–63.

Thompson, R. C. A., A. Houghton and V. Zaman 1982. A study of the microtriches of adult *Echinococcus granulosus* by scanning electron microscopy. *Int. J. Parasitol.* **12**, 579–83.

Thompson, R. C. A., L. M. Kumaratilake and J. Eckert 1984. Observations on *Echinococcus granulosus* of cattle origin in Switzerland. *Int. J. Parasitol.* **14**, 283–91.

Vanek, M. 1980. A morphological study of hydatids of *Echinococcus granulosus* (Batsch, 1786) from pigs. *Fol. Parasitol.* **27**, 37–46.

Varela-Diaz, V. M. and J. M. Torres 1977. Antigenic characterization of *Echinococcus granulosus* cysts. *Boll. 1st Sieroter, Milanese* **56**, 303–9.

Verheyen, A. 1982. *Echinococcus granulosus*: the influence of mebendazole therapy on the ultrastructural morphology of the germinal layer of hydatid cysts in humans and mice. *Z. ParasitKde* **67**, 55–65.

Verster, A. J. M. 1965. Review of *Echinococcus* species in South Africa. *Onderstepoort J. Vet. Res.* **32**, 7–118.

Vogel, H. 1957. Über den *Echinococcus multilocularis* Süddeutschlands. I. Das Bandwurm-Stadium von Stämmen menschlicher und tierischer Herkunft. *Z. Tropenmed. Parasitol.* **8**, 404–54.

Vogel, H. 1978. Wie wächst der Alveolarechinokokkus? *Tropenmed. Parasitol.* **29**, 1–11.

Walters, T. M. H. and M. J. Clakson 1980. The development of *Echinococcus granulosus* in sheep dogs, beagles and foxes. *Trans. R. Soc. Trop. Med. Hyg.* **74**, 118.

Wardle, R. A., J. A. McLeod and S. Radinovsky 1974. *Advances in the zoology of tapeworms*. Minneapolis: University of Minnesota Press.

Webster, G. A. and T. W. M. Cameron 1961. Observations on experimental infections with *Echinococcus* in rodents. *Can. J. Zool.* **39**, 877–91.

Whitfield, P. J. 1979. *The biology of parasitism: an introduction to the study of associating organisms*. London: Edward Arnold.

Whitfield, P. J. and N. A. Evans 1983. Pathogenesis and asexual multiplication among parasitic platyhelminths. *Parasitology* **86**, 121–60.

Williams, J. F. and C. W. Colli 1970. Primary cystic infection with *Echinococcus granulosus* and *Taenia hydatigena* in *Meriones unguiculatus*. *J. Parasitol.* **56**, 509–13.

Williams, R. J. and G. K. Sweatman 1963. On the transmission, biology and morphology of *Echinococcus granulosus equinus*, a new subspecies of hydatid tapeworm in horses in Great Britain. *Parasitology* **53**, 391–407.

Wilson, J. F. and R. L. Rausch 1980. Alveolar hydatid disease. A review of clinical features of 33 indigenous cases of *Echinococcus multilocularis* infection in Alaskan Eskimos. *Am. J. Trop. Med. Hyg.* **29**, 1340–55.

Wilson, J. F., A. C. Diddams and R. L. Rausch 1968. Cystic hydatid disease in Alaska. A review of 101 autochthonous cases of *Echinococcus granulosus* infection. *Am. Rev. Resp. Dis.* **98**, 1–15.

Willis, J., I. V. Herbert and T. C. Elliott 1981. Some factors affecting the survival and transmission of *Taenia multiceps* eggs. *Proc. 9th Int. Conf. W.A.A.V.P., Budapest*, 126.

Yamashita, J., M. Ohbayashi and S. Konno 1956. Studies on echinococcosis. III. On experimental infection in dogs, especially on the development of *Echinococcus granulosus* (Batsch, 1786). *Jap. J. Vet. Res.* **4**, 113–22.

2 Life-cycle patterns and geographic distribution of *Echinococcus* species

ROBERT L. RAUSCH

INTRODUCTION

Most of our knowledge concerning the biology of cestodes of the genus *Echinococcus* Rudolphi, 1801 has been acquired during the last 30 years, after fundamental studies provided the means for distinguishing taxa at the infrageneric level. The cycle of *E. granulosus* (Batsch, 1786) had been determined experimentally by von Siebold (1853) not long before Virchow (1855) recognised that the condition earlier designated alveolar colloid, or colloid carcinoma, of the liver in man was caused by a larval cestode of the genus *Echinococcus*. During the following century, a great number of works were published concerning the structure and development of *E. granulosus*, and clinical and pathological findings were reported for many cases of cystic and alveolar forms of hydatid disease, but investigations were hampered by growing controversy surrounding the identity of the aetiologic agent of alveolar hydatid disease. The 'unicist' view, that only a single species, *E. granulosus*, caused both forms of disease in man, gained adherents world-wide on the authority of F. Dévé and H. R. Dew, and prevailed.

The investigations eventually leading to a vindication of the 'dualist' concept of the causality of hydatid disease in man in Europe, as maintained by A. Posselt, C. Mangold and others, began in the 1950s, after a cestode identified as the aetiologic agent of alveolar hydatid disease among Eskimos in North America (arctic Alaska) was described (as *E. sibiricensis* Rausch and Schiller, 1954), its natural cycle elucidated, and its possible causal relationship to classical alveolar hydatid disease recognised. On the grounds that the question could be resolved without doubt only in Europe, the late Professor Hans Vogel undertook similar investigations in southern Germany. Preliminary findings were reported at the Sixth International Congress of Hydatidosis, with the conclusion (Vogel 1957, p. 522), '*Damit . . . dürfte die seit fast hundert Jahren umstrittene Natur des europäischen Alveolar-Echinococcus geklärt sein. Die Entscheidung ist im Sinne der dualistischen Auffassung von Posselt gefallen.*' Vogel also determined that the applicable name for the cestode causing alveolar hydatid disease is *E. multilocularis* Leuckart, 1863. The beginning of intensive studies of that cestode in the Soviet Union was marked by a paper by Leikina (1957), which reviewed relevant Russian literature, acknowledged the validity of the findings in Alaska and Germany, but expressed uncertainty about the significance of alveolar-like lesions sometimes found in the liver of domestic ungulates. Although such lesions, which represent an anomalous growth-form of the larval *E. granulosus*, remained a source of confusion, the two taxa had been clearly distinguished by the 1960s.

A third member of this group, *Taenia oligarthra* Diesing, 1863, from the cougar, *Felis concolor* L., in Brasil, was redescribed by Lühe (1910), and transferred to the genus *Echinococcus*. The cycle of *E. oligarthrus* was determined experimentally by Sousa and Thatcher in 1969. The genus includes a fourth species, *E. vogeli* Rausch and Bernstein, 1972, of which the strobilar stage was described from the bush dog, *Speothos venaticus* (Lund), from Ecuador.

The purpose of the present work, based on the comprehension provided by these recent studies, is to define parasite–host interactions, i.e. patterns of cycles, of cestodes of the four species, to list final and intermediate hosts, and to discuss geographic ranges. The specific identity of these taxa has been based on standard taxonomic procedure for cestodes, with the exception that two biologically distinct forms of *E. granulosus* have been recognised. Local strains of this cestode are not considered here (see Ch. 1). Because of limitations of space, citations of literature have been kept to a minimum. Scientific names for domestic animals, to indicate their derivation, follow Herre and Röhrs (1973); those of wild mammals are mainly according to Honacki *et al.* (1982); identities of small mammals reported under common names in the Russian literature have been determined from Vinogradov and Gromov (1952).

ECHINOCOCCUS GRANULOSUS (BATSCH, 1786)

Two biological forms of *Echinococcus granulosus* have been recognised on the basis of differences in host-specificity in the larval stage (Rausch 1967a). In this stage as well, the two forms differ developmentally, and in pathogenicity and quality of immune response in man (Wilson *et al.* 1968, and unpublished). The Northern Form is indigenous to the holarctic zones of tundra and boreal forest, or taiga, and occurs also under favourable conditions at lower latitudes. I consider this form to be ancestral to the second, the European Form, which became adapted to synanthropic hosts with the development of animal husbandry. For mammals (wolf and ungulates), the times of habituation to controlled life differed with species and geographic region, but most of the ungulates apparently were domesticated within the past 10 000 years (see Herre & Röhrs 1973, p. 64, for details). Regardless of time and place of adaptation, the European Form of *E. granulosus* must have occurred in domestic animals throughout Europe by the end of the 15th century, when the period of conquest and colonisation began. By then that taeniid and others, similarly adapted, were dispersed with their hosts to widely separated regions of the world.

The Northern Form of *Echinococcus granulosus*

In the larval stage, the Northern Form of *E. granulosus* occurs almost exclusively in ungulates of the family Cervidae; no evidence indicates that its development takes place in domestic ungulates (excluding the domesticated reindeer). The dog, *Canis lupus* f. *familiaris*, may replace the wolf as final host.

PATTERNS OF CYCLES

Natural cycle In the zones of tundra and taiga, where natural conditions usually have not been disrupted, the Northern Form of *E. granulosus* is perpetuated primarily by the predator–prey relationship existing between the wolf, *Canis lupus* L., and large deer – elk, *Alces alces* L. (called 'moose' in North America); reindeer (including the semidomesticated form), *Rangifer tarandus* (L.); and others. Based on surveys in North America, rates of infection in wolves may be relatively high: 60 (30 per cent) of 200 animals in Alaska (Rausch & Williamson 1959); 103 (20 per cent) of 520 in Ontario (Freeman *et al.* 1961); 71 (72 per cent) of 98 in Alberta (Holmes & Podesta 1968); and 24 (14 per cent) of 171 in the Yukon and Northwest Territories (Choquette *et al.* 1973). The numerous records from wolves and cervids in northern Eurasia indicate a comparable magnitude. Ten (42 per cent) of 24 wolves from the Soviet Far East were infected (Kikot' 1980); 11 per cent of wolves examined harboured *E. granulosus* in Kazakhstan (Panin & Lavrov 1962).

The intermediate hosts overlap in geographic range and, at least seasonally, in habitat. Wild reindeer migrate with season, from summer range on the tundra to winter range in the taiga, and the reverse (for patterns of migration in Siberia, see Geptner *et al.* 1961, Fig. 109). Elk are primarily inhabitants of taiga, but may occur in substantial numbers beyond the northern forest, along rivers and streams bordered by dense stands of willow and alder. In deer, the larval stage of the Northern Form of *E. granulosus* consists of a subspherical to spherical cyst, in which the germinal layer is covered by contiguous, firmly attached brood capsules, and occurs typically in the lungs; those found rarely in other organs (liver, heart) are anomalous and usually lack protoscoleces. Findings in experimentally infected reindeer and elk have shown that the larval stage of the Northern Form develops more slowly than that of the European Form in domestic ungulates (R. L. Rausch, unpublished).

In North America, rates of infection in wild reindeer are low. In the central Brooks Range (arctic Alaska), cysts were found in three (*c.* 5 per cent) of 63 animals (predominantly adults) examined during October 1962, and in two (3 per cent) of 79 during April 1963 (unpublished). As in elk, the rates evidently increase with age (see Ovsiukova 1966, for domesticated reindeer). R. A. Rausch (1959) reported that of 101 elk of all ages examined within a small area in south-central Alaska 24 per cent were infected, but that of the 16 animals between 7 and 9 years of age, 62 per cent were infected. A similar pattern was observed by Addison *et al.* (1979) in a reserve in northeastern Ontario, where all 14 animals between 7 and 9 years of age were infected. The larval cestode has been reported in elk from widely separated areas of Eurasia (see Nazarova 1967 for a review). Kikot' (1980) reported that of 31 elk examined in the Soviet Far East 22 (71 per cent) were infected. In North America, the larval cestode has also been reported in wapiti or red deer (called 'elk' in North America), *Cervus elaphus* L. (holarctic in distribution); mule deer or black-tailed deer, *Odocoileus hemionus* (Rafinesque); and white-tailed deer, *O. virginianus* (Zimmermann). Data concerning findings in these deer have been summarised by Leiby and Dyer (1971).

A variant of the natural cycle of the Northern Form may also involve the coyote, *Canis latrans* Say, as final host. This canid, which usually preys on mammals up to the size of hares, could only become infected by scavenging. Few large series of coyotes have been examined within the geographic range of the cestode. In Ontario, of 339 animals examined seven (2 per cent) were infected (Freeman *et al.* 1961); in Alberta, of 75 examined six (8 per cent) were infected (Holmes & Podesta 1968). Liu *et al.* (1970) found that of 173 coyotes examined in California, seven (4 per cent) were infected.

Wild ungulate–dog In arctic and subarctic regions where indigenous peoples subsist mainly by hunting wild reindeer, dogs kept as a means of transportation may be fed the lungs of infected deer or, if unrestrained, may scavenge on viscera left by hunters. Where reindeer herding is not practised, such a pattern alone must account for the infection of dogs. The risk of transmission to nomadic hunters is usually low if habitations are moved before the environs become grossly contaminated by dog faeces. In permanent settlements, the risk is much higher.

A variant of this pattern was noted in the Matanuska Valley, south-central Alaska, where large numbers of elk (moose) overwintered in habitat interspersed among cleared or cultivated areas. Many animals were killed annually by hunters, who left the viscera in the field. Dogs from nearby farms scavenged on the remains and thereby became infected.

Wolf–domesticated reindeer In some regions, as in western Alaska, domesticated reindeer may utilise range that is frequented by wolves. Where dogs are not used in herding, eggs dispersed by wolves serve as the source of infection for reindeer.

Dog–domesticated reindeer In Eurasia, the cycle of *E. granulosus* is completed where dogs are used for herding reindeer. In North America, Choquette *et al.* (1957) examined 1664 reindeer from range east of Aklavik (mouth of Mackenzie River), North West Territories, and found 158 (9.5 per cent) to be infected. They considered dogs, especially those used for herding, to be the source of infection. Hadwen and Palmer (1922), in Alaska, recognised that the larval stage of taeniid cestodes did not occur in domesticated reindeer in the absence of dogs.

On the collective farms of northern Siberia, the cycle of the cestode appears to be essentially synanthropic, with little involvement of hosts other than dogs and domesticated reindeer. Griuner (1927), in one of the first reviews of the status of the infection in reindeer, considered *E. granulosus* to be widespread in the north of the Tobolsk region and in Iakutia, Kamchatka and Chukotka. A single example of more recent findings in Siberia is that of Ovsiukova (1966) in Chukotka, who examined the viscera of 16 878 domesticated reindeer, and found 4310 (25.5 per cent) infected [lungs in all; liver of 506 (3 per cent) as well]. Ovsiukova also examined 586 dogs, of which 33 (5.6 per cent) harboured the strobilar stage, in numbers ranging from 59 to 52 582. A recent review of the problem of hydatid disease *sensu lato* in the Russian Soviet Federal Socialist Republic (RSFSR) by Nemurovskaia *et al.* (1980) indicated that the prevalence of cystic hydatid disease (involving the Northern Form) was highest in north eastern Siberia. When data for cystic hydatid disease and alveolar hydatid disease were combined, rates as great as 50–70 per thousand were determined among herders, hunters, fur-farmers and fur-workers in Iakutia.

The pattern of the cycle in western Eurasia is similar. Skjenneberg (1959) examined 2204 reindeer in Finmark (northern Norway) over a period of two years, 1956–58, 9 per cent of which were infected; he assumed that dogs used by the Lapps for herding served as the final host. Information about cystic hydatid disease in northern Fennoscandia has been provided also by Söderhjelm (1945, 1946) and Rein (1957). In Sweden (north of latitude 67 °N), Ronéus (1974) examined the lungs of 1453 reindeer and found only 23 (1.6 per cent) infected.

HOSTS OF THE NORTHERN FORM

The host-range of the Northern Form of *E. granulosus* in the strobilar stage is relatively restricted. The wolf is the usual final host, but it is often replaced by its domestic derivative. In North America, the coyote is a final host of minor importance. The extent of involvement of canids of other species in the cycle in Eurasia is not clear, since cestodes of the two forms are not distinguishable in the strobilar stage. The jackal, *Canis aureus* L., which occurs widely in southern Asia, has been found to be a host of *E. granulosus* in Georgia (Soviet Union) (Rodonaia 1951, cited in Petrov & Delianova 1962); in Azerbaidzhan (Sadykhov 1953); in the Kazakh SSR (Ul'ianov 1957, cited in Asadov 1960); and in Uzbekistan (Sultanov *et al.* 1971). The red wolf, *Cuon alpinus* (Pallas), occurs in the eastern regions of southern Asia, where it preys on large ungulates, including the maral, *Cervus elaphus sibiricus* Sev. (Geptner *et al.* 1967). Le Van Hoa and Vu Ngoc Tan (1967) reported *E. granulosus* in this canid from the Democratic Republic of Vietnam. Sweatman (1952) reported *E. granulosus* from a fisher, *Martes pennanti* (Erxleben), in Ontario (Canada). That report, however, was based on an error in records (T. W. M. Cameron, personal communication). *Echinococcus* species have not been found in mammals of the family Mustelidae, and attempts to infect them have been unsuccessful.

The reindeer and elk are the primary intermediate hosts in northern regions. In Eurasia, the range of the elk extends southward to about latitude 50°N. According to Kadenatsii and Zinov'ev (1973), infected elk have been found as far south as the Omsk Oblast', the Tuvinsk ASSR, and Khabarovsk Krai. A third holarctic species, the red deer or wapiti, has an extensive range southward from about latitude 60°N. A rate of infection of 28 per cent was reported by Liubimov (1956, cited in Asadov 1960) in the Siberian red deer (maral) in the Altai Krai. Green (1949) examined the lungs of 1073 wapiti over a 4-year period in Alberta and found 57 (5 per cent) infected. Both the mule deer and the white-tailed deer serve as intermediate hosts in North America; rates of infection are generally low. Brunetti and Rosen (1970) found only 26 (1.3 per cent) infected of 2049 mule deer examined in California over a 25-year period. In coastal areas of southeastern Alaska, the cycle of the cestode involves the wolf and a small form of mule deer. The roe deer, *Capreolus capreolus* (L.), which has a range similar to that of the red deer in Eurasia, has been listed as intermediate host of *E. granulosus* by Gagarin (1960) in Kirgizia, and by Abuladze (1964). The larval stage of the Northern Form was reported from a mountain goat, *Oreamnos americanus* (Blainville) in southeastern Alaska (Rausch & Williamson 1959). Gibbs and Tener (1958) found a single cyst in the lung of a muskox, *Ovibos moschatus* (Zimmermann) in the Thelon Game Sanctuary, North West Territory; protoscoleces were not present. The lack of any records of larval *E. granulosus* from wild sheep within the known range of the Northern Form, e.g. northeastern Siberia and Alaska, seems significant.

GEOGRAPHIC DISTRIBUTION OF THE NORTHERN FORM

Distributions of the two forms of *E. granulosus* in Eurasia are difficult to define precisely, particularly beyond the southern limits of the boreal forest, where the European Form occurs widely in domestic animals. Definition is less complex in North America, where the two forms are usually separated geographically.

The geographic range of the Northern Form in North America encompasses most of the continent, where the requisite hosts occur, north of approximate latitude 45°N. The cestode is commonly present across southern Canada, from Ontario to British Columbia (see Leiby & Dyer 1971). In the east, the extent of its range southward is delineated approximately by the southern limit of boreal forest. In the north-central United States, the Northern Form is present in Minnesota, where *E. granulosus* was recorded for the first time from elk and wolves in North America by Riley (1933). The same hosts are involved in the cycle on Isle Royale in Lake Superior (Mech 1966). In the western United States, where the wolf has been exterminated, deer and wapiti are numerous in the southward extensions of coniferous forest along mountain ranges. Records of the larval cestode from cervids in the western states appear to be only those of Hall (1925), Rosen (1951), and Brunetti and Rosen (1970) in

Oregon and California. Completion of the cycle would depend on involvement of coyotes or dogs.

The Northern Form of *E. granulosus* is evidently widespread in Eurasia, wherever the requisite hosts are present. In the north, its range appears to be continuous throughout the zones of tundra and taiga, from Fennoscandia to the Bering Strait. To the south, in central and southern Europe and across the Soviet Union, cestodes of both forms may be present. The infection of cervids in central Europe has long been recognised, as in Belgium, where Jansen (1961) found two of 53 red deer to have the larval stage in the lungs. In some parts of Europe, wolves are still a part of the natural fauna. Cervids are frequently found to be infected in the southern regions of the Soviet Union. In the Soviet Far East, Krotov (1953, cited in Asadov 1960) found the larval stage in 4.7 per cent of domesticated reindeer on the island of Sakhalin. Apparently no data are available concerning findings in wild ungulates in the Mongolian People's Republic (see Ivashkin 1955). Nor has information been obtained concerning occurrence of the larval cestode in natural hosts in the People's Republic of China, where the requisite hosts exist in some regions. In Ceylon, the presence of the Northern Form is indicated by the finding of the larval stage of *E. granulosus* in the lungs of a sambur, *Rusa unicolor* [*Cervus unicolor* (Kerr)] (Dissanaike & Paramananthan 1962).

The Northern Form of *E. granulosus* evidently has not become established following the introduction of potentially infected animals to other regions of the world. In New Zealand, for example, where cervids of numerous species from Eurasia and North America have thrived, Sweatman and Williams (1962) examined 181 deer representing five species from various localities there and found none infected, although the larval *E. granulosus* occurred in feral goats and swine. They subjected to experimental infection two fallow deer, *Cervus dama* L., and four red deer, using eggs of the local (European) form of *E. granulosus*; one fallow deer had a small, necrotic cyst, only one cyst in a red deer showed indication of normal development, but sheep used as controls became infected.

The European Form of *Echinococcus granulosus*

Here, the designation 'European Form' is applied to *E. granulosus* wherever the cycle primarily involves synanthropic hosts. A single geographic origin is not implied by this term, since involvement of the cestode in synanthropic cycles must have occurred at different times and places from the very beginnings of animal husbandry in Eurasia and Africa. Consequently, genetic homogeneity of the cestodes is not to be expected, and indeed, practices of animal husbandry no doubt resulted in selection pressures to which local 'populations' of cestodes responded. Infraspecific variation in *Echinococcus* spp. has been considered recently by Thompson (1979), Krotov (1979), and Thompson and Kumaratilake (1982), among others (see Ch. 1).

The cycle of the European Form of *E. granulosus* typically involves the domestic dog and domestic ungulates of various species as final and intermediate hosts. Wild ungulates of the family Bovidae commonly appear to be a part of the cycle in Africa. Fox-like canids are frequently found to be infected by the strobilar stage in some regions of South America. Other variants of the cycle have been reported from other regions.

PATTERNS OF CYCLES

The synanthropic cycle of the European Form is distinguished from the natural cycle of the Northern Form in that it exists almost invariably under conditions modified by man.

Synanthropic cycle, *sensu stricto* Throughout most of its geographic range, the European Form of *E. granulosus* is perpetuated by domestic animals, with the incidental infection of man being frequent. The dog is the only final host of significance in most regions, becoming infected by the strobilar stage when fed offal or through scavenging. Feral dogs, e.g. the dingo, may be important final hosts under some conditions.

Domestic ungulates of apparently every species may serve as intermediate host for this form of *E. granulosus*, but the relative importance of each varies with regional conditions that govern animal husbandry. Differences exist among ungulates in degree of compatibility with the larval cestode, as indicated by polymorphism. These are well reflected in the series of binomials formerly applied to larvae of the diverse morphological types. Localisation of oncospheres in the body is related to species of ungulate. Another variable is breed or strain, since breeds may differ from one another as much as do subspecies of wild mammals (Rausch 1967b).

Data concerning findings in equine animals are scarce, since smaller numbers are slaughtered. Unilocular cysts, usually multiple, predominate in horses, asses and their hybrids. The liver appears to be a typical locus, but the lungs may be involved; pulmonary cysts alone seem to be rare. Dixon *et al.* (1973) reported the distribution of cysts in 1318 horses from England, Scotland and Wales during 1971–72: 1003 (76 per cent) had cysts only in the liver; 271 (20 per cent), in both the liver and lungs; and 44 (3 per cent) in the lungs only. Findings elsewhere have been similar. Nieberle and Cohrs (1949) stated that the larval cestodes in horses usually die at an early age, while still small, and that the equine liver does not provide a favourable environment for development. However, according to Fiebiger (1947), about 70 per cent of cysts from horses contain protoscoleces. Cysts were fertile in seven of nine horses examined by Biocca and Massi (1952).

In swine, numerous, disseminated, simple cysts are characteristic. The liver is often involved, sometimes in combination with other organs. According to Lichtenheld (1904), localisation of oncospheres is influenced by the age of the animal when it is exposed to infection. The liver:lung ratio for swine under 2 years of age was 12.8:82; for animals over 2 years, 39.3:36. Fairley and Wright-Smith (1929) observed the distribution of 727 cysts from 20 swine to be 55 per cent in liver, 40 per cent in lungs, 4 per cent in kidneys, 0.3 per cent in spleen, and 0.1 per cent in heart. Bailenger (1957) reported for swine from Bayonne (Basses Pyrénées) that organs affected were the liver in 59.8 per cent, the lungs in 40.2 per cent, the liver alone in 32.9 per cent, and both liver and lungs in 67.1 per cent.

Multiple, sometimes massive, infections are characteristic of sheep, and the cysts, typically pleomorphic, localise predominantly in the lungs and liver. The respective rates for these organs in Australian sheep were given by Dew (1926) as 52 and 42 per cent. Data on more than 400 000 sheep slaughtered in the municipal abattoir of Concepción (Chile) over a 12-year period were summarised by Wilhelm (1953), who reported hepatic and pulmonary infections to be 67.8 and 38.2 per cent. Cysts had the following distribution in 101 108 sheep from abattoirs in Spain during 1948–49: lungs, 36 124 (35.72 per cent); liver 33 187 (32.82 per cent); both organs, 31 997 (31.44 per cent) (Talavera 1955). Of 215 infected sheep at Armavir, Northern Caucasus, both the lungs and liver were affected in 130 (60.5 per cent), the lungs only in 42 (19.5 per cent), and the liver only in 43 (20 per cent) (Kuznetzov 1958).

Little specific information is available concerning goats, since these animals often have not been distinguished from sheep in reports. From a given area, goats are usually infected to a lesser degree, which Cousi (1951) attributed to different feeding habits. Eugster (1978) also remarked that the relatively low prevalence in Kenya might be explained in that goats usually browsed on shrubs and bushes, whereas sheep grazed on pasture. Cysts in goats are predominantly unilocular and occur in the lungs and liver. Eugster (1978) usually found only single cysts, in one or the other of these organs. A fertility rate of only 2.68 per cent was reported (Tanda 1960) for cysts from 112 infected goats at the abattoir of Sassari (Sardinia), but the average number of protoscoleces was unusually high in local goats in Ceylon (Paramananthan 1961). In Europe, rates of infection in goats are often low; only 3.64 per cent were infected of 95 053 adult animals examined in Greece in 1955–56 (Papachristophilou 1957), but Suić (1957) found 23.8 per cent infected of an unspecified number examined during 1952–53 in Sarajevo (Yugoslavia).

In cattle, cysts are often multiple, and most are unilocular. Multilobular cysts are not uncommon, but the multicystic form is rare. Localisation of oncospheres may be in the spleen, heart or other organs, but is most frequent in the liver and lungs. In Australia, Pullar and Marshall (1958) examined 2074 infected cattle in Victoria, and found that the liver was involved in 1833 (88.4 per cent); the lungs in 1508 (72.7 per cent); and the spleen in 149 (7.2 per cent). In 24 719 cattle slaughtered during 1948–49 in Spanish abattoirs, cysts were present in the lungs in 30.24 per cent, in the liver in 34.69 per cent, and in both organs in 35.06 per cent (Talavera 1955). El Kordy (1946), in Egypt, reported rates of 61.96 and 36.62 per cent for the liver and lungs, respectively. Of 220 951 cattle slaughtered in Uruguay during 1948–50, 71 525 were infected, 23 per cent with hepatic, and 17 per cent with pulmonary cysts; cardiac locations were noted in six animals (Bregante 1951). In cattle, as with ungulates of other species, rates of infection increase with age (Pullar & Marshall 1958, for Victoria; Vitale 1954, for Sicily). A rather high proportion of degenerated or otherwise abnormal cysts in cattle seems indicative of a relatively unfavourable parasite–host relationship. Of 158 infected cattle, all more than 5 years of age, only 24 (15 per cent) had fertile cysts (Biocca & Massi 1951).

Dog–wild ungulate Data published by Eugster (1978) and others suggest that eggs dispersed by dogs might be ingested by wild ungulates under the conditions existing in East Africa, but wild carnivores are probably more important hosts in this region. A comparable situation might exist locally in southern Asia, wherever wild bovids occur in areas frequented by dogs.

Feral dog–macropodids An independent cycle of *E. granulosus*, involving the dingo and marsupials of the family Macropodidae, has been documented in Australia. Durie and Riek (1952) found the larval cestode in one of four specimens of *Thylogale* sp. and in 12 of 55 wallabies representing four species in Queensland. There also, the strobilar stage was present in nine of 11 dingoes. In southeastern Australia, it was found in 88 per cent of 120 dingoes (Anon. 1980). Thompson and Kumaratilake (1982) noted that *E. granulosus* might have been introduced with dogs (dingoes) that accompanied the aboriginal colonisers of Australia, where the presence of suitable intermediate hosts made possible its perpetuation.

Wild canid–hare That an independent cycle, involving fox-like canids of the genus *Dusicyon* and European hares, *Lepus europaeus* (= *L. capensis* L.) (an introduced species), exists in Argentina is conceivable. In 1960–61, Szidat (1971) found *E. granulosus* (designated *E. patagonicus* Szidat, 1960) in 12 per cent of more than 200 preserved intestines of *Dusicyon culpaeus* (Molina). Blood *et al.* (1963) examined 250 specimens of *D. gymnocercus* (Fischer), finding 15 per cent to be infected. Blood and Lelijveld (1969) reported overall rates of 3.6 per cent for 442 specimens of *D. gymnocercus* from the Azul region, and 15.5 per cent for 360 specimens of *D. griseus* (Gray) in Patagonia. Schantz and Lord (1972) investigated possible intermediate hosts of *E. granulosus* among wild animals in the Province of Neuquén, and found four of 71 European hares infected. Cysts from hares produced large numbers of cestodes when fed to dogs. That a cycle involving wild canids and hares would exist independently was questioned by Schantz *et al.* (1975), who considered that the canids usually became infected by scavenging on carcasses of sheep. Schantz *et al.* (1976) made the significant observation that cestodes reared experimentally in *D. culpaeus* and *D. griseus* from cysts from domestic sheep exhibited host-induced morphological variation.

Fox–domestic ungulate Several investigators have suggested that the red fox, *Vulpes vulpes* (L.), is an important final host for *E. granulosus* in

Great Britain and, with dogs, may be a source of infection for domestic ungulates. Records, including information about presence of eggs in gravid segments, have been reviewed by Thompson (1977). Foxes can only become infected by scavenging, and particularly important are discarded carcasses of sheep (Cook & Crewe 1963), since those of horses appear rarely to be accessible to them.

Wild carnivore–wild ungulate Investigations in East Africa, most undertaken in Kenya, have shown that the cycle of *E. granulosus* involves both wild and domestic animals. The interactions among these are complex, but the cycle probably is completed independently in wild mammals. In the Turkana District, Nelson and Rausch (1963) identified the adult cestode from domestic dogs [27 (63 per cent) of 43] as well as from wild carnivores [three of four hunting dogs, *Lycaon pictus* (Temminck); one of nine black-backed jackals, *Canis mesomelas* Schreber; and three of nine hyaenas, *Crocuta crocuta* (Erxleben)]. Among wild ungulates and other herbivores examined, only one wildebeest, *Connochaetes taurinus* (Burchell), was infected. In the Kajiado District Eugster (1978) found 45 (27.3 per cent) of 165 dogs to harbour the strobilar stage, which he also obtained from a lion, *Panthera leo* (L.), and from five black-backed jackals. Of 1446 cattle from the same district, 676 (46.7 per cent) were infected, while rates in sheep and goats were 29.5 and 9 per cent, respectively. Of particular interest was Eugster's finding of the larval cestode in 69 (12 per cent) of 576 wildebeests. In the Turkana District, Macpherson *et al.* (1983) recorded relatively low rates in cattle, sheep and goats, but a high rate in camels (33 per cent). They found the cestode in 11 (22 per cent) of 49 black-backed jackals, and six (27 per cent) of 28 golden jackals, *Canis aureus* L. These small canids obviously can become infected only through scavenging. Macpherson *et al.* studied cestodes from various hosts, including some reared in jackals following feeding of cysts of human origin, and found no indications of morphological or biological differences. They concluded that their findings supported evidence for the existence of an independent cycle in wild mammals.

Wild/domestic carnivore–man Customs concerning disposal of the dead or dying as practised by some Africans provide access to corpses by dogs and wild carnivores, and under such conditions, man may have a significant role as intermediate host of *E. granulosus.* Evidence for this has been obtained only recently; in northwestern Kenya, Macpherson (1983) compared cysts obtained surgically from 97 Turkana tribesmen with those from domestic ungulates, and determined that a high degree of fertility and viability was characteristic of the larval cestode in man, as well as in sheep, goats and camels. Based on surgical data, rates of infection among the Turkana ranged up to 220 cases per 100 000, but the actual rate is probably much higher (Macpherson 1983). Since the Turkana either do not bury the dead, or they place them only in shallow graves that may be excavated by carnivores, Macpherson concluded that most persons who die of hydatid disease are likely to be consumed by such mammals. Because cysts in man are characteristically large (greater than 15 cm in diameter, according to Macpherson), they may contain abundant protoscoleces. Man would thus appear to be an important source of infection for a considerable range of carnivores under conditions existing in some districts of Kenya.

HOSTS OF THE EUROPEAN FORM

Since *E. granulosus* in the strobilar stage is easy to identify, most published records of the parasite from carnivores are probably reliable. Some records of the larval stage, particularly those involving mammals in captivity, appear to be questionable. A list of known hosts, related to some extent to geographic region, will be given here.

The domestic dog is the ubiquitous final host of the European Form of *E. granulosus* wherever the practice of animal husbandry provides the requisite conditions for completion of the cycle. With few exceptions, other final hosts are of little significance. Besides the dog, only wild canids are known to serve as final host in the Northern Hemisphere. Circumstantial evidence suggests that the wolf may become infected by this form in some regions of the Soviet Union particularly. Similarly, the coyote in the southwestern United States may scavenge on carcasses of sheep in endemic areas (Liu *et al.* 1970). The golden jackal may harbour *E. granulosus* throughout its range in Eurasia (records reviewed by Macpherson *et al.* 1983). The red fox is considered to be important as a final host in Great Britain; findings elsewhere indicate that cestodes in this canid usually do not attain full development. Shumakovich and Nikitin (1959) reported *E. granulosus* from the corsac fox, *Vulpes corsac* (L.), in the Soviet Union. The domestic cat is not a suitable host for *E. granulosus* (see Thompson 1977 for a review).

The widest range of final hosts has been reported from Africa, where the presence of the cestode probably long antedated the comparatively recent introductions from Europe. Records from African carnivores have been reviewed by Round (1968), Eugster (1978), and Macpherson *et al.* (1983). The cestode has been reported from carnivores representing three families, among which members of the Canidae predominate, including the golden jackal, black-backed jackal and hunting dog, of which only the last is capable of killing larger ungulates. Records from black-backed jackals and hunting dogs indicate that these canids commonly become infected in the vast geographic region south of the Sahara. The role of jackals in the transmission of *E. granulosus* has been discussed by Macpherson and Karstad (1981). In South Africa, one of 24 Cape foxes, *Vulpes chama* (Smith) was found to be infected (Verster & Collins 1966).

The sole record for members of the family Hyaenidae appears to be that of Nelson and Rausch (1963), who identified *E. granulosus* from three of 19 spotted hyaenas in northwestern Kenya. Among members of the family Felidae, only the lion appears frequently to harbour cestodes now considered to represent *E. granulosus*. Some evidence indicates that the cycle involves only the lion and wart-hog, *Phacochoerus aethiopicus* (Pallas) (see Macpherson *et al.* 1983). If so, the species may indeed be distinct, and the name *Echinococcus felidis* Ortlepp, 1937 would be applicable. Otherwise, in felids *E. granulosus* has been reported from one of 15 wild cats, *Felis libyca* (= *F. silvestris* Schreber) in South Africa (Verster & Collins 1966).

Elsewhere in the Southern Hemisphere, the domestic dog (including the dingo and other feral forms; see Herre & Röhrs 1973, p. 183) is the characteristic and usually the only final host of the European Form of *E. granulosus*. Fox-like canids of the genus *Dusicyon* harbour the cestode in Argentina.

Wherever they are kept, domestic animals of the common species serve as intermediate host of the European Form: horse and ass (Equidae); pig (Suidae); camels, *Camelus bactrianus* L. and *C. dromedarius* L. (Camelidae); cattle, yak, *Bos grunniens* L., buffalo, *Bubalus bubalis* (L.), goats and sheep (Bovidae). The larval stage has been reported from wild ungulates representing numerous species of the family Bovidae.

In Eurasia, the wild boar, *Sus scrofa* L. (from which domestic swine are derived), is widely known as an intermediate host of this cestode (Wetzel & Rieck 1962). Records include boars from the Pribalkhash region and the Astrakhansk Reserve (Rukhliadev 1952); boars in different biotic zones in Kazakhstan (Shol' 1963); and seven infected of 34 animals in Azerbaidzhan (Ialiev 1975). The records from wild ruminants other than cervids must be presumed to involve the European Form until experimental studies show otherwise. The reports of hosts include the European bison, *Bison bonasus* (L.) (Zablontskii 1939, cited in Geptner *et al.* 1961); an antelope, *Procapra gutterosa* (Pallas), in the Soviet Far East (Geptner *et al.* 1961); one of 10 goral, *Nemorhaedus goral* (Hardwicke), also in the Soviet Far East (Shul'ts & Kadenatsii 1950); the saiga, *Saiga tatarica* (L.), in western Siberia (range-maps given in Geptner *et al.* 1961) (Radionov 1971); and chamois, *Rupicapra rupicapra* (L.), in the Caucasus Reserve (Rukhliadev 1959, cited in Geptner *et al.* 1961). Wild sheep and goats seem rarely to be infected in Eurasia. Pershinym (1949, cited in Badaev *et al.* 1977) reported the larval cestode from the Turkmen wild sheep, *Ovis ammon cycloceros* Hutton, in Turkmenia. Feral swine perhaps serve as intermediate host of the European Form of *E. granulosus* in the southeastern United States (Hutchison 1960).

The widest range of intermediate hosts has been recorded in Africa, south of the Sahara. The following list of species (not including captive animals) is based mainly on the reviews by Round (1968), Eugster (1978), and Macpherson *et al.* (1983): Equidae – zebra, *Equus burchelli* (Gray) and *Equus* spp.; Suidae – wart-hog, *Phacochoerus aethiopicus* (Pallas); Hippopotamidae – hippopotamus, *Hippopotamus amphibius* L.; Giraffidae – *Giraffa camelopardalis* (L.) (including *G. reticulata*); Bovidae – Grant's gazelle, *Gazella granti* Brooke; Thomson's gazelle, *G. thomsoni* Gunther; impala, *Aepyceros melampus* (Lichtenstein); puku, *Kobus vardoni* (Livingstone); waterbuck, *K. ellipsiprymnus* (Ogilby) (including *K. defassa*); oryx,

Oryx sp. (probably *O. gazella* (L.), based on distribution); gerenuk, *Litocranius walleri* (Brooke); topi, *Damaliscus lunatus* (Burchell) (including *D. korrigum*); blue duiker, *Cephalophus monticola* (Thunberg); common duiker, *Sylvicapra grimmia* L.; eland, *Tragelaphus oryx* (Pallas); hartebeest, *Alcelaphus buselaphus* (Pallas); wildebeest, *Connochaetes taurinus* (Burchell); buffalo, *Syncerus caffer* (Sparrman); Cercopithecidae – baboon, *Papio* spp.

In South America, camelids of the genus *Lama* are important in regions at high elevation. Cysts of *E. granulosus* were found in alpacas, *Lama pacos* (L.), in Peru by Santiváñez and Cuba (1949). There also, Roman (1956) found 90 (19 per cent) infected of 470 animals examined. The occasional records of the larval *E. granulosus* from European hares in Argentina have been noted.

On the mainland of Australia, macropodids of several species serve as intermediate hosts of *E. granulosus*: eastern grey kangaroo, *Macropus giganteus* Shaw; whiptail, *M. parryi* Bennett; walleroo, *M. robustus* Gould; red-necked wallaby, *M. rufogriseus* (Desmarest); tammar, *M. eugenii* (Desmarest); black-striped wallaby, *M. dorsalis* (Gray); red-necked pademelon, *Thylogale thetis* (Lesson); red-legged pademelon, *T. stigmatica* (Gould); and swamp wallaby, *Wallabia bicolor* (Desmarest) (for review of records, see Kumaratilake & Thompson 1982). Series of all three species of macropodids occurring in Tasmania were examined by Howkins (1966), with negative results.

GEOGRAPHIC DISTRIBUTION OF THE EUROPEAN FORM

Numerous publications document that the form of *E. granulosus* for which domestic ungulates serve as intermediate host has nearly cosmopolitan distribution (Suić 1952, Herrera & Cranwell 1960, Volokh 1965, Lupaşcu & Panaitescu 1968, Acha & Szyfres 1980, and others). The most detailed review of recent information was that of Schantz and Schwabe (1969). Only a few supplemental remarks need be included here.

In Eurasia, the cestode occurs widely in the Soviet Union (see geographic review by Asadov 1960). In the Mongolian People's Republic, the larval cestode has been reported from various domestic animals (Ivashkin 1955). Kan (1966) cited 29 papers, mainly concerning clinical hydatid disease, published in the People's Republic of China during 1949–64. According to Dr Lin Yuguang, Xiamen University (personal communication), the cestode occurs widely in that country. Le-Van-Hoa and Vu-Ngoc-Tan (1967) reviewed records of *E. granulosus* in the Democratic Republic of Vietnam. Its occurrence in Malaya was reported by Euzeby (1957). Shamsul Islam (1979) obtained an overall rate of 56.3 per cent in 523 sheep slaughtered at Mymensingh, Bangaladesh. The cestode appears to be uncommon in the Philippines (Arambulo 1974).

In the Middle East and Africa, an absence of records of *E. granulosus* from some countries seems to suggest that investigations are yet to be made. In Kuwait, the first examination of dogs for this cestode disclosed 23 per cent of 204 animals to be infected (Hassounah & Behbehani 1976). Cysts were also found commonly in domestic ungulates, particularly sheep (Behbehani & Hassounah 1976). Extensive investigations by Larbaui *et al.* (1980) in Algeria revealed high rates of infection in domestic animals and man (5305 human cases since 1960).

In North America, the European Form of *E. granulosus* is known to have been more widespread during the last century (Rausch 1967a) and was believed to have become rare in the United States. Endemic areas are now known to exist in California, Utah, Arizona and New Mexico (Schantz *et al.* 1977, Sawyer *et al.* 1969, Kahn *et al.* 1972, Crellin *et al.* 1982). A cyst obtained from the lung of an Indian child in Washington was consistent morphologically and pathologically with the European Form (R. L. Rausch, unpublished). An endemic area exists also in the southeastern United States (Hutchison 1960).

ECHINOCOCCUS MULTILOCULARIS LEUCKART, 1863

Since establishment of its specific independence, *Echinococcus multilocularis* has been intensively studied in the field and in the laboratory. The cycle typically involves foxes (genera *Vulpes* and *Alopex*) as final host. Rodents of many species are susceptible to infection by the larval stage. Larvae with abundant protoscoleces have been obtained experimentally in such diverse rodents as *Calomys callosus* (Rengger) (Cricetidae), from the highlands of Bolivia, and *Acomys cahirinus* (Desmarest) (Muridae) from the Egyptian desert (R. L. Rausch unpublished). In the intermediate host, the embryo seems invariably to localise and develop in the liver. In chronic infections, spread to other loci by extension or by metastasis is typical. Compatible with its occurrence in short-lived hosts, development of the larval cestode is rapid; in arvicolids, larvae may produce infective protoscoleces within 60 days of establishment of the embryo. As with *E. granulosus* and *E. vogeli*, the domestic dog can readily replace the natural final host of *E. multilocularis*, and indeed dogs appear to be the only significant source of infection for man. House cats, *Felis silvestris* f. *catus*, also serve as final host.

PATTERNS OF CYCLES

The natural cycle of *E. multilocularis* is universally uniform in pattern, although the host-assemblages differ in accordance with faunal changes southward from the Arctic.

Natural cycle Throughout the holarctic zone of tundra, the natural cycle is completed by means of the predator–prey relationship existing between foxes [primarily the arctic fox, *Alopex lagopus* (L.)] and rodents (mainly of the genera *Microtus, Lemmus* and *Clethrionomys*). Helminth–host interactions might be best exemplified on St Lawrence Island, in the Bering Sea, where investigations have been conducted since 1950. There, the incidence of infection in both arctic foxes and northern voles, *Microtus* *oeconomus* (Pallas), varied seasonally. The highest prevalence of infection in foxes was in autumn, following the several months when their diet consisted mainly of voles. By October, the rate was at least 90 per cent in adult animals and about 10 per cent higher in the young of the year, nearly all of which had become infected by the time they left the maternal den. With onset of winter, accumulating snow prevented effective hunting of voles, and the foxes utilised alternative food resources, e.g. carcasses of marine mammals. A gradual loss of cestodes by the foxes took place during winter. By spring, the rate of infection declined to about 30 per cent, the lowest for the year. In voles, of which 2795 were examined prior to 1964, the maximum rate of infection, about 15 per cent, was observed in spring before the onset of seasonal reproduction. Beginning in late May, production of successive litters greatly modified the population structure of the voles, with the result that the overall prevalence of the larval cestode was lowest in late summer, when reproduction ceased (Fay & Rausch 1966, and unpublished). On St Lawrence Island also, northern red-backed voles, *Clethrionomys rutilus* (Pallas), had a high rate of infection. They inhabit rocky slopes where they are not easily captured by foxes.

An important factor in the interaction of *E. multilocularis* and its hosts on St Lawrence Island is the relatively high numerical density sustained by the populations of voles, as compared with findings in regions where the rodents undergo strongly defined, cyclic fluctuations in density. On the arctic coast of Alaska near Point Barrow, the brown lemming *Lemmus sibiricus* (Kerr), occurs with a varying lemming (genus *Dicrostonyx*), but voles are absent. Arctic foxes produce large litters in years when lemmings are abundant; they are numerous along the coast by autumn. Red foxes may be present in smaller numbers. In this area, the sustained interaction of *E. multilocularis* and its hosts required to maintain a high prevalence of the cestode does not exist. The varying lemming, rarely numerous, is not a suitable intermediate host (Ohbayashi *et al.* 1971). On the arctic coast of Siberia (Chaunsk Gulf), where colleagues and I examined large series of brown lemmings, northern voles and northern red-backed voles, the larval cestode likewise was rare. We did not examine arctic foxes. Ovsiukova (1966) found 60 (33 per cent) infected of 178 animals from other localities in Chukotka. Seasonal variation in prevalence of *E. multilocularis* in arctic foxes was not strongly defined in Iakutia (Isakov 1982). In that region also, Gubanov (1964) reported a decline from 71 per cent infected in November to 59 per cent in February; in red foxes, prevalence declined from 18 per cent in November–December to 5.2 per cent in February. At the same time, both species exhibited a decrease in intensity of infection. Saffronov (1966) found that maximum prevalence in dogs in Iakutia was in August.

In central Europe, the natural cycle involves the red fox and arvicolid rodents of various species. Vogel (1961) reported 40 per cent of red foxes examined in southern Germany and northern Switzerland to be infected. During May 1974–December 1980, Zeyhle (1982), in 4441 red foxes in Württemberg, found 598 (13.5 per cent) to be infected. Of 60 animals in the Massif Central of France, five (7 per cent) harboured the cestode (Petavy & Deblock 1980). Prevalences in rodents in Europe have been generally low. Vogel (1961) found only four (0.8 per cent) of 496 field voles, *Microtus arvalis* (Pallas), to be infected. Zeyhle (1982) obtained an overall rate of 0.5 per cent in 6168 field voles from five districts of Württemberg; among many rodents of other species, only muskrats were infected. Houin *et al.* (1982) found the larval cestode in five (0.02 per cent) of 2010 water voles, *Arvicola terrestris* (L.), in France.

In central North America, where *E. multilocularis* has become established relatively recently, the cycle involves the red fox and the coyote as final host. In the winter of 1965 in northern North Dakota, 70 (67 per cent) of 96 red foxes were infected (Rausch & Richards 1971); over a larger region, Leiby *et al.* (1970) found the cestode in 131 (8.5 per cent) of 1540 red foxes and in seven (4 per cent) of 171 coyotes. There, the meadow vole, *M. pennsylvanicus* (Ord), and the white-footed mouse, *Peromyscus maniculatus* (Wagner), serve as intermediate hosts. Leiby *et al.* found the larval cestode in 20 (1.94 per cent) of 1033 voles and in 204 (5.84 per cent) of 4209 white-footed mice. In the latter, few protoscoleces are produced, a condition that may account for the relatively low numbers of cestodes in foxes.

Dog–vole In villages in the Arctic, northern voles often occur as commensals and, when dogs are present, a hyperendemic focus may develop. Such an interaction was observed in Alaska, on the mainland and on St Lawrence Island, before dogs had been mostly replaced by machines for winter travel. The Eskimos have begun to keep dogs as pets; such animals also may be important in the cycle of *E. multilocularis*. At one village on St Lawrence Island, investigations during late May–early June in 1980 and 1981 disclosed that about 25 per cent of voles were infected (unpublished).

Dog/cat–wild rodent Wherever the cycle of *E. multilocularis* is completed in natural hosts in agricultural or semirural areas, dogs and cats may capture and eat infected voles. While they may not contribute significantly to the cycle, such carnivores are potentially important as sources of infection for man.

Cat–house mouse Vogel (1960) recognised that a cycle involving cats and house mice, *Mus musculus* L., might exist on farms, where mice are often abundant. The question has been discussed by Leiby and Kritsky (1972), who found infected cats on a farm in North Dakota. The larval *E. multilocularis* has been reported infrequently from house mice, local populations of which appear to differ in susceptibility to infection. In endemic areas, the potential importance of house mice is probably much less than that of wild rodents, which are also commonly captured by cats.

HOSTS OF *ECHINOCOCCUS MULTILOCULARIS*

In the summary below, only naturally infected wild mammals are considered. The list of species known to serve as intermediate host may be incomplete, since some of the relevant literature has not been available from the Soviet Union, where the most comprehensive surveys have been made. The citations of records for rodents of species found commonly to be infected are so numerous that all cannot be included here.

As noted, the occurrence of the multicystic larva of *E. granulosus* in ungulates has caused confusion concerning the host-range of *E. multilocularis*. Following the recognition by Shul'ts (1961, in Shul'ts 1962) of a subspecies of this cestode capable of developing in ungulates (in Kazakhstan), several papers concerning this problem have been published in the Soviet Union. It suffices here to cite Lukashenko (1978), who concluded (p. 37), concerning ungulates, that '*Eta gruppa zhivotnykh, kak i dikie kopytnye, v tsikle al'veokokka ne prinimaet uchastiia.*' [This group of animals, as well as wild ungulates, takes no part in the cycle of alveococcus (= *E. multilocularis*).]

Many records also document the occurrence of *E. multilocularis* in the arctic fox and the red fox. It occurs as well in the corsac fox, *V. corsac* (L.), first reported by Petrov (1957). Prior to 1962, it had been recorded but twice from this canid in the Soviet Union, in Tadzhikistan and the Volgogradsk Oblast' (Petrov & Delianova 1962). Sokolov (1972), in the Altai, found five (12 per cent) of 41 animals to be infected. A single record from a grey fox, *Urocyon cinereoargenteus* (Schreber), exists (from Minnesota, USA) (Vande Vusse *et al.* 1978). *E. multilocularis* occurs rarely in the wolf; the first record was apparently that of Kadenatsii (cited in Petrov 1958), in the Omsk Oblast'. Lazarev (cited in Iakovleva *et al.* 1973) found two wolves infected near Ust'-Bol'sheretsk (Kamchatka). Farther west, on the Taimyr Peninsula, Savel'ev (1972) reported the cestode in 9.7 per cent of wolves examined. Lukashenko (1978) noted that the typical diet of the wolf is not conducive to infection by *E. multilocularis.* The coyote appears to have a significant role in the cycle in the endemic region of central North America. The only record of *E. multilocularis* from felids other than the domestic cat appears to be that of Bondareva (1966), who found that three of six wild cats, *Felis libyca* (= *F. silvestris*), were infected near Lake Balkhash (Kazakhstan), where muskrats were numerous. Bondareva reviewed negative findings in numerous wild felids in the Soviet Union.

Considering the many species of rodents and of other small mammals that occur within the geographic range of *E. multilocularis*, the number known to serve as intermediate host seems remarkably small. The larval cestode has been reported from mammals representing at least eight families: Soricidae (shrews) (one genus); Talpidae (moles) (one genus); Sciuridae (squirrels) (three genera); Cricetidae (hamsters and gerbils) (five genera); Arvicolidae (voles and lemmings) (six genera); Muridae (rats and mice) (two genera); Dipodidae (jerboas) (one genus); and Ochotonidae (pikas) (one genus).

Soricidae The larval cestode in *Sorex jacksoni* Hall and Gilmore on St Lawrence Island was reported by Thomas *et al.* (1954). Others have found this shrew to be rather commonly infected on the island; vesicles attain relatively large size, but protoscoleces may be few or lacking (Ohbayashi *et al.* 1971).

Talpidae The larval cestode was reported from *Talpa altaica* Nikol'skii in the Altai Krai by Marchenko (1967, cited in Diveeva-Mogila 1969).

Sciuridae Gubanov (1964) found the larval *E. multilocularis* in the common squirrel, *Sciurus vulgaris* L., in Iakutia. On St Lawrence Island, Thomas *et al.* (1954) reported well developed larvae in two of 12 ground squirrels, *Citellus undulatus* (Pallas) [= *C. parryi* (Richardson); chromosomal comparisons have shown that the holarctic ground squirrel around Bering Strait, *C. parryi*, is distinct from the palaearctic *C. undulatus*]. Of 217 specimens of *C. parryi* examined by others on that island, eight had hepatic lesions macroscopically like those produced by *E. multilocularis*, but histological sections revealed other causes (Fay 1973). Attempts to infect *C. parryi* have been uniformly unsuccessful (Rausch & Schiller 1956, Rausch & Richards 1971, Ohbayashi *et al.* 1971). The larval cestode in *C. undulatus* in Buriat-Mongolia was reported by Machul'skii (1958). Six were infected of 130 marmots, *Marmota bobak* (Müller), in the Pavlodarsk Oblast' (Kazakhstan) (Logachev & Bat'kaev 1979). Protoscoleces were present.

Cricetidae Few cricetids are known to serve as intermediate host of *E. multilocularis*. Protoscoleces were lacking in an infected hamster, *Cricetus cricetus* (L.), noted by Petrov (1958) in western Siberia. Infections have been reported in the Mongolian gerbil, *Meriones unguiculatus* (Milne-Edwards), in Burait-Mongolia (Machul'skii 1958); in *M. erythrourus* (= *M. libycus* Lichtenstein) in Kazakhstan (Boev *et al.* 1971); in *Meriones* sp. in Iran (Rausch 1967a); and in the great gerbil, *Rhombomys opimus* (Lichtenstein), in the Aktiubinsk Oblast' (Chun-Siun & Alekseev 1960) and Kazakhstan (Boev *et al.* 1971). Boev *et al.* also listed the mole-rat, *Myospalax myospalax* (Laxmann), as a host in Kazakhstan. *Peromyscus maniculatus* is an important host in central North America. The larval cestode (without calcareous corpuscles and protoscoleces) was identified in a woodrat, *Neotoma cinerea* (Ord), in Wyoming (Kritsky *et al.* 1977).

Arvicolidae Arvicolid rodents have the greatest importance as intermediate host of *E. multilocularis*. Reported rates of infection have varied widely, perhaps depending in part on the season when animals were collected. The first record in *Microtus arvalis* was from southern Germany (Vogel 1955); there, Zeyhle (1982) observed rates from 0.1 to 2.7 per cent in voles from different districts. An infected vole obtained in Switzerland by Professor J. G. Baer (in Rausch 1952) probably was of this species. In the Soviet Union, *M. arvalis* has been found infected in the Tselinogradsk

Oblast' (Pleshchev 1978); Novosibirsk Oblast' (Lukashenko & Zorikhina 1961); and in Georgia (Matsaberidze 1966). The earliest record from *M. oeconomus*, an holarctic species, was that of Ishino (1941) from Sumishir Island (Kurile Islands). Records from this vole in the Soviet Union are numerous: Trans-Ural and Ob' regions (Petrov & Chertkova 1959); Novosibirsk Oblast' (Leikina *et al.* 1959); Tselinogradsk Oblast' (Pleshchev 1978); Tuvinsk Autonomous Oblast' (Sulimov 1963); and Bering Island (Nadtochii 1970). The larval cestode from *M. oeconomus* in North America was first identified on St Lawrence Island (Rausch & Schiller 1951); subsequently, it has been found in this host on the Alaskan mainland (unpublished). *M. socialis* (Pallas) was found infected in Georgia (Soviet Union) by Kurashvili (1961, 1962) and Matsaberidze (1966), who also reported *M. roberti* Thomas to be a host. Records from *M. hyperboreus* [= *M. middendorffi* (Poliakov)] have been reported by Gubanov (1964) and by Gubanov and Fedorov (1970) in Iakutia. Several records exist from the narrow-skulled vole, *M. gregalis* (Pallas): Trans-Ural and Ob' regions (Petrov & Chertkova 1959); Kirgiz SSR (Gagarin *et al.* 1957, Tokobaev 1959, 1960); Novosibirsk Oblast' (Lukashenko & Zorikhina 1961); Iamal Peninsula (Kopein 1959, cited in Luzhkov 1963); and Iakutia (Gubanov 1964). *M. pennsylvanicus* has been found infected frequently in central North America, since the first report by Leiby (1965) in North Dakota. The first record from a water vole, *Arvicola terrestris*, was that of Petrov (1958) in western Siberia; Pleshchev (1978) found one infected of 65 in the Tselinogradsk Oblast'. Findings by Houin *et al.* (1982) in France have been noted.

Of particular interest are the numerous records from the muskrat, *Ondatra zibethicus* (L.), a nearctic rodent that has become widely established in Eurasia. In southern Germany, Zeyhle (1982) found eight (2.2 per cent) infected of 371 examined. Infections in muskrats have been extensively reported in the Soviet Union, where introductions date from 1929 (Korsakov 1963), the first record apparently by Spasskii *et al.* (1951) in the Kurgansk Oblast' and Kzyl-Orda, where infected animals also were reported by Lavrov (1953). Other records include the Ruzaevsk region of Moldavia (Machinskii & Semov 1972); Tiumensk Oblast' (Koval'chuk 1979); Cheliabinsk Oblast' (Salmatin 1958, cited in Leikina *et al.* 1959); Trans-Ural and Ob' regions (Petrov & Chertkova 1959); Novosibirsk Oblast' (Leikina *et al.* 1959, Lukashenko & Zorikhina 1961); Kazakhstan (various regions) (Zikeeva & Arslanova 1961, Arslanova 1962, Romazanov 1963, Gvozdev 1969, Pleshchev 1978). In the Kazakh SSR, the findings of Arslanova disclosed prevalences in muskrats ranging from 1.2 per cent (Uialy River) to 9.4 per cent (Lake Kashkarul'). In North America, where muskrats have an extensive geographic distribution, two (1 per cent) were infected of 196 examined in Montana (USA) (Eastman & Worley 1979). In Alaska, muskrats are not present in the zone of tundra, where arctic foxes are abundant. Muskrats trapped in Alaska were infected experimentally (Ohbayashi *et al.* 1971). None of more than 12 000 animals from North Dakota was infected (Rausch & Richards 1971).

One was infected of 57 steppe voles, *Lagurus lagurus* (Pallas), in the Tselinogradsk Oblast' (Pleshchev 1978). The northern mole-vole *Ellobius talpinus* (Pallas), was found to be infected in Kirgizia (Tokobaev 1959, 1960). The brown lemming, *Lemmus sibiricus*, appears to be an important host in tundra of the Trans-Ural and Ob' regions (Petrov & Chertkova 1959), Iamal Peninsula (Kopein 1959, cited in Luzhkov 1963), Taimyr Peninsula (Savel'ev 1972), Iakutia (Gubanov 1964), and Chaunsk Gulf (Chukotka) (L. V. Smirnova, unpublished); one infected animal was reported from St George Island, Bering Sea (Rausch 1967a).

Red-backed voles, *Clethrionomys* spp., also are important intermediate hosts in Eurasia; records have included one bank vole, *C. glareolus* (Schreber), in Latvia (Lesin'sh 1959), and red-grey voles, *C. rufocanus* (Sundevall), in Iakutia (Gubanov & Fedorov 1970) and on Sakhalin Island (Surkov 1974). Since the report of Iogansen (1934) on Bering Island, records from the northern red-backed vole, *C. rutilus*, have been numerous, and include the Novosibirsk Oblast' (Leikina *et al.* 1959, Lukashenko & Zorikhina 1961), Iakutia (Gubanov 1964), and Karaginsk Island, off the eastern coast of Kamchatka (46 per cent infected of 113 animals) (Nadtochii 1970). Comparatively low prevalences were recorded on Sakhalin Island, where the highest rate occurred in red-backed voles (two species) in October (Surkov 1974). Yorozuya *et al.* (1968) found the larval cestode in a northern red-backed vole in the Nemuro District, Hokkaido, Japan. Infection in *C. rutilus* has not been reported on the North American mainland.

Muridae Records include the field mouse, *Apodemus agrarius* (Pallas) in the Belorussian SSR (one) (Merkusheva 1958, cited in Leikina *et al.* 1959), in Kazakhstan (Boev *et al.* 1971), and in the Pavlodarsk Oblast' (Bat'kaev 1973); the wood mouse, *A. sylvaticus* (L.), in Tselinogradsk Oblast' (Pleshchev 1978) and in Pavlodarsk Oblast' (Bat'kaev 1973); and the short-tailed mole-rat, *Nesokia indica* (Gray and Hardwicke), in Iran (Rausch 1967a). Otherwise, records from murids involve only the commensal house mouse (not listed here).

Dipodidae The larval cestode has been reported from a jerboa, *Allactaga elater* (Lichtenstein), in Azerbaidzhan (Mamedov 1964).

Ochotonidae Pikas of two species, *Ochotona daurica* (Pallas) and *O. pricei* [*O. pallasi* (Gray)], have been reported as intermediate hosts of *E. multilocularis* in the Tuvinsk Autonomous Oblast' (Sulimov 1963, 1972), as was a specimen of *O. roylei* (Ogilby) in Kirgizia (Dzhumadilov 1966).

GEOGRAPHIC DISTRIBUTION OF *ECHINOCOCCUS MULTILOCULARIS*

Attempts to delineate the approximate geographic range of *E. multilocularis* have been made by Rausch (1967a), Lukashenko (1975), and others, but distributional data are incomplete. In western Eurasia, a disjunct endemic region encompasses southern Germany, eastern France, and parts of

Switzerland and Austria. In the zone of tundra, the cestode evidently occurs from Kil'din Island, in the White Sea, east to Bering Strait, corresponding to the range of the arctic fox. Similarly, in North America, the cestode occurs in foxes in tundra from the western coast of Alaska (south to the mouth of the Kuskokwim River) to Hudson Bay. In the polar basin, it may be present wherever wandering foxes are found on the sea-ice, but completion of the cycle on arctic islands depends on the presence of intermediate hosts. The rodent fauna of the northernmost islands comprises only lemmings of the genus *Dicrostonyx*, of which the various species differ in degree of susceptibility to infection (Ohbayashi *et al.* 1971, and unpublished). *E. multilocularis* has not been found in foxes on Greenland (Rausch *et al.* 1983). The cestode is present on subarctic islands, including St Lawrence Island, St George Island (Pribilof Group) (Fay & Williamson 1962), Bering Island (Komandorskie Islands) (introduced; Rausch 1967a) and the Kurile Islands.

The southern limits of the range of *E. multilocularis* on the Eurasian continent are difficult to define. The map shown by Lukashenko (1975, Fig. 49) indicated that it is not known from extensive central and eastern regions. Little information is available for regions farther to the south, where the composition of the mammalian fauna generally would seem to favour completion of the cycle. Ninety human cases of alveolar hydatid disease have been diagnosed in the north-west of the People's Republic of China (Jiang 1981), and 11 in Qinghai Province (Han *et al.* 1981). The identity of intermediate hosts there has not been reported (Dr Lin Yuguang, personal communication). One human case, diagnosed *post mortem*, occurred in northern India (Aikat *et al.* 1978).

In the Middle East, *E. multilocularis* has been found in Turkey (Tahsinoğlu & Hacihanefioğlu 1962) and Iran (Alavi & Maghami 1964, Mobedi & Sadighian 1971). Robbana *et al.* (1981) reported a case of alveolar hydatid disease in man in northern Tunisia, providing the first indication of the occurrence, and potential spread, of *E. multilocularis* in northern Africa.

The cestode occurs naturally on the island of Sakhalin. In Japan, it was introduced on Rebun Island, off the northern coast of Hokkaido, by means of foxes from the Kuriles (Rausch 1967a), and has spread into northeastern Hokkaido, evidently again from the Kurile Islands (Iida 1969). Kamiya and Ohbayashi (1975) found 328 (19 per cent) infected of 1724 red foxes in the Nemuro and Kushiro districts of Hokkaido during 1966–73. Further spread southward in Japan seems inevitable.

In North America, *E. multilocularis* is indigenous in the zone of tundra, extending southward along the western shore of Hudson Bay (Choquette *et al.* 1962). Following its discovery in North Dakota (Leiby & Olsen 1964), the cestode has been recorded from seven additional (contiguous) states and in the adjacent Canadian provinces of Manitoba, Saskatchewan, and Alberta. The recent report from the states of Illinois and Nebraska (Ballard & Vande Vusse 1983) suggests that continuing, peripheral spread is taking place. Arctic foxes are known to disperse southward at intervals from the tundra along Hudson Bay (Wrigley & Hatch 1976); eggs expelled by such migrants might have been the origin of an endemic focus involving red foxes and local rodents (Rausch 1985). Spread of *E. multilocularis* in Manitoba would have been favoured by changes in land-use that provide habitat for rodents and red foxes. Such a pattern of dispersal of the cestode could account for the otherwise inexplicable case of alveolar hydatid disease in Manitoba (James & Boyd 1937). Because the requisite host-assemblages exist widely in the northern and eastern United States, continuing dispersal in natural hosts seems probable.

ECHINOCOCCUS OLIGARTHRUS (DIESING, 1863)

Echinococcus oligarthrus was described from a cougar, *Felis concolor*, L., collected by Johann Natterer in Brasil during the early 19th century, and notwithstanding the 120 years that have elapsed since it was recognised, its biological characteristics are not well known. As concluded by Cameron (1926), the larval stage of *E. oligarthrus* from an agouti (Rodentia: Dasyproctidae), also in Brasil, was described as *E. cruzi* Brumpt and Joyeux 1924. The study of paratype material of *E. cruzi* has confirmed Cameron's assessment of that relationship (Rausch *et al.* 1984). The larval *E. oligarthrus* occurs in subcutaneous muscle as well as in the liver and other organs in the intermediate host.

PATTERNS OF CYCLES

The strobilar stage of *E. oligarthrus* develops only in carnivores of the family Felidae. The larval stage occurs typically in rodents, of which agoutis, *Dasyprocta* spp., appear to be the most important. Host specificity evidently is not strongly expressed in the larval stage.

Natural cycle Wild felids of several species serve as final host of *E. oligarthrus*, indicating that a proportional size range must also prevail in the rodents on which they prey and that function as intermediate host. The large cats evidently also extensively prey on agoutis, *Dasyprocta* spp., and pacas, *Cuniculus paca* L. (Dasyproctidae).

Experimental studies (Sousa & Thatcher 1969) have shown that *E. oligarthrus* develops well in the domestic cat. Establishment of a partially synanthropic cycle is thus conceivable.

HOSTS OF *ECHINOCOCCUS OLIGARTHRUS*

In addition to the type-host, the cougar, felids of various species are known to harbour *E. oligarthrus*: jaguar *Panthera onca* (L.) (Thatcher & Sousa 1967); ocelot, *Felis pardalis* L. (D'Alessandro *et al.* 1981); jaguarundi, *F. yagouaroundi* Geoffroy (Cameron 1926, D'Alessandro *et al.* 1981); Geoffroy's cat, *F. geoffroyi* d'Orbigny and Gervais (Schantz & Colli 1973); and pampas cat, *F. colocolo* Molina (reported as *Echinococcus pampeanus* Szidat, 1967). The data are meagre concerning prevalence of the cestode in these hosts. In

Colombia, one of 11 ocelots and two of nine jaguarundis were found to be infected (D'Alessandro *et al.* 1981). In southern Argentina, seven (15 per cent) were infected of 46 Geoffroy's cats (Schantz & Colli 1973).

Natural infections have been reported in rodents of comparatively few species: agoutis, *Dasyprocta leporina* (L.) (Brumpt & Joyeux 1924) and *D. punctata* Gray (Sousa & Thatcher 1969); paca, *Cuniculus paca* (Rausch *et al.* 1978); spiny rat, *Proechimys* cf. *guyannensis* (Geoffroy) (Thatcher 1972, Rausch *et al.* 1978). Thatcher (1972) also cited a record for *Proechimys semispinosus* (Tomes) and reported the larval cestode from an opossum, *Didelphis marsupialis* L. Rodents of several species have been infected experimentally (Sousa & Thatcher 1969). The larval *E. oligarthrus* has not been found in man; earlier apparent records involved instead *E. vogeli*.

GEOGRAPHIC DISTRIBUTION OF *ECHINOCOCCUS OLIGARTHRUS*

Echinococcus oligarthrus is a neotropical species, occurring from Central America (Costa Rica and Panama) (Sousa & Thatcher 1969, Brenes *et al.* 1973), southward as far as the Subantarctic; it has been identified in Ecuador (Thatcher 1972), Colombia (Rausch *et al.* 1978), Brasil (Brumpt & Joyeux 1924, Rausch *et al.* 1984) and Argentina (Szidat 1967, Schantz & Colli 1973). The known distribution of suitable hosts indicates that *E. oligarthrus* can be expected to occur over most of South America. The cestode has been collected from mammals mainly in tropical forest, but the record from Geoffroy's cat was from the temperate zone (southern Argentina).

ECHINOCOCCUS VOGELI RAUSCH AND BERNSTEIN, 1972

Echinococcus vogeli was described from the bush dog, *Speothos venaticus* (Lund), from Ecuador, and is known to occur elsewhere in South America and in Central America, but its distribution and host-range are very inadequately understood. In Colombia, the typical intermediate host of *E. vogeli* is the paca, *Cuniculus paca* L. (Rodentia: Dasyproctidae) (Rausch *et al.* 1981). In the paca, the larval cestode occurs usually in the liver. Results of experimental infections and findings in animals in zoos have shown a relative lack of host specificity in the larval stage (D'Alessandro *et al.* 1981, O'Grady *et al.* 1982). The cestode is the cause of polycystic hydatid disease in man (D'Alessandro *et al.* 1979).

PATTERNS OF CYCLES

In addition to the natural cycle, the domestic dog can replace the bush dog as final host; thus, a partial synanthropic cycle may exist. A dog–wild rodent cycle conceivably could become established outside the neotropical regions if the cestode were introduced under favourable circumstances. Its transmission outside the endemic region has occurred thus far only among animals in zoos.

Natural cycle In nature, the cycle of *E. vogeli* is completed by means of the predator–prey relationship existing between the bush dog and the paca. The bush dog is the only known natural final host of *E. vogeli*. Pacas inhabit gallery forest in northern South America and take refuge in the associated streams when pursued. They are hunted by bush dogs on land or in water. The occasional infection of other rodents in the habitat of the bush dog, such as spiny rats, *Proechimys* spp., and agoutis, *Dasyprocta* spp., is perhaps incidental. The neotropical canids of smaller size (genus *Dusicyon*), which do not hunt in packs and which feed mainly on small animals, including insects, in open country, appear to be incapable of killing mammals as large as pacas. The maned wolf, *Chrysocyon brachyurus* (Illiger), is a steppe-inhabiting canid that also preys on animals of small size.

Wild rodent–dog Experimentally, domestic dogs have been found to be a suitable final host of *E. vogeli*. In northern South America, pacas are utilised as a food resource by people in rural areas, and the viscera (including the liver, the principal locus of the larval cestode) are often fed to domestic dogs. Few dogs have been examined in such areas; gravid specimens of *E. vogeli* (and undeveloped strobilae of *E. oligarthrus*) were found in a hunter's dog in Colombia (D'Alessandro *et al.* 1981). Domestic dogs appear to be the source of infection in the human population. The natural final host, the bush dog, is wary of man and rarely seen; it thus would seem to have no significance as a direct source of infection for man.

HOSTS OF *ECHINOCOCCUS VOGELI*

The strobilar stage of *E. vogeli* has not been reported from naturally infected carnivores other than the bush dog. The helminths of that canid are poorly known, and since animals have rarely been available for examination, information has not been obtained concerning prevalence of the cestode. The larval stage occurs commonly in the paca; rates of infection, determined only in Colombia, ranged from 19 to 23 per cent in large series of animals (D'Alessandro *et al.* 1981). The larval cestode was found also in six (0.5 per cent) of 1168 spiny rats in Colombia. Helminths reared in dogs by Dr G. E. Vogelsang, who fed them cysts from an agouti, *Dasyprocta leporina*, in Venezuela, were identified as *E. vogeli* (Rausch *et al.* 1984). Rodents of several species have been infected experimentally (unpublished).

GEOGRAPHIC DISTRIBUTION OF *ECHINOCOCCUS VOGELI*

E. vogeli is a neotropical species that, like *E. oligarthrus*, appears to have an extensive geographic range. The northernmost record is based on a case of polycystic hydatid disease in Panama (Sousa & Lombardo 1965, Rausch *et al.* 1978). It has been reported from Ecuador (Rausch & Bernstein 1972), Colombia and Venezuela (Rausch *et al.* 1978, D'Alessandro *et al.* 1981), and Brasil (Rausch *et al.* 1984). Considering the geographic range of the bush dog and the ubiquity of suitable intermediate hosts, the occurrence of

E. vogeli southward in tropical and subtropical forest to about latitude 25°S would seem to be a reasonable expectation.

CONCLUDING REMARKS

Investigations conducted during the last three decades have greatly expanded our knowledge of the biology of *Echinococcus* spp. Such knowledge is fundamental to the definition and implementation of measures that may ultimately lead to an acceptable level of control or prevention of hydatid disease, *sensu lato*, in man.

Nevertheless, many questions remain concerning these organisms under both natural and synanthropic conditions. Not yet established is the taxonomic status of the cestode that may be perpetuated by a predator–prey relationship existing between the lion and the wart-hog. Whether the apparent lack of human cases of hydatid disease caused by *E. oligarthrus* is attributable to some specific characteristic of the larval cestode, or only to the low probability of exposure, is unknown. *E. multilocularis* is expanding its range in Japan and in central North America, and its further spread geographically would seem to depend on inadvertent introductions of infected carnivores. In North America, red foxes are known to have been captured in the endemic region in the north-central United States and released some hundreds of kilometres to the south-east, for purposes of hunting. The distributional status and host-range of *E. multilocularis* in southern Eurasia, including the People's Republic of China, are poorly understood. Based on our findings in experimental animals and in animals in zoos, *E. vogeli* is known to have a wide range of potential intermediate hosts. With the extensive destruction of tropical forest and settlement in the Amazon basin, given a significant population of dogs, the involvement of *E. vogeli* in a partially synanthropic cycle seems possible. The potential risk involved in importation of infected canids was amply demonstrated by severe losses caused by polycystic hydatid disease among large primates at the Los Angeles Zoo, following indirect association with a bush dog from Ecuador.

It is evident that this highly successful group of cestodes will provide opportunities for productive research in the field and in the laboratory for a long time in the future. Indeed, the problem of hydatid disease may well be intensified as a consequence of the ever-increasing disruption of ecosystems by the expanding human population, combined with the seemingly inevitable deterioration of living standards worldwide. We must re-assess our priorities in the training of students, if we are to have in the future sufficient numbers of parasitologists competent to undertake the kinds of field investigations that in the past have been so productive.

REFERENCES

Abuladze, K. I. 1964. *Teniaty – lentochnye gel'minty zhivotnykh i cheloveka i vyzyvaemye imi zabolevaniia.* Moskva: Nauka.

Acha, P. N. and B. Szyfres 1980. *Zoonoses and communicable diseases common to man and animals.* Washington, D.C.: Pan American Health Organisation.

Addison, E. M., A. Fyvie and F. J. Johnson 1979. Metacestodes of moose, *Alces alces, of the Chapleau Crown Game Preserve, Ontario. Can. J. Zool.* **57**, 1619–23.

Aikat, B. K., S. R. Bhusnurmath, M. Cadersa, P. N. Chhuttani and S. K. Mitra 1978. *Echinococcus multilocularis* infection in India: first case report proved at autopsy. *Trans. R. Soc. Trop. Med. Hyg.* **72**, 619–21.

Alavi, A. and G. Maghami 1964. L'échinococcose hydatidose en Iran. *Arch. Inst. Razi* **16**, 76–81.

Anonymous 1980. Dingo – parasites. *Div. Wildl. Res., CSIRO*, 1978–80, 48.

Arambulo, P. V. 1974. The natural nidality of zoonoses in the Philippines. *Int. J. Zoonoses* **1**, 58–74.

Arslanova, A. Kh. 1962. Enzooticheskii ochag al'veoliarnogo ekhinokokkoza v Alma-Atinskoi Oblasti. *Med. Parazitol.* **31**, 88–91.

Asadov, S. M. 1960. *Gel'mintofauna zhvachnykh zhivotnykh SSSR i ee ekologo-geograficheskii analiz.* Baku: Skad. Nauk Azerbaid. SSR.

Badaev, Ia., M. I. Dobrynin, M. Meredov, B. Badaev, D. Annaev, L. M. Shagalina and S. A. Alakhverdiants 1977. *Gel'minty cheloveka, zhivotnykh i rastenii Turkmenii.* Ashkhabad: Ylym.

Bailenger, J. 1957. Une zone française d'endémie hydatique: les Basses Pyrénées. *Annls Parasitol. Hum. Comp.* **32**, 21–7.

Ballard, N. B. and J. Vande Vusse 1983. *Echinococcus multilocularis* in Illinois and Nebraska. *J. Parasitol.* **69**, 790–1.

Bat'kaev, A. I. 1973. O prirodnykh ochagakh al'veokokkoza v Pavlodarskoi oblasti. *Voprosy prirodnoi ochagovosti boleznei* **6**, 202–7.

Behbehani, K. and O. Hassounah 1976. The role of native domestic animals in the dissemination of *Echinococcus* infection among dogs in the State of Kuwait. *J. Helminthol.* **50**, 275–80.

Biocca, E. and O. Massi 1951. Ricerche preliminari sulla diffusione dell'echinococcosi in Italia. *Atti Soc. Ital. Sci. Vet.* **5**, 262–4.

Biocca, E. and O. Massi 1952. Il problema della echinococcosi in Italia: indagini e considerazioni. *Revta Parassitol.* **13**, 235–40.

Blood, B. D. and J. L. Lelijveld 1969. Studies on sylvatic echinococcosis in southern South America. *Z. Tropenmed. Parasitol.* **20**, 475–82.

Blood, B. D., J. L. Lelijveld and R. D. Lord 1963. Nota preliminar sobre equinococosis en el zorro gris pampeano *Dusicyon gymnocercus. Bol. Ofic. Sanit. Panam.* **54**, 127.

Boev, S. N., V. I. Bondareva and Z. Kh. Tazieva 1971. Vospriimchivost' nekotorykh vidov gryzunov k al'veokokky. *Voprosy prirodnoi ochagovosti boleznei* **4**, 152–9.

Bondareva, V. I. 1966. Piatnistaia koshka (*Felis libyca*) – novyi definitivnyi khoziain al'veokokka. *Mat. Nauch. Konf. VOG* (3), 47–50.

Bregante, J. L. 1951. Fréquence de l'hydatidose chez les bovins (*Bos taurus*) en Uruguay. *Afr. Fr. Chir.* **4**, 375–8.

Brenes, R. R., E. Monge, G. Muñoz and G. Rojas 1973. Presencia en Costa Rica de *Echinococcus oligarthrus* Diesing, 1863, colectado en el intestino delgado de *Felis concolor costaricensis. Rev. Biol. Trop.* **21**, 139–41.

Brumpt, E. and Ch. Joyeux 1924. Description d'un nouvel échinocoque: *Echinococcus cruzi* n.sp. *Annls Parasitol. Hum. Comp.* **2**, 226–31.

Brunetti, O. A. and M. N. Rosen 1970. Prevalence of *Echinococcus granulosus* hydatid in California deer. *J. Parasitol.* **56**, 1138–40.

Cameron, T. W. M. 1926. Observations on the genus *Echinococcus* Rudolphi, 1801. *J. Helminthol.* **4**, 13–22.

Choquette, L. P. E., G. G. Gibson, E. Kuyt and A. M. Pearson 1973. Helminths of wolves, *Canis lupus* L., in the Yukon and North West Territories. *Can. J. Zool.* **51**, 1087–91.

Choquette, L. P. E., A. H. Macpherson and J. G. Cousineau 1962. Note on the occurrence of *Echinococcus multilocularis* Leuckart, 1863 in the arctic fox in Canada. *Can. J. Zool.* **40**, 1167.

Choquette, L. P. E., L. K. Whitten, G. Rankin and C. M. Seal 1957. Note on parasites found in reindeer (*Rangifer tarandus*) in Canada. *Can. J. Comp. Med.* **21**, 199–203.

Chun-Siun, F. and V. K. Alekseev 1960. Al'veoliarnyi ekhinokokk u bol'shoi peschanki (*Rhombomys opimus* Licht.) v Kazakhstane. *Med. Parazitol.* **29**, 482.

Cook, B. R. and W. Crewe 1963. The epidemiology of *Echinococcus* infection in Great Britain. I. Abnormal behaviour of sheep in the mining valleys of South Wales and its relation to hydatid disease in man. *Ann. Trop. Med. Parasitol.* **57**, 150–6.

Cousi, D. 1951. L'échinococcose en Tunisie. *Afr. Fr. Chir.* **4**, 379–86.

Crellin, J. R., F. L. Andersen, P. M. Schantz and S. J. Condie 1982. Possible factors influencing distribution and prevalence of *Echinococcus granulosus* in Utah. *Am. J. Epidemiol.* **116**, 463–74.

D'Alessandro, A., R. L. Rausch, C. Cuello and N. Aristizabal 1979. *Echinococcus vogeli* in man, with a review of polycystic hydatid disease in Colombia and neighboring countries. *Am. J. Trop. Med. Hyg.* **28**, 303–17.

D'Alessandro, A., R. L. Rausch, G. A. Morales, S. Collet and D. Angel 1981. *Echinococcus* infections in Colombian animals. *Am. J. Trop. Med. Hyg.* **30**, 1263–76.

Dew, H. R. 1926. Observations on hydatid disease in the domestic herbivora (Echinococcus multilocularis) and its relationship with Echinococcus alveolaris. *Med. J. Aust.* **2**, 301–9.

Dissanaike, A. S. and D. C. Paramananthan 1962. On the occurrence and significance of hydatid cysts in the Ceylon sambhur *Rusa unicolor unicolor*. *Ceylon J. Med. Sci. (D)* **11**, 1–7.

Diveeva-Mogila, Iu. A. 1969. Prirodnoochagovye gel'mintozy Altaica. In *Problemy prirodnoi ochagovosti gel'mintozov cheloveka*, V. N. Shpil'ko (ed.), 80–1. Tiumen': Minist. Zdravookhr. RSFSR.

Dixon, J. B., J. K. Baker-Smith and J. C. Greatorex 1973. The incidence of hydatid cysts in horses in Great Britain. *Vet. Rec.* **93**, 255.

Durie, P. H. and R. F. Riek 1952. The role of the dingo and wallaby in the infestation of cattle with hydatids (*Echinococcus granulosus* (Batsch, 1786) Rudolphi, 1805) in Queensland. *Aust. Vet. J.* **28**, 249–54.

Dzhumadilov, Sh. D. 1966. Nekotorye dannye po izucheniiu al'veokokkoza v Kirgizii. In *Gel'minty zhivotnykh Kirgizii i sopredel'nykh territorii*, 138–46. Frunze: Ilim.

Eastman, K. L. and D. E. Worley 1979. The muskrat as an intermediate host of *Echinococcus multilocularis* in Montana. *J. Parasitol.* **65**, 34.

El Kordy, M. I. 1946. On the incidence of hydatid disease in domestic animals in Egypt. *J. R. Egypt. Med. Ass.* **29**, 265–79.

Eugster, R. O. 1978. *A contribution to the epidemiology of echinococcosis/hydatidosis in*

Kenya (East Africa) with special reference to the Kajiado District. Doctoral thesis, University of Zürich.

Euzeby, J. 1957. Les helminthes du bétail et du porc dans la Fédération de Malaya. *Rev. Élev. Med. Vet. Pays Trop.* **10**, 15–23.

Fairley, N. H. and R. J. Wright-Smith 1929. Hydatid infestation (*Echinococcus granulosus*) in sheep, oxen and pigs, with special reference to daughter cyst formation. *J. Pathol.* **32**, 309–35.

Fay, F. H. 1973. The ecology of *Echinococcus multilocularis* Leuckart, 1863 (Cestoda: Taeniidae) on St Lawrence Island, Alaska. *Annls Parasitol. Hum. Comp.* **48**, 523–42.

Fay, F. H. and R. L. Rausch 1966. The seasonal cycle of abundance of *Echinococcus multilocularis* in naturally infected arctic foxes. *Proc. First Int. Congr. Parasitol.* **2**, 765–6.

Fay, F. H. and F. S. L. Williamson 1962. Studies on the helminth fauna of Alaska. XXXIX. *Echinococcus multilocularis* Leuckart, 1863, and other helminths of foxes on the Pribilof Islands. *Can. J. Zool.* **40**, 767–72.

Fiebiger, J. 1947. *Die tierischen Parasiten der Haus- und Nutztiere, sowie des Menschen.* Vienna: Urban and Schwarzenberg.

Freeman, R. S., A. Adorjan and D. H. Pimlott 1961. Cestodes of wolves, coyotes, and coyote–dog crosses in Ontario. *Can. J. Zool.* **39**, 527–32.

Gargarin, V. 1960. Gel'mintofauna dikikh zhvachnykh Kirgizii. *Helminthologia* **2**, 9–12.

Gagarin, V. G., V. M. Steshenko and M. M. Tokobaev 1957. Rol' gryzunov v rasprostranenii gel'mintozoonozov. *Trudy̆ Inst. Zool. Parazitol.* **6**, 159–60.

Geptner, V. G., A. A. Nasimovich and A. G. Bannikov 1961. *Mlekopitaiushchie Sovetskogo soiuza. 1. Parnokopytnye i neparnokopytnye.* Moskva: Vysshaia Shkola.

Geptner, V. G., N. P. Naumov, P. B. Iurgenson, A. A. Sludskii, A. F. Chirkova and A. G. Bannikov 1967. *Mlekopitaiushchie Sovetskogo soiuza. 2. Morskie korovy i khishchnye.* Moskva: Vysshaia Shkola.

Gibbs, H. C. and J. S. Tener 1958. On some helminth parasites collected from the musk ox (*Ovibos moschatus*) in the Thelon Game Sanctuary, North West Territories. *Can. J. Zool.* **36**, 529–32.

Green, H. U. 1949. Occurrence of *Echinococcus granulosus* in elk (*Cervus canadensis nelsoni*), Banff National Park. *Can. Field-Nat.* **63**, 204–5.

Griuner, S. A. 1927. Ekhinokokki u severnykh olenei. *Trudy̆ Sibirsk. Vet. Inst.* **8**, 55–9.

Gubanov, N. M. 1964. *Gel'mintofauna promyslovykh mlekopitaiushchikh Iakutii.* Moskva: Nauka.

Gubanov, N. M. and K. P. Fedorov 1970. Fauna gel'mintov myshevidnykh gryzunov Iakutti. In *Fauna sibiri*, A. I. Cherepanov (ed.), 18–47. Novosibirsk: Nauka.

Gvozdev, E. V. 1969. Gel'mintofauna ondatry (*Ondatra zibethica*), akklimatizirovannoi v Kazakhstan. In *Raboty po gel'mintologii v Kazakhstane*, Sh. E. Esenov (ed.), 66–76. Alma-Ata: Nauka.

Hadwen, S. and L. J. Palmer 1922. *Reindeer in Alaska.* Washington, D.C.: US Government Printing Office.

Hall, M. C. 1925. Parasites of deer, *Odocoileus* sp. *J. Parasitol.* **12**, 105.

Han, F., R. Liu, T. Zhong and Zh. Zhang 1981. Echinococcus alveolaris in Quinghai Province. *Chinese Med. J.* **94**, 391–5.

Hassounah, O. and K. Behbehani 1976. The epidemiology of *Echinococcus* infection in Kuwait. *J. Helminthol.* **50**, 65–73.

Herre, W. and M. Röhrs 1973. *Haustiere – zoologisch gesehen.* Stuttgart: Gustav Fischer.

Herrera, M. and D. J. Cranwell 1960. *Los quistes hidatídicos en la Republica Argentina.* Buenos Aires.

Holmes, J. C. and R. Podesta 1968. The helminths of wolves and coyotes from the forested regions of Alberta. *Can. J. Zool.* **46**, 1193–204.

Honacki, J. H., K. E. Kinman and J. W. Koeppl 1982. *Mammal species of the world.* Lawrence, Kan: Allen Press and the Association of Systematics Collections.

Houin, R., M. Deniau, M. Liance and F. Puel 1982. *Arvicola terrestris* an intermediate host of *Echinococcus multilocularis* in France: epidemiological consequences. *Int. J. Parasitol.* **12**, 593–600.

Howkins, A. B. 1966. The role of macropodidae in Tasmania as intermediate hosts in hydatid disease. *Aust. Vet. J.* **42**, 240–1.

Hutchison, W. F. 1960. Studies on the hydatid worm, *Echinococcus granulosus.* II. Prevalence in Mississippi. *Am. J. Trop. Med. Hyg.* **9**, 612–5.

Iakovleva, T. A., A. A. Lazarev, L. V. Smirnova and G. A. Mikhailov 1973. O rasprostranenii ekhinokokkoza i al'veokokkoza y zhivotnykh Kamchatki. *Gel'mintozy Dalnego vostoka,* (2), 47–8.

Ialiev, S. M. 1975. K izucheniiu gel'mintofauny kabanov v Zakatal'skom zapovednike. In *Issledovaniia po gel'mintologii v Azerbaidzhane,* S. M. Asadov *et al.* (eds), 150–5. Baku: Elim.

Iida, H. 1969. Epidemiology of multilocular echinococcosis in Hokkaido, Japan. In *Multilocular echinococcosis in Hokkaido, Japan,* 7–15. Sapporo: Hokkaido Institute of Public Health.

Iogansen, G. Kh. 1934. Ptitsy Komandorskikh Ostrovov. *Trudỹ Tomsk. Gosudarst. Univ.* **86**, 222–66.

Isakov, S. I. 1982. Ob ochage al'veokokkoza v Iakutii. *Parazitologiia* **16**, 330–3.

Ishino, E. 1941. Discussion about the development of alveolar type of Echinococcus. (In Japanese.) *J. Anim. Hlth Ass.* **9**, 115–28.

Ivashkin, V. M. 1955. *Gel'minty sel'skokhoziaistvennykh zhivotnykh Mongol'skoi narodnoi respubliki.* Moskva: Akad. Nauk SSSR.

James, E. and. W. Boyd 1937. Echinococcus alveolaris (with the report of a case). *Can. Med. Ass. J.* **36**, 354–6.

Jansen, J. 1961. *Echinococcus granulosus* bij het edelhert (*Cervus elaphus*). *Tijdschr. Diergeneesk.* **86**, 82–4.

Jiang, C. 1981. Liver alveolar echinococcosis in the North West. Report of 15 patients and a collective analysis of 90 cases. *Chinese Med. J.* **91**, 771–8.

Kadenatsii, A. N. and L. I. Zinov'ev 1973. Gel'mintofauna losia v svete izucheniia prirodnoi ochagovosti gel'mintozov. *Voprosy prirodnoi ochagovosti boleznei* **6**, 139–43.

Kahn, J. B., S. Spruance, J. Harbottle, P. Cannon and M. G. Schultz 1972. Echinococcosis in Utah. *Am. J. Trop. Med. Hyg.* **21**, 185–8.

Kamiya, H. and M. Ohbayashi 1975. Some helminths of the red fox, *Vulpes vulpes schlencki* Kishida, in Hokkaido, Japan, with a description of a new trematode, *Massaliatrema yamashitai* n.sp. *Japan. J. Vet. Res.* **23**, 60–7.

Kan, L.-B. 1966. *Parasitic infections of man and animals. A bibliography of articles in Chinese medical periodicals 1949–64.* Hong Kong: Hong Kong University.

Kikot', V. I. 1980. Prirodnaia ochagovost' ekhinokokkoza v gornotaezhnoi zone Dal'nego vostoka. *Med. Parazitol.* **49**, 60–4.

Korsakov, G. K. 1963. Results of acclimatization of muskrats in the USSR. In *Akklimatizatsiia zhivotnykh v SSSR,* A. I. Ianushevich (ed.), 75–6. Alma-Ata: Akad. Nauk Kazakh. SSR.

Koval'chuk, E. S. 1979. Gel'minty dikikh promyslovykh mlekopitaiushchikh Tiumenskoi oblasti i nekotorye voprosy ikh ekologicheskogo analiza. In *Ekologiia i morfologiia gel'mintov zapadnoi Sibiri*, V. E. Sudarikov (ed.), 56–93. Novosibirsk: Nauka.

Kritsky, D. C., P. D. Leiby and G. E. Miller 1977. The natural occurrence of *Echinococcus multilocularis* in the bushy-tailed woodrat, *Neotoma cinerea rupicola*, in Wyoming. *Am. J. Trop. Med. Hyg.* **26**, 1046–7.

Krotov, A. I. 1979. K voprosu o podvidakh i shtammakh predstavitelei roda *Echinococcus* Rudolphi, 1801. *Med. Parazitol.* **48**, 22–6.

Kumaratilake, L. M. and R. C. A. Thompson 1982. Hydatidosis/echinococcosis in Australia. *Helminthol. Abstr. A* **51**, 233–52.

Kurashvili, B. E. 1961. O roli polevok i zakavkazskoi stepnoi lisitsy v epizootologii i epidemiologii al'veoliarnogo ekhinokokkoza v vostochnoi Gruzii. *Soobshch. Akad. Nauk Gruz. SSR* **26**, 309–15.

Kurashvili, B. E. 1962. Ekhinokokkoz i al'veokokkoz v Gruzii. *Tez. Doklad. Nauch. Konf. VOG* (2), 91–2.

Kuznetsov, M. I. 1958. K voprosu o rasprostranenii ekhinokokkoza i finnoza u zhivotnykh, zabitykh na Armavirskom miasokombinate. *Biull. Nauchno-Tekh. Inform. Vsesoiuz. Inst. Gel'mintol.* **4**, 47–8.

Larbaui, D., R. Alliulia, L. V. Osiiskaia, I. Iu. Osiiskii and M. Benel'muffok 1980. Ekhinokokkoz v Alzhire. *Med. Parazitol.* **49**, 21–3.

Lavrov, N. P. 1953. Vnutrennie i naruzhnye parazity ondatry. *Trudy̆ VNII Okhot. Promysla* (12), 132–5.

Le-Van-Hoa and Vu-Ngoc-Tan 1967. Sur la présence des cestodes, *Echinococcus granulosus* (Batsch, 1786), chez un chien sauvage, *Cyon primaerus* (Hodgs.) au Sud-Viet-Nam. *Bull. Soc. Pathol. Exot.*, No. 1.

Leiby, P. D. 1965. Cestode in North Dakota: *Echinococcus* in field mice. *Science* **150**, 763.

Leiby, P. D. and W. G. Dyer 1971. Cyclophyllidean tapeworms of wild carnivora. In *Parasitic diseases of wild mammals*, J. W. Davis and R. C. Anderson (eds), 174–234. Ames, Iowa: Iowa State University.

Leiby, P. D. and D. C. Kritsky 1972. *Echinococcus multilocularis*: a possible domestic life cycle in central North America and its public health implications. *J. Parasitol.* **58**, 1213–5.

Leiby, P. D. and O. W. Olsen 1964. The cestode *Echinococcus multilocularis* in North Dakota. *Science* **145**, 1066.

Leiby, P. D., W. P. Carney and C. E. Woods 1970. Studies on sylvatic echinococcosis. III. Host occurrence and geographic distribution of *Echinococcus multilocularis* in the north central United States. *J. Parasitol.* **56**, 1141–50.

Leikina, E. S. 1957. K voprosu o prirodnoi ochagovosti nekotorykh gel'mintozov. *Med. Parazitol.* **26**, 140–52.

Leikina, E. S., N. P. Lukashenko, V. I. Zorikhina, B. K. Lavrenov and M. M. Mamedov 1959. K voprosu o prirodnykh ochagakh mnogokamernogo ekhinokokka v Novosibirskoi Oblasti. *Med. Parazitol.* **28**, 206–13.

Lesin'sh, K. P. 1959. Izuchenie gel'mintofauny evropeiskoi ryzhei polevki (*Clethrionomys glareolus*) v Latviiskoi SSR. *Fauna Latviiskoi SSR i sopredel'nykh territorii* **2**, 273–82.

Lichtenheld, G. 1904. Ueber die Fertilität und Sterilität der Echinokokken beim Rind, Schwein, Schaf, und Pferd. Histologischer Teil. *Zentbl. Bakt. Orig.* **37**, 64–73.

Liu, I. K. M., C. W. Schwabe, P. M. Schantz and M. N. Allison 1970. The occurrence of *Echinococcus granulosus* in coyotes (*Canis latrans*) in the central valley of California. *J. Parasitol.* **56**, 1135–6.

Logachev, E. D. and A. I. Bat'kaev 1979. Surok-baibak – novyi promezhutochnyi khoziain al'veokokka. *Voprosy prirodnoi ochagovosti boleznei* **10**, 133–41.

Lühe, M. 1910. Cystotänien südamerikanischer Feliden. *Zool. Jahrb.* Suppl. 12, 687–710.

Lukashenko, N. P. 1975. *Alveokokkoz (al'veoliarnyi ekhinokokkoz).* Moskva: Meditsina.

Lukashenko, N. P. 1978. Al'veokokkoz – prirodnoochagovyi antropozoonoz. *Voprosy prirodnoi ochagovosti boleznei* **9**, 29–49.

Lukashenko, N. P. and V. I. Zorikhina 1961. Epidemiologiia al'veokokkoza (al'veoliarnogo ekhinokokkoza) v tsentral'nykh raionakh Barabinskoi lesostepi Novosibirskoi oblasti. *Med. Parazitol.* **30**, 159–68.

Lupașcu, Gh. and D. Panaitescu 1968. *Hidatidoza.* București: Acad. Rept. Soc. Romania.

Luzhkov, A. D. 1963. K epizootologii i epidemiologii al'veokokkoza na Poluostrove Iamal. *Med. Parazitol.* **32**, 180–3.

Machinskii, A. P. and V. N. Semov 1972. Gel'minty lisits Mordovii. In *VIII Vsesoiuz. Konf. po prirodnoi ochagovosti boleznei zhivotnykh i okhrane ikh chislennosti*, S. N. Boev (ed.), 111. Kirov: Akad. Nauk SSSR.

Machul'skii, S. N. 1958. Gel'mintofauna gryzunov Buriatskoi ASSR. In *Raboty po gel'mint. k 80-let. Akad. K. I. Skriabina*, N. P. Shikhobalova (ed.), 219–24. Moskva: Akad. Nauk SSSR.

Macpherson, C. N. L. 1983. An active intermediate host role for man in the life cycle of *Echinococcus granulosus* in Turkana, Kenya. *Am. J. Trop. Med. Hyg.* **32**, 397–404.

Macpherson, C. N. L. and L. Karstad 1981. The role of jackals in the transmission of *Echinococcus granulosus* in the Turkana District of Kenya. In *Wildlife disease research and economic development: proceedings of a workshop held in Kabete, Kenya*, L. Karstad, B. Nestel and M. Graham (eds), 53–6. Ottawa: International Development Research Centre.

Macpherson, C. N. L., L. Karstad, P. Stevenson and J. H. Arundel 1983. Hydatid disease in the Turkana District of Kenya. III. The significance of wild animals in the transmission of *Echinococcus granulosus*, with particular reference to Turkana and Masailand in Kenya. *Ann. Trop. Med. Parasitol.* **77**, 61–73.

Mamedov, M. M. 1964. K. voprosu o rasprostranenii ekhinokokkoza i al'veokokkoza v Azerbaidzhanskoi SSR. *Med. Parazitol.* **33**, 278–83.

Matsaberidze, G. V. 1966. Gel'minty myshevidnykh gryzunov v raionakh Kartli. (In Georgian.) *Parazitol. Sbornik, Inst. Zool., Akad. Nauk Gruzinsk. SSR* **1**, 65–90.

Mech, L. D. 1966. *The wolves of Isle Royale.* Washington, D.C.: US Government Printing Office.

Mobedi, I. and A. Sadighian 1971. *Echinococcus multilocularis* Leuckart, 1863, in red foxes, *Vulpes vulpes* Linn., in Moghan, Azerbaijan Province, north-west of Iran. *J. Parasitol.* **57**, 493.

Nadtochii, E. V. 1970. Fauna gel'mintov gryzunov Dal'nego vostoka. *Dal'nevostoch. Gosudarst. Univ., Uchenie Zapiski* **16**, 62–84.

Nazarova, N. S. 1967. Gel'mintofauna losia v Sovetskom soiuze. In *Biologiia i promysel losia*, A. G. Bannikov (ed.), 288–312. Moskva: Rossel'khozizdat.

Nelson, G. S. and R. L. Rausch 1963. *Echinococcus* infections in man and animals in Kenya. *Ann. Trop. Med. Parasitol.* **57**, 136–49.

Nemurovskaia, A. I., V. Ia. Nekipelov, T. A. Iakovleva and A. A. Iasinskii 1980. Problema ekhinokokkoza i al'veokokkoza v RSFSR. *Med. Parazitol.* **49**, 17–21.

Nieberle, K. and P. Cohrs 1949. *Lehrbuch der speziellen pathologischen Anatomie der Haustiere.* Jena: Gustav Fischer.

O'Grady, J. P., C. H. Yeager, G. N. Esra and W. Thomas 1982. Ultrasonic evaluation of echinococcosis in four lowland gorillas. *J. Am. Vet. Med. Ass.* **181**, 1348–50.

Ohbayashi, M., R. L. Rausch and F. H. Fay 1971. On the ecology and distribution of *Echinococcus* spp. (Cestoda: Taeniidae), and characteristics of their development in the intermediate host. II. Comparative studies on the development of larval *E. multilocularis* Leuckart, 1863, in the intermediate host. *Jap. J. Vet. Res.* **19**, 1–53.

Ovsiukova, N. I. 1966. *Gel'minty i osnovnye gel'mintozy mlekopitaiushchikh Chukotki.* Doctoral dissertation, Vsesoiuz. Inst. Gel'mint. im K. I. Striabina, Moskva.

Panin, V. Ia. and L. I. Lavrov 1962. K gel'mintofaune volkov Kazakhstana. *Trudy̆ Inst. Zool., Alma-Ata* **16**, 57–62.

Papachristophilou, P. 1957. L'hydatidose en Grece chez les ruminants et les porcs. *Bull. Off. Int. Epizootiol.* **47**, 469–85.

Paramananthan, D. C. 1961. Some observations on brood capsules of hydatid cysts from local animals. *Ceylon J. Med. Sci. D* **10**, 57–9.

Petavy, A. F. and S. Deblock 1980. Helminthes du renard commun (*Vulpes vulpes* L.) dans la région du Massif Central (France). *Annls Parasitol. Hum. Comp.* **55**, 379–91.

Petrov, A. M. 1957. Sovremennye vozzreniia na epizootologiu i epidemiologiiu ekhinokokkozov. *Tez. Doklad. Nauch. Konf. VOG* (2), 12-4.

Petrov, A. M. 1958. K obnaruzheniiu vozbuditelia al'veoliarnogo ekhinokokkoza (*Echinococcus multilocularis*) u domashnikh i dikikh zhivotnykh v SSSR. *Biull. Nauchno-Tekh. Inform. Vsesoiuz. Inst. Gel'mintol* **3**, 36–8.

Petrov, A. M. and A. N. Chertkova 1959. Otlichitel'nye priznaki odnokamernogo i al'veoliarnogo ekhinokokkov po lichinochnym i polovozrelyn formam. *Trudy̆ Vsesoiuz. Inst. Gel'mintol.* **7**, 129–39.

Petrov, A. M. and R. Sh. Delianova 1962. Rasprostranenie vozbuditelei ekhinokokkoza i al'veokokkoza u domashnikh i dikikh plotoiadnykh v SSSR. *Trudy̆ Vsesoiuz. Inst. Gel'mintol.* **9**, 67–87.

Pleshchev, V. S. 1978. Rol'gryzunov v rasprostranenii al'veokokkoza na territorii Tselinogradskoi oblasti. *Voprosy prirodnoi ochagovosti boleznei* **9**, 50–2.

Pullar, E. M. and W. K. Marshall 1958. The incidence of hydatids in Victorian cattle. *Aus. Vet. J.* **34**, 193–201.

Radionov, P. V. 1971. Rol' saigakov i khishchnikov v epizootiologii gel'mintozov sel'skokhozaistvennykh zhivotnykh v Kustanaiskoi oblasti. *Prirodnaia ochagovost' boleznei i voprosy parazitol. zhivotnykh* **6**, 96–9.

Rausch, R. A. 1959. Notes on the prevalence of hydatid disease in Alaskan moose. *J. Wildl. Mgmt* **23**, 122–3.

Rausch, R. L. 1952. Hydatid disease in boreal regions. *Arctic* **5**, 157–74.

Rausch, R. L. 1967a. On the ecology and distribution of *Echinococcus* spp. (Cestoda: Taeniidae), and characteristics of their development in the intermediate host. *Annls Parasitol. Hum. Comp.* **42**, 16–93.

Rausch, R. L. 1967b. A consideration of infraspecific categories in the genus *Echinococcus* Rudolphi, 1801 (Cestoda: Taeniidae). *J. Parasitol.* **53**, 484–91.

Rausch, R. L. 1985. Parasitology: retrospect and prospect. *J. Parasitol* 71, 139–51.

Rausch, R. L. and J. J. Bernstein 1972. *Echinococcus vogeli* sp.n. (Cestoda: Taeniidae) from the bush dog, *Speothos venaticus* (Lund). *Z. Tropenmed. Parasitol.* **23**, 25–34.

Rausch, R. L. and S. H. Richards 1971. Observations on parasite–host relationships of *Echinococcus multilocularis* Leuckart, 1863, in North Dakota. *Can. J. Zool.* **49**, 1317–30.

Rausch, R. L. and E. L. Schiller 1951. Hydatid disease (echinococcosis) in Alaska and the importance of rodent intermediate hosts. *Science* **113**, 57–8.

Rausch, R. L. and E. L. Schiller 1956. Studies on the helminth fauna of Alaska. XXV. The ecology and public health significance of *Echinococcus sibiricensis* Rausch and Schiller, 1954, on St Lawrence Island. *Parasitology* **46**, 395–419.

Rausch, R. L. and F. S. L. Williamson 1959. Studies on the helminth fauna of Alaska. XXXIV. The parasites of wolves, *Canis lupus* L. *J. Parasitol.* **45**, 395–403.

Rausch, R. L., A. D'Alessandro and M. Ohbayashi 1984. The taxonomic status of *Echinococcus cruzi* Brumpt and Joyeux, 1924 (Cestoda: Taeniidae) from an agouti (Rodentia: Dasyproctidae) in Brazil. *J. Parasitol.* **70**, 295–302.

Rausch, R. L., A. D'Alessandro and V. R. Rausch 1981. Characteristics of the larval *Echinococcus vogeli* Rausch and Bernstein, 1972 in the natural intermediate host, the paca, *Cuniculus paca* L. (Rodentia: Dasyproctidae). *Am. J. Trop. Med. Hyg.* **30**, 1043–52.

Rausch, R. L., F. H. Fay and F. S. L. Williamson 1983. Helminths of the arctic fox, *Alopex lagopus* (L.), in Greenland. *Can. J. Zool.* **61**, 1847–51.

Rausch, R. L., V. R. Rausch and A. D'Alessandro 1978. Discrimination of the larval stages of *Echinococcus oligarthrus* (Diesing, 1863) and *E. vogeli* Rausch and Bernstein, 1972 (Cestoda: Taeniidae). *Am. J. Trop. Med. Hyg.* **27**, 1195–202.

Rein, K. 1957. Echinokokksykdommens forekomst i Kautokeino. *Nord. Med.* **57**, 375–80.

Riley, W. A. 1933. Reservoirs of Echinococcus in Minnesota. *Minn. Med.* **16**, 744–5.

Robbana, M., M. S. Ben Rachid, M. M. Zitouna, N. Heldt and M. Hafsia 1981. Première observation d'échinococcose alvéolaire autochtone en Tunisie. *Arch. Anat. Cytol. Pathol.* **29**, 311–2.

Roman, C. 1956. Nota sobre incidencia de hidatidosis en alpacas y ovinos de la Sierra del Peru. *Rev. Med. Exper.* **10**, 85–7.

Romazanov, V. T. 1963. Endemicheskii ochag al'veokokkoza v Alma-Atinskoi oblasti i rol' sobak v rasprostranenii etoi invazii. In *Gel'minty cheloveka, zhivotnykh i rastenii i bor'ba s nimi*, N. P. Shikhobalova (ed.), 51–3. Moskva: Akad. Nauk SSSR.

Ronéus O. 1974. Prevalence of echinococcosis in reindeer (Rangifer tarandus) in Sweden. *Acta Vet. Scand.* **15**, 170–8.

Rosen, M. N. 1951. A noticeable absence of bladder worms in Catalina deer. *Calif. Fish Game* **37**, 217.

Round, M. C. 1968. *Check list of the helminth parasites of African mammals*. Farnham Royal, Slough: Commonwealth Bureau of Helminthology.

Rukhliadev, D. P. 1952. K izucheniiu gel'mintofauny dikogo kabana. *Trudȳ Gel'mint. Lab.* **6**, 330–3.

Sadykhov, I. A. 1953. K izucheniiu gel'mintofauny shakalov Azerbaidzhana. In *Raboty pol gel'mint. k 75-let. Akad. K. I. Skriabina*, A. M. Petrov (ed.), 620–1. Moskva: Akad. Nauk SSSR.

Saffronov, M. G. 1966. *Gel'minty i gel'mintozy zhivotnykh Iakutii*. Iakutsk: Iakutskoe Knizhnoe.

Santiváñez, J. and A. Cuba 1949. Quiste hidatico en *Lama glama pacos* o alpaca. *Rev. Fac. Med. Vet., Lima* **4**, 22–4.

Savel'ev, V. D. 1972. O rasprostranenii vozbuditelei ekhinokokkoza i al'veokokkoza sredi mlekopitaiushchikh Taimira. In *VIII Vsesoiuz. Konf. po prirodnoi ochagovosti boleznei zhivotnykh i okhrane ikh chislennosti*, S. N. Boev (ed.), 120. Kirov: Akad. Nauk SSSR.

Sawyer, J. C., P. M. Schantz, C. W. Schwabe and M. W. Newbold 1969.

Identification of transmission foci of hydatid disease in California. *Publ. Hlth Rep., Wash.* **84**, 531–41.

Schantz, P. M. and C. Colli 1973. *Echinococcus oligarthrus* (Diesing, 1863) from Geoffroy's cat (*Felis geoffroyi* d'Orbigny y Gervais) in temperate South America. *J. Parasitol.* **59**, 1138–40.

Schantz, P. M. and R. D. Lord 1972. *Echinococcus* in the South American red fox (*Dusicyon culpaeus*) and the European hare (*Lepus europaeus*) in the Province of Neuquén, Argentina. *Ann. Trop. Med. Parasitol.* **66**, 479–85.

Schantz, P. M. and C. Schwabe 1969. Worldwide status of hydatid disease control. *J. Am. Vet. Med. Ass.* **155**, 2104–21.

Schantz, P. M., C. Colli, A. Cruz-Reyes and U. Prezioso 1976. Sylvatic echinococcosis in Argentina. II. Susceptibility of wild carnivores to *Echinococcus granulosus* (Batsch, 1786) and host-induced morphological variation. *Tropenmed. Parasitol.* **27**, 70–8.

Schantz, P. M., A. Cruz-Reyes, C. Colli and R. D. Lord 1975. Sylvatic echinococcosis in Argentina. I. On the morphology and biology of strobilar *Echinococcus granulosus* (Batsch, 1786) from domestic and sylvatic animal hosts. *Tropenmed. Parasitol.* **26**, 334–44.

Schantz, P. M., C. F. von Reyn, T. Welty, F. L. Andersen, M. G. Schultz and I. G. Kagan 1977. Epidemiologic investigation of echinococcosis in American Indians living in Arizona and New Mexico. *Am. J. Trop. Med. Hyg.* **26**, 121–6.

Shamsul Islam, A. W. M. 1979. Hydatid disease in sheep of Mymensingh District, Bangladesh. *J. Parasitol.* **65**, 37.

Shol', V. A. 1963. Fauna gel'mintov kabanov (*Sus scrofa* L.) Kazakhstana. In *Parazity dikikh zhivotnykh Kazakhstana*, I. G. Galuzo (ed.), 97–100. Alma Ata: Akad. Nauk Kazakh. SSR.

Shul'ts, R. S. 1962. O nekotorykh voprosakh epidemiologii ekhinokokkozov i metodakh bor'by s nimi. *Med. Parazitol.* **31**, 272.

Shul'ts, R. S. and A. N. Kadenatsii 1950. Gel'minty dal'nevostochnogo gorala. *Trudӯ Gel'mintol. Lab.* **3**, 152–60.

Shumakovich, E. E. and V. F. Nikitin 1959. K obnaruzheniiu *Echinococcus granulosus* (Batsch, 1786) u korsaka. *Biull. Nauchno-Tekh. Inform. Vsesoiuz. Inst. Gel'mintol.* **5**, 98–9.

Skjenneberg, S. 1959. Ekinokokkose hos rein i Kautokeino. *Nord. Vet.-Med.* **11**, 110–23.

Söderhjelm, L. 1945. Förekomsten av Echinococcus hydatidosus hos människa och ren (Rangifer tarandus). *Svenska Läkartid.* **28**, 1–7.

Söderhjelm, L. 1946. Echinococcus hydatidosis hos ren (Rangifer tarandus). *Skand. Veterinartid.* **36**, 378–81.

Sokolov, V. A. 1972. K izucheniiu gel'mintov kanid na Altae. In *VIII Vsesoiuz. konf. po prirodnoi ochagovosti boleznei zhivotnykh i okhrane ikh chislennosti*, S. N. Boev (ed.), 122–3. Kirov: Akad. Nauk SSSR.

Sousa, O. E. and J. D. Lombardo 1965. Informe de un caso de hidatidosis en sujeto nativo panameño; primer case autóctono. *Arch. Med. Panam.* **14**, 79–86.

Sousa, O. E. and V. E. Thatcher 1969. Observations on the life-cycle of *Echinococcus oligarthrus* (Diesing, 1863) in the Republic of Panama. *Ann. Trop. Med. Parasitol.* **63**, 165–75.

Spasskii, A. A., N. P. Romanova and N. V. Naidenova 1951. Novye dannye o faune paraziticheskikh chervei ondatry – *Ondatra zibethica* (L.). *Trans. Gel'mintol. Lab.* **5**, 42–52.

Suić, M. 1952. *Ehinokokoza*. Zagreb: Jugoslav. Akad. Znanosti i Umjetnosti.

Suić, M. 1957. L'échinococcose animale en Yougoslavie. *Arch. Int. Hidatidosis* **16**, 143–6.

Sulimov, A. D. 1963. Gel'mintofauna gryzunov tuvinskoi ASSR. *Materialy Nauch. Konf. VOG* (2), 111–5.

Sulimov, A. D. 1972. Ob ekhinokokkoze i al'veokokkoze v Tuve. In *VIII Vsesoiuz, konf. prirodnoi ochagovosti boleznei zhivotnykh i okhrane ikh chislennosti*, S. N. Boev (ed.), 125–6. Kirov: Akad. Nauk SSSR.

Sultanov, M. A., P. A. Muminov, N. Davlatov and E. Koshchanov 1971. Rol' dikikh zhivotnykh v rezervatsii i rasprostranenii gel'mintozov domashnikh zhivotnykh i cheloveka v usloviiakh Uzbekistana. *Prirodnaia ochagovost' boleznei i voprosy parazitologii zhivotnykh* **6**, 119–21.

Surkov, V. S. 1974. Sezonnaia dinamika zarazhennosti lesnykh polevok gel'mintami na Sakhaline. *Zool. Zh.* **53**, 184–8.

Sweatman, G. K. 1952. Distribution and incidence of *Echinococcus granulosus* in man and other animals with special reference to Canada. *Can. J. Publ. Hlth* **43**, 480–6.

Sweatman, G. K. and R. J. Williams 1962. Wild animals in New Zealand as hosts of *Echinococcus granulosus* and other taeniid tapeworms. *Trans. R. Soc. N.Z. (Zool.)* **2**, 221–50.

Szidat, L. 1967. *Echinococcus pampeanus* una nueva especie de la Argentina, parasita de *Felis colocolo pajeros* Desmarest, 1916 (Cestoda). *Neotropica* **13**, 90–6.

Szidat, L. 1971. Neue Aspekte des Echinococcen-Problems. *Angew. Parasitol.* **12**, 133–43.

Tahsinoğlu, M. and U. Hacihanefioğlu 1962. Echinococcus alveolaris' in Türkiyede bugünkü durumu. *Ist. Tip Fak. Mec.* **25**, 289–94.

Talavera, J. 1955. Les maladies parasitaires du bétail en Espagne. *Bull. Off. Int. Epizootiol.* **43**, 214–32.

Tanda, S. 1960. Osservazioni sull'echinococcosi (idatidosi) degli animali macellati a Sassari. *Parassitologia* **2**, 315–20.

Thatcher, V. E. 1972. Neotropical echinococcosis in Colombia. *Ann. Trop. Med. Parasitol.* **66**, 99–105.

Thatcher, V. E. and O. E. Sousa 1967. *Echinococcus oligarthrus* (Diesing, 1863) from a Panamanian jaguar (*Felis onca* L.). *J. Parasitol.* **53**, 1040.

Thomas, L. J., B. B. Babero, V. Gallicchio and R. J. Lacey 1954. Echinococcosis on St Lawrence Island, Alaska. *Science* **120**, 1102–3.

Thompson, R. C. A. 1977. Hydatidosis in Great Britain. *Helminthol. Abstr. A* **46**, 837–61.

Thompson, R. C. A. 1979. Biology and speciation of *Echinococcus granulosus*. *Aust. Vet. J.* **55**, 93–8.

Thompson, R. C. A. and L. M. Kumaratilake 1982. Intraspecific variation in *Echinococcus granulosus*: the Australian situation and perspectives for the future. *Trans. R. Soc. Trop. Med. Hyg.* **76**, 13–6.

Tokobaev, M. M. 1959. Gel'mintofauna gryzunov Kirgizii. *Trudȳ Inst. Zool. Parazitol.* **7**, 133–42.

Tokobaev, M. M. 1960. Gel'mintofauna gryzunov Kirgizii. *Trudȳ Gel'mintol. Lab.* **10**, 235–47.

Vande Vusse, F. J., D. E. Little, R. B. Callaway and N. B. Ballard 1978. Incidence and distribution of *Echinococcus multilocularis* in fox from southern Minnesota. In *Program and Abstracts, 53rd Annual Meeting, American Society of Parasitologists*, 93.

Verster, A. and M. Collins 1966. The incidence of hydatidosis in the Republic of South Africa. *Onderstepoort J. Vet. Res.* **33**, 49–72.

Vinogradov, B. S. and I. M. Gromov 1952. *Gryzuny fauny SSSR.* Moskva–Leningrad: Akad. Nauk SSSR.

Virchow, R. 1855. Die multiloculäre, ulcerirende Echinokokkengeschwulst der Leber. *Verh. Physiol.-Med. Ges. Würzburg* **6**, 428–9.

Vitale, G. 1954. Sulla frequenza della echinococcosi, distomatosi e cisticercosi nei bovini macellati in Messina. *Atti Soc. Ital. Sci. Vet.* **8**, 689–92.

Vogel, H. 1955. Über den Entwicklungszyklus und die Artzugehörigkeit des europäischen Alveolarechinococcus. *Dt. Med. Wschr.* **80**, 931–2.

Vogel, H. 1957. Über die spezifische Natur und die Entwicklung des Alveolar-Echinococcus in Europa. *Arch. Int. Hidatidosis* **16**, 517–22.

Vogel, H. 1960. Tiere als natürliche Wirte des *Echinococcus multilocularis* in Europa *Z. Tropenmed. Parasitol.* **11**, 36–42.

Vogel, H. 1961. Biologie und Parasitologie des Alveolarechinokokkus. *Chir. Praxis* **5**, 407–12.

Volokh, Iu. A. 1965. *Ekhinokokkoz i al'veokokkoz cheloveka.* Frunze: Kyrgyzstan.

von Siebold, C. T. E. 1853. Über die Verwandlung der Echinococcus-Brut in Taenien. *Z. Wiss. Zool.* **4**, 409–25.

Wetzel, R. and W. Rieck 1962. *Krankheiten des Wildes.* Hamburg: Parey.

Wilhelm, O. 1953. La hidatidosis equinococosica en la provincia de Concepción (Chile). *Arch. Int. Hydatidosis* **13**, 379–92.

Wilson, J. F., A. C. Diddams and R. L. Rausch 1968. Cystic hydatid disease in Alaska. A review of 101 autochthonous cases of *Echinococcus granulosus* infection. *Am. Rev. Resp. Dis.* **98**, 1–15.

Wrigley, R. E. and D. R. M. Hatch 1976. Arctic fox migrations in Manitoba. *Arctic* **29**, 147–58.

Yorozuya, K., T. Kosaka, A. Ichikawa, T. Sato and T. Ida 1968. Epizootiological consideration on multilocular echinococcosis in eastern Hokkaido, Japan. *J. Jap. Vet. Med. Assoc.* **21**, 471–6 [In Japanese].

Zeyhle, E. 1982. Die Verbreitung von *Echinococcus multilocularis* in Südwestdeutschland. In *Probleme der Echinokokkose unter Berücksichtigung parasitologischer und klinischer Aspekte*, R. Bähr (ed.), 26–33. Bern: Hans Huber.

Zikeeva, A. I. and A. Kh. Arslanova 1961. Nekotorye sravnitel'nye dannye po patomorfologii al'veokokkoza (al'veoliarnogo ekhinokokkoza) ondatry i cheloveka. *Helminthologia* **3**, 440–7.

3 Current status of hydatid disease: a zoonosis of increasing importance

CALVIN W. SCHWABE

INTRODUCTION

Hydatid disease was one of the earliest consequences of an infectious process described. In an apparent reference to hydatid anaphylaxis in his *Aphorisms*, Hippocrates noted that 'in cases where the liver is filled with water and bursts into the epiploon, the belly fills with water and the patient dies' (Jones 1948–53). Assuming such human deaths resulted from a phenomenon he actually had observed in other species, he stated further:

> I will demonstrate the formation of dropsy by tumours using cattle, sheep [variant translation: dogs] and hogs as examples; actually it is principally among these quadrupeds that aqueous tumours are produced in the lung; you will at once be convinced of this when you cleave them, for water will issue forth (Littré 1962 (1851), Laclainche 1936).

Aretaeus of Cappodocia noted that secondary cysts sometimes occur within these hydatid tumours (Hoeppli 1959).

Continuing into more modern times to intrigue such other comparative medical observers as Edward Jenner, Rudolph Virchow and William Osler (Schwabe 1978), hydatid infection became a subject for study by a long list of eminent parasitologists of medical, veterinary and zoological backgrounds, including Redi, Rudolphi, Goeze, von Siebold, Leuckart, Krabbe and Cameron. It also afforded an unusual research diversion among infectious diseases for such leading surgeons of their day as Harold Dew and Louis Barnett. Numerous synopses of then current information appeared during the past century, among them book-length accounts by Thomas (1884, 1894), Graham (1891), Dew (1928), Hosemann *et al.* (1928), Dévé (1946, 1949), Suić (1952), Volokh (1965), Coudert and Goinard (1967), Deineka (1968), Lupascu and Panaitescu (1968), Euzéby (1971), Lukashenko (1975) and Bähr (1981). The history of no disease demonstrates better than does hydatidosis the potential fruits of interactive medical and veterinary co-operation. In this chapter, we shall review the current public health and economic importance of hydatid infection, indicating areas where information is especially deficient, and suggesting factors that may be partly responsible for changing patterns of infection and disease in some parts of the world.

MODERN KNOWLEDGE OF HYDATID DISEASE*

In 1960, Dr Martin Kaplan, then chief of the Veterinary Public Health Unit of the World Health Organisation (WHO), asked the author to respond to WHO's first request (from the newly independent government of Cyprus) for assistance in combating hydatid disease (Schwabe 1961a). At that time only a handful of widely scattered investigators in New Zealand, Alaska, Chile, Japan and Lebanon were pursuing sustained programmes of research on the *Echinococcus* parasite or the infection it caused. While Iceland had effectively reduced the incidence of surgical cases in man through a quite unique effort, widespread misunderstanding by public health officials of this Icelandic success had resulted in initiation of innumerable 'control' efforts elsewhere, virtually all of them ineffective. Only in New Zealand was a rational, but little publicised, model for control then being pursued. The WHO effort in Cyprus led to the UN Food and Agricultural Organization undertaking, with WHO aid, planning for the pilot stage of hydatid control on the island (LeRiche & Jorgensen 1971). This also resulted in creation of a formal WHO hydatid disease programme which emphasised promotion of essential research, and identification and promotion of effective methods for control. In the initial phase, the author undertook several visits to widely scattered laboratories to establish a 'working network' among the few investigators then doing significant hydatid research (Schwabe 1961b). The first result was that Rausch was brought into contact with Nelson in Kenya, enabling him to study the latter's extensive collection of *Echinococcus* material from African mammals (Nelson & Rausch 1963). As one consequence, international attention was focused for the first time on an unusually serious hydatidosis situation among Kenya's isolated Turkana people (Schwabe 1964, O'Leary 1976, and see below).

During that period the Pan American Health Organisation (PAHO) also asked the author to assist its new Pan American Zoonoses Center, in Argentina, to initiate an hydatid disease research programme for Latin America. This far-reaching effort was staffed eventually by Williams and Varela-Diaz from Soulsby's laboratory at Pennsylvania, Schantz and Thakur from the University of California and others. Between 1964 and 1966 these communicating and co-ordinating activities were pursued by the author full-time from WHO headquarters in Geneva. It was just before this that Desmond Smyth, to whom this volume is dedicated, transferred his laboratory from Dublin to Canberra, with a highly profitable redirection of his pioneering successes with *in vitro* cultivation of Pseudophyllidean cestodes to *Echinococcus*. A working relationship between Smyth and Gemmell was soon initiated with WHO assistance, as was another between Gemmell and Yamashita in Japan. Such exchanges of ideas and personnel reached major fruition in 1966 with the convening in

*A bibliography of the literature on *Echinococcus* and hydatid infection prior to initiation of the WHO programme was published by Powers and Churchill (1959).

Geneva of the first WHO Scientific Group Meeting on Hydatid Disease Research [attended by Yamashita, Rausch, Kagan, Gemmel (rapporteur), Agosin (vice-chairman) and the author (chairman), with Smyth invited but unfortunately unable to attend because of illness]. Participation by Abdussalam and other WHO and PAHO staff resulted in a joint memorandum which detailed research needs and priorities in echinococcosis (WHO 1968), a document that has seen periodic revisions, the more recent also in connection with research on taeniasis/cysticercosis. Many valuable contacts continued to be made under these auspices, as for example, when parasites collected by Bernstein at the Los Angeles Zoo were sent to Rausch, resulting in the description of *E. vogeli* (Rausch & Bernstein 1972). A WHO Inter-regional Seminar on Hydatid Disease Control was convened in Buenos Aires in 1970 and a manual for surveillance and control, the first of a WHO series of guidelines for combating important zoonoses, was prepared through the efforts of an international committee (WHO/FAO/UNEP 1981).

Today the hydatidosis research situation is vastly different from that in the 1950s and 1960s. In place of only a few investigators, a relatively large number of laboratories now are directing attention to the varied aspects of *Echinococcus* and hydatid disease discussed in this volume, and others, and notable progress is being made not only in some research areas, but also in control of the disease (Laing 1961, Meldrum & McConnell 1968, Schantz & Schwabe 1969, Polydorou 1980, Pappaioanou 1982, Schwabe 1984, and see Ch. 7).

HYDATID DISEASE IN MAN

Unilocular hydatid disease

No parasite produces lesions in as many anatomical sites as does *E. granulosus*. In approximately 30 000 human cases included in 11 published case series summarised by Schantz (1972a), 52–77 per cent of cysts occurred in the liver, 8.5–44 per cent in the lungs and the remaining 13–19 per cent in virtually every other bodily location. The reasons for this distribution are still uncertain. Some investigators hold that all penetrating oncospheres enter venules of the intestinal villi, hence the hepatic portal circulation (Dew 1925, Dévé 1949). Whether they are then trapped in the hepatic sieve would depend upon the rapidity of their passage to the liver and the extent to which they have grown by then. This explanation assumes that a few oncospheres also squeeze through the vascular bed of the lungs and are then randomly distributed. An alternative view is that the organ site of cysts is determined by whether the particular oncosphere enters the venule of the intestinal villus, or its lymphatic lacteal, in which case it would bypass the liver entirely (Tenhaeff & Ferwerda 1935, Heath 1971, see also Ch. 1). The growth rate of individual cysts is highly variable, even in experimental infections with multiple cysts of the same age (Schwabe *et al.* 1964, 1970). Moreover, cysts in different host species and among certain human populations appear to grow at different rates. Thus, a slow rate of cyst growth has been reported in infections of indigenous peoples in Alaska (Wilson *et al.* 1968), while in the Turkana area of Kenya 5–10 cm cysts are frequently observed in children between 3 and 5 years old and secondary cysts may reach that size within a few years of a first operation (Macpherson 1983). As one consequence of these variety of sites and differential growth rates, the documented incubation period in unilocular hydatidosis in man has been as long as 53 years (Spruance 1974) and the range of clinical manifestations is enormous (Amir-Jahed *et al.* 1975, Little 1976, Bähr 1981).

Despite the relative immensity of the clinical literature on human hydatid disease, its bulk, until recently, has reflected more preoccupations with details of surgical or radiological technique than a systematic medical workup of patients, with refinement of a range of diagnostic aids. Errors about the morphology of cysts and epidemiology of the infection have been oft repeated in the process (Barnett 1939), including a belief recently restated that 'the eating of raw meat undoubtedly contributes [to failure of hydatid control programmes]' (Editorial 1976). Diagnostic limitations of conventional radiography, plus, until recently, the use of non-standardised and poorly described immunodiagnostic techniques, meant that diagnoses of hydatidosis often were forthcoming only after pathological examination of surgical specimens or at autopsy. This situation has begun to change rapidly with the advent of such newer diagnostic aids as scintigraphy (Front & Israel 1981), angiography (Rivera & Delcan 1980), tomography (Grabbe *et al.* 1981) and ultrasound (Vicary *et al.* 1977, Niron & Özer 1981), as well as better standardised and more sensitive and specific serological techniques (see Ch. 8).

Most commonly, unilocular hydatid disease in man simply reflects the results of pressure and other space-occupying effects of an isolated and well delineated, but growing, mass. A cellular immune response, with subsequent pericystic fibrosis, is prominent in all but cysts of the brain (Schwabe *et al.* 1959, Yusuf & Frayha 1975). Complications most frequently encountered include multiple cysts in the same and other organs; or ruptured cysts resulting in anaphylactoid responses (Jakubowski & Barnard 1971), daughter cyst formation and/or secondary bacterial infection (Panner & Leonard 1960). In the latter case, cyst death and calcification often follow.

LIVER

Unilocular hydatid cysts in man occur most frequently in the liver. In a number of published case series, hepatic cysts have been of approximately equal frequency in both lobes, while other surgeons have reported a preponderance of cysts in the right lobe. The range of clinical complications encountered was well summarised by Barros (1978) in his recent series of 212 cases. Upper abdominal pain was the most common presenting symptom and a palpable mass or hepatomegaly was detectable in two-thirds of patients. In about 34 per cent there was more than one cyst present in the liver, while in about 10 per cent of cases there were also cysts elsewhere in the abdominal cavity. Rupture into the biliary tree occurred in about 17 per cent of patients. In patients with additional cysts, especially large ones, there were communications between the biliary passages with the pericystic space. Secondary bacterial infections were present in 75 per cent of ruptured cysts. Traumatic cyst rupture with acute abdominal pain and anaphylactic symptoms was the cause of hospitalisation in two patients (see also Berenson *et al.* 1974). Over 9 per cent of Barros' patients presented with large cysts of the dome of the liver extending into the thoracic cavity through the diaphragm. In 11 of these 20 individuals, this cyst was intact, while three had ruptured into the bronchial tree. Biliary and bronchial communications both occurred in another four instances, with bile present in sputum.

LUNGS

Lung cysts may be underdiagnosed especially in countries where tuberculosis is prevalent and diagnostic facilities are meagre. As Barnett (1939) put it, 'deep seated lung cysts, so commonly associated with cough and hemoptysis, have been treated for long months, and even for years, as cases of pulmonary tuberculosis'. When diagnostic and treatment facilities were non-existent in the Turkana area of Kenya, hydatid patients had to walk very long distances for help. Under such conditions, no lung cysts at all were seen.

On the other hand, relative over-estimation of the proportions of lung cases in a geographical area may result from patient-finding through use of mass chest radiography in anti-tuberculosis campaigns (Wilson *et al.* 1968). Infections of the lungs caused by the arctic sylvatic strain (Northern Form; see Ch. 2) of *E. granulosus* are said to be more benign clinically than are those resulting from the pastoral dog–sheep strain (European Form; see Ch. 2) of the parasite occurring in most other areas of high hydatidosis endemicity (Pinch & Wilson 1973). However, the site predilections of both geographical types are similar; Cuthbert's (1975) series of 75 arctic cases involved the right lung in 58 per cent, while 60 per cent of the 50 pastoral cases reported by Balikian and Mudarris (1974) from the Middle East also occurred in that site. Communication of the pericystic cavity with a bronchus is common and cyst rupture into the bronchial tree is a fairly frequent finding (Tomb & Matossian 1976, Pieters *et al.* 1976). Serological tests are generally less sensitive for lung than liver cysts, while ordinary radiology has seen its most extensive applications in diagnosis of the former.

HEART

From 1 to 1.5 per cent of hydatid patients have cysts in the heart. The first successful surgery for cysts in that location was performed in 1932. Data from Ivanissevich and Rivas's series of 194 cardiac cysts (cited by Calamai *et al.* 1974) indicate that about 60 per cent occurred in the left ventricular myocardium, 17 per cent in the right, 9 per cent in the interventricular septum, 8 per cent in the right atrium, with the remaining few in the left atrium and the interatrial septum. Symptoms are frequently absent, but precordial pain is a fairly common complaint. About 10 per cent of fatal cardiac cysts rupture into the pericardial sac and 40 per cent into the heart cavities. Anaphylactoid reactions of varying severity may accompany either type of rupture. Other consequences of the latter are arterial emboli and valvular obstruction (Perez-Gomez *et al.* 1973, Chin 1981), including coronary insufficiency from occlusions of coronary arteries (Rivera & Delcan 1980).

CENTRAL NERVOUS SYSTEM

In 10 published series, between 0.2 and 2.4 per cent of diagnosed hydatid patients had cysts of the brain (Schantz 1972b). Because of generalised intracranial pressure or local pressure on the brain, cerebral cysts are probably diagnosed at a much earlier age than cysts in other locations. The fact that over 60 per cent have been found in children 15 years of age or less lends support to Dew's much quoted statement that 'an hydatid cyst is just about as old as the patient', a contention which Beard (1978) has presented evidence to show is frequently not the case. Brain cysts most often localise in the parietal or occipital areas and are chiefly right-sided. Young patients most frequently present with convulsions and some degree of hemiparesis, often followed by headache and vomiting (Begg *et al.* 1957). In contrast, cases in adolescents generally reflect a generalised increase in intracranial pressure with cortical sensory loss and visual changes. In both cases, there is severe bilateral papilloedema. In some reported series of cerebral cysts, epilepsy has been a clinical feature of up to 35 per cent (Arseni & Marinescu 1974). Brain cysts may become quite large prior to surgical intervention. Simpson and Verco (1976) noted that a 114 mm ($4\frac{1}{2}$ inch) diameter cyst was removed surgically from an Australian boy in 1888, and in a case operated upon by Haddad in Lebanon much more recently a cerebral cyst removed from a totally incapacitated patient, weighed 1.8 kg (see Schwabe *et al.* 1959). Because there is no host tissue reaction to most cysts of the brain, they may often be removed intact either by simply tipping out the exposed cyst or by injecting saline between the cyst wall and the brain, causing the cyst to be extruded.

SKELETAL SYSTEM

Approximately 1–2.5 per cent of hydatid cysts are believed to occur in the skeletal system. Of 19 cases reported by Duran *et al.* (1978), involving the spine, pelvis or femur, several affected more than one of these sites and resulted in irreparable bone destruction. Osseous cysts, particularly those present in the cavities of long bones, are often diagnosed only following a pathological fracture. About 3–4 per cent of osseous cysts are in the skull and some 42 such cases have been well described in the literature

(Teymoorian & Bagheri 1976). Diagnosis usually follows evidence of skull deformity. These cysts may break through the boney plates producing a typical unilocular cyst either extra- or intracranially. In the latter case, there may be cranial nerve involvement or intracranial hypertension (see central nervous system).

OTHER SITES

Kidney cysts may be primary or secondary to hydatid infections in other locations, and are found in about 2 per cent of human cases (Kirkland 1966). Most are single and there may or may not be renal pain. Ureteral obstruction and destruction of the organ may result. Death and calcification of cysts often occurs and cyst debris may be passed in the urine. Cysts of the spleen occur with similar frequency (Golematis 1983). The thyroid is occasionally involved. Subcutaneous cysts are most frequently secondary and result from spillage of hydatid sand in the incision during hydatid surgery (Sapunar & Cancino 1974). Cysts free in the peritoneal, pelvic (Shanbhag *et al.* 1974) and thoracic cavities and in the musculature are often of similar origin (Freedman 1974, Harris 1976). Bickers (1970) reviewed a series of pelvic hydatids, including cysts of the ovary and uterus (one of which eventually passed via the vagina), and a case of obstructed labour (see also Shanbhag *et al.* 1974). Rare infections, such as an apparently primary cyst of the tongue (Goel *et al.* 1974), a retroperiteonal cyst involving the prostate and seminal vesicles (Deklotz 1976) and similar instances have been described from practically every other part of the body (Amir-Jahed *et al.* 1975, Bähr 1981).

Polycystic hydatid disease

Human polycystic hydatid disease, characterised by formation of clusters of relatively small cysts, has been reported from Argentina, Colombia, Ecuador, Panama and Venezuela. While the most frequent primary site is the liver, primary polycystic infections have also occurred elsewhere in the abdominal cavity, and in the lungs and other thoracic organs (D'Alessandro *et al.* 1979). Originally thought to represent infections by *E. oligarthrus* (Thatcher 1972), experimental infections have caused D'Alessandro *et al.* (1979) to identify the responsible parasite as *E. vogeli.*

Alveolar hydatid disease

Alveolar hydatidosis is caused by *E. multilocularis*, a discovery by Rausch and Schiller (1956) and Vogel (1957), which settled a century-old debate (see introduction to Ch. 2). A comprehensive review of the infection and disease, based largely upon Soviet literature, was published by Lukashenko (1975). The site for primary development of alveolar cysts in man is far more consistent than for *E. granulosus*, with the liver being virtually the sole location for primary cyst growth. (This fact supports the theory that the *Echinococcus* oncosphere always enters venules of the intestinal villi; see above.) Rather than being well delineated and relatively isolated from the tissues of its host, the alveolar lesion is a proliferating, invasive mass of hydatid germinal layer tissue, which in man rarely contains islands of brood capsules with protoscoleces (see Ch. 1). Frequently this parasitic mass is partitioned by often thin and incomplete bands of laminated layers of variable thickness, plus ribbons of the host tissues which proliferate on the periphery of the developing cystic mass (Baron & Tanner 1977, Ali-Khan 1978). In cysts of any size, the centre may degenerate and contain a turbid fluid with fragments of necrotic tissues. Metastasis, presumably haematogenous, may result in secondary alveolar cyst formation, almost always in the lungs or brain.

The patient usually presents with a complaint of right hypochondrial or epigastric pain and some evidence of hepatomegaly, although symptoms referable to the lungs or brain may be the first indication of illness (Miguet *et al.* 1976, Thierry *et al.* 1978, Wilson & Rausch 1980). Complications include obstructive jaundice and oedema, including terminal anasarca. The diagnostic approach is similar to that for unilocular cysts and the case fatality rate, with or without surgery, is between 50 and 75 per cent (Wilson & Rausch 1980).

HYDATID DISEASE IN OTHER INTERMEDIATE HOSTS

The then known natural intermediate hosts of *E. granulosus* were listed by Smyth and Smyth in 1964 and this information is brought up to date in Chapter 2. Hydatid infections in domestic animals in the families Bovidae, Camelidae, Suidae and Equidae are of most significance economically. It is reasonable to believe that all, if not more of the clinical conditions in human hydatid disease, also occur among domestic animals, but published evidence for this is scarce. The principal explanations for this paucity of literature are that the life-spans of most domestic food animals are truncated, thus not allowing many infections to run their natural courses. Infections occur frequently in species like sheep, goats and pigs that possess little individual value and in consequence, rarely receive veterinary clinical attention. Moreover, the most common presenting complaint for human hydatidosis is pain, a reaction in animals frequently overlooked or ignored by farmers. As a result, clinical case reports in animals have been forthcoming almost entirely from individually valuable draft or multipurpose species such as cattle or buffaloes which may live out more fully their natural life-spans. The prevalence of infection appears to increase with age in all animal species, reflecting no doubt an extended period of exposure to contaminated environments (Dixon *et al.* 1973). A markedly different average age for slaughter is probably responsible for camels and cattle, for example, appearing to be at higher risk of infection compared to sheep or goats in some areas than may actually be the case. Only a few studies have been undertaken of the effects of very heavy cystic burdens in sheep or swine, as compared to man, or of infections of different intensities, upon such things as weight gains, milk or wool production. Virtually the only reasonably reliable measurements of the economic costs of hydatid infection in domestic animals for any country concern condemnations of organs, chiefly livers, and even these data are frequently absent or incomplete (see below). In ruminant animals, cysts are found more frequently in the lungs than the liver, while in non-ruminants, including man, the reverse is true.

Sheep

Sheep at slaughter frequently exhibit massive multicystic infections with extensive involvement of the lungs and liver. Rarely do detailed descriptions of individual infections enter the literature, however. In one rare example, Larsson *et al.* (1983) reported what they believed to be the first recorded instance of an ovine subcutaneous hydatid cyst in a sheep.

Clinically manifest hydatidosis has been described very rarely in sheep or goats and most knowledge of cyst site in these species has come from routine examinations of animals at slaughter, with examinations often limited to the animals' livers and lungs. However, of 524 slaughter sheep from an area of Bangladesh, of which over 56 per cent were infected, careful laboratory examination of all viscera found that cysts also occurred in the spleens of 1.36 per cent of infected sheep, in the heart of 1.02 per cent, in the kidneys of 0.67 per cent and the omentum of 0.34 per cent (Shamsul Islam 1979). Clinical and pathophysiological changes characteristic of anaphylaxis have followed intravenous injections of hydatid cyst fluid into sheep infected with *E. granulosus* (Schantz 1977), but sudden deaths of infected sheep ascribable to the parasite apparently have not been recorded in the literature.

Cattle and buffaloes

More information is available on individual infections in cattle and buffaloes. During a period of 8 years the author daily examined all hydatid cysts noted in cattle of unknown origin slaughtered in the Beirut Municipal Abattoir. Numerous observations, both *ante* and *post mortem*, suggested how fairly commonplace instances of clinical hydatidosis must be in older cattle, such as those outlined below. Cattle cysts frequently are non-fertile (sterile), but this is not always the case, as is implied by some authors. Much of what is known about clinical hydatidosis in these species originates in India where cattle and buffaloes generate 54 per cent of the energy consumed in agriculture and provide a full 32 per cent of all energy for that country's rural economy (Odend'hal 1972, Schwabe 1984). This is not surprising given the important multiple roles of cattle and buffaloes as work animals, and as providers of dung, for fuel and fertiliser, and milk; plus the presence in India of a well developed veterinary profession.

Prevalence of bovine hydatidosis in the Indian subcontinent varies considerably from survey to survey and has been reported to be as high as 90 per cent among cattle examined in the Punjab (Sami 1938). Arora and Dixit (1970) reported a fatal case of generalised hydatidosis in an $11\frac{1}{2}$ year old bullock complicated by tympanites. This animal harboured multiple fertile, sterile, intact, infected and ruptured primary cysts, many with daughter cysts, in the liver and lungs, with an additional cyst in an enlarged spleen (see below). The liver was enormously enlarged but possessed negligible functional tissue. The lungs presented the same multicystic appearance, with little normal parenchyma, complicated by extensive adhesions between the pleura, lungs, thoracic wall and pericardium. In another case reported by Pal and Sinha (1970), a markedly cachectic bullock died following a progressive 4-month illness characterised by anorexia and icterus. A greatly enlarged liver, with about 80 per cent of its parenchyma replaced by 35 or more coalescing hydatid cysts, contrasted strikingly with other abdominal organs which were highly atrophied. An estimated 30 per cent of the animal's lung tissue had been similarly replaced by numerous cysts for which many of the pericystic spaces were confluent.

Serious, far more localised hydatid infections have also been reported in cattle in India and elsewhere. One, which suggests that the splenic cyst in the case above may have been related to the animal's tympanites, was described by Awachat and Iyer (1971). This bullock presented with inanition and chronic recurrent tympanites. Surgical exploration revealed an hydatid cyst five litres in volume on the lower border of the spleen and pressing on the rumeno-reticular wall. Rumenotomy disclosed a resultant rumeno-reticular stenosis leading to loss of rumen motility, digestive malfunction and pronounced malaise. Another localised cyst with a significant consequence was reported by Bali *et al.* (1978) in a 10 year old bullock which presented with a 7 year history of an enlarging swelling in the brisket region. At the time of examination this animal had great difficulty walking and displayed marked pain in attempting to lie down. Surgical exploration revealed six egg-sized hydatid cysts subcutaneously. Post-mortem examination revealed chronic myositis in the ventral sternal region and an additional hydatid cyst of the spleen, plus pulmonary tuberculosis.

At slaughter, a large cyst in a cow was observed in the left ventricular wall which protruded into the ventricle. This cow also had smaller cysts of the liver and lungs (Boko & Barašić 1963). A case of cardiac insufficiency resulting from a right ventricular cardiac cyst in a Yugoslavian cow was reported by Čaklovisa *et al.* (1981). Dent (1960) described a case of cerebral hydatidosis (left lateral ventricle) in a Hereford cow in Australia manifested by fixed rotation of the head, tight circling and apparent visual disturbance. The cyst had degenerated and there was a marked inflammatory reaction. Of 21 osseous cysts in cattle noted in the literature (Baldelli 1947), three each were in the femur and tibia, four in the sternum and five in the spine. Baldelli described a further case in a 9 year old bovine incapacitated by a cyst in the pubis which had eroded through the bone and involved adjacent musculature. The original cyst had degenerated but viable daughter cysts were present, as were other primary cysts in the liver and lungs. Prenatal hepatic hydatidosis has been reported in a calf (Gluhovschi *et al.* 1970).

Hydatid infections in the buffalo have been described in the spleen, kidney, heart and uterus, in addition to the liver and lungs, with the latter organ their most common site. In contrast to cattle, up to 90 per cent of buffalo cysts are fertile. Two fatal cases in 7–8 year old female buffaloes reported by Mandal (1977) were attributed to replacement of virtually the total parenchyma of one lung by cysts and pericystic connective tissue, with substantial but lesser involvement of the other lung. Both cows displayed severe brisket and generalised oedema and one exhibited greatly impaired respiration. In one animal there were also apparently embolic secondary cysts in the cerebrum. Another case was described by Gupta and Singh (1975) in a 7 year old female buffalo which died of congestive heart failure caused by massive development of several thousand secondary cysts in the pleural cavity following apparent rupture of a primary lung cyst. Only a single additional primary cyst was present in one of this animal's lungs. The clinical diagnosis in this case had been traumatic pericarditis ('hardware disease'). In a similar fatal case, Bali and Chhabra (1978) collected masses of secondary cysts weighing 30 kg in total from the animal's pleural cavity. Extensive abdominal secondary hydatidosis, involving especially the diaphragm and omentum, was seen in another 16 year old female buffalo by Gill (1968). The author witnessed the necropsy of a working buffalo in India that had died suddenly from a rupture of a cardiac cyst into the right ventricle.

In Sikkim, 80 per cent of another large bovid, the yak, were found infected, as compared to 25 per cent of cattle and 50 per cent of sheep, but clinical manifestations have not been described.

Horses

In horses, cysts occur most frequently in the liver, followed by the lungs. Two instances of hepatic hydatidosis leading to clinical hepatic insufficiency in the horse, both manifested by chronic emaciation, anaemia and congestive heart failure with generalised oedema have been described (Florio & Benoit 1938, Barvaux & Derzelle 1947). Several individual case reports of equine hydatidosis also appear in the literature of the last century. In one, a suppurative osseous cyst of the cranium, containing daughter cysts, had eroded into the cranial vault of an 18 year old London cart-horse causing pressure on the cerebrum and cranial nerves 1–3, 5 and 6. The horse presented with anorexia, diminished ability to work and a swelling over the eye (Kirkman 1863). Rare cysts also have been recorded in the brain, heart, pericardium, pleura, spleen, kidneys, muscles and uterus of horses (Pierotti 1954, Thompson 1977). As compared to some other hosts, horse cysts appear to be quite slow-growing. Ronéus *et al.* (1982) noted that fertile cysts 11–16 years of age rarely exceeded 4 cm in diameter, with only one cyst seen as large as 10 cm. This may explain why, despite the age to which many horses live, so few reports of clinical hydatid disease in this species have been noted in the recent literature.

Swine

The literature describing individual cases of hydatidosis in swine is practically as scarce as that for sheep. In a series of 727 infected swine detected at slaughter in Australia (Fairley & Wright-Smith 1929), 3.8 per cent were in the kidneys (up to 50 cysts in one kidney), 0.29 per cent in the spleen and 0.14 per cent in the heart. Cysts also were seen in the musculature. Other reported sites of swine infections include testes (Holgado Rivas 1969).

Camels

Cysts in camels occur most commonly in the lungs. However, individual case reports comparable to those cited for draught cattle and buffaloes are absent from the literature, probably a partial result of the poor development of veterinary services in most areas where camels are important animals. In Kenya's Turkana District, very high infection rates in man more nearly parallel those in camels than those in sheep, goats or cattle, in which they are fairly low (Macpherson 1983). Substantial infection rates in camels have also been reported from across North Africa and throughout the continent's Sudanic belt (Sudan, Chad, Central African Republic, northern Cameroons, northern Nigeria) (Graber *et al.* 1969, Dada & Belino 1978, Dada *et al.* 1979). As with cattle, these high prevalence rates can be explained, at least in part, by the older average ages at which these animals often are slaughtered. In the few surveys in which animal age is recorded and younger camels are well represented, prevalence increases strikingly with age (Afshar *et al.* 1971). Camel infections are also commonplace in the Middle East. Dailey and Sweatman (1965) reported a 100 per cent infection rate among animals probably raised in Syria. In an area of eastern Iran where human hydatid infection is prevalent, one study revealed that camel meat constituted 70 per cent of all meat locally consumed (Nasseh & Khadivi 1975) indicating that that species could, therefore, be an important source of infection for local dogs.

Alveolar, multicystic and multilobular hydatidosis in animals

There is no convincing evidence from pathological studies or experimental infections that larval *E. multilocularis* occurs in domestic animals. So-called 'alveolar or multilocular hydatidosis' in cattle and some other species represents either multicystic infections (see Pal & Sinha 1970) or multilobular cysts caused by *E. granulosus*. The former superficial resemblance results when multiple unilocular cysts become confluent through growth. This is common when secondary daughter cysts develop within the rigid and frequently distorted pericystic cavity of a large dead or dying mother cyst, a circumstance often seen in cattle. Multilobular cysts, on the other hand, are individual, non-spherical, primary or secondary cysts which have been distorted in shape, sometimes bizarrely, by the uneven resistance to their growth offered by the surrounding normal or reactive tissues of their host (Cameron 1927, Dew 1953, 1958, Slais 1980). The extremes encountered among such irregularly shaped cysts are those developing within the spongiosa of bones.

PUBLIC HEALTH IMPORTANCE OF HYDATID DISEASE

The public health importance of hydatidosis to any country is reflected not only in deaths among untreated and treated patients, but in diminished capacity to function optimally during a portion of the often prolonged prodromal period, the direct and indirect costs of hospitalisation and recovery from surgery, and any residual disability or clinical sequellae. A further less tangible factor is anxiety related to knowledge about, and justifiable fear of, the disease among certain heavily infected populations. Recently, Matossian *et al.* (1977) have expressed the view that hydatidosis is increasing in global public health importance and that 'there have been many [recent] reports of hydatid disease in previously free countries'. A Working Group of the Office International des Epizooties (OIE 1979) came to a similar conclusion. However, Gemmell (1979) raised the question of whether this apparently changing situation in some areas reflects recent spread or simply improved surveillance. Increasing public health importance would be indicated by clearly demonstrated increases in human deaths attributable to hydatidosis, increases in prevalence of human infection or incidence of clinical cases, or instances where there is markedly increased anxiety or fear among a population concerning the disease. Potential problems would be indicated by proven spread of infections into new domestic or wild animal populations of domestic definitive hosts, or by clearly increased prevalences of infections among these reservoir hosts. Few of these parameters have been even reasonably measured in any country.

Nevertheless, high hydatidosis death rates have been estimated fairly recently for a few areas in which nothing was previously known. The most notable instance is Kenya's Turkana District (Macpherson 1983 and see below), where medical attention was formerly non-existent and is currently sparse. Beyond such fairly striking evidence of major public health effects of hydatidosis, the numbers of clinical cases of human hydatid actually diagnosed underestimates considerably the potential problem for many countries. This is because in any country clinically diagnosed infections reflect only a relatively small proportion of existing human hydatid infections. This is partly because the incubation period for onset of signs or symptoms is variable and frequently long, and partly because clinical infection is often misdiagnosed. Uruguay and Rio Negro province in Argentina are virtually the only areas in which this relationship between infection and disease has been well estimated (Purriel *et al.* 1973, Schantz *et al.* 1973). As compared to 17.7 new surgical cases per 100 000 persons per year revealed by a nationwide reporting system in Uruguay, extrapolations from mass radiography results indicate that at least 150 hydatid infections are actually present per 100 000 persons at any given time. Similarly, in Argentina's Rio Negro, where the annual incidence of surgical cases is 143 per 100 000, 460 pulmonary infections alone per 100 000 people can be demonstrated radiographically.

In most countries hydatid disease is not even legally reportable, as in the above examples. Therefore, many diagnosed cases may go unreported or may not be recorded even in special hospital surveys. Moreover, in some Third World countries many clinical cases are never seen by a physician. Of those that are, not all are diagnosed correctly, at least initially. The range of such possibilities for less than reliable data, from country to country and within countries, is enormous. One known extreme is surely the isolated Turkana area of Kenya where diagnostic facilities are meagre. There, a known high risk of infection causes virtually every tumour seen by medical personnel to be diagnosed as hydatid disease. However, lung cysts are still rarely diagnosed among Turkana, and were never diagnosed a few decades ago, presumably because all such patients died without obtaining any medical attention. Even where medical facilities are more available, as in Iraq, one local surgeon has opined that 'if you diagnose a lump anywhere in the body as hydatid disease you are 50 per cent correct'. In contrast, in California, in the years before hydatid disease was recognised as endemic, use of relatively excellent diagnostic facilities by unsuspecting physicians resulted in hydatid cysts not being considered at all in the admission diagnoses of 44 of 69 hospitalised patients in which hydatid cysts were eventually found (Miller *et al.* 1971).

Apart from the value of mortality rates, morbidity rates or infection rates in describing the public health importance of hydatidosis, are data reflecting time lost from work, cost of hospitalisation, convalescence, etc. Here, information is almost completely lacking for any country. Exceptions include a study in Chile where 1528 patients were hospitalised for hydatidosis during a 2 year period. Their average hospital stay was 40.4 days (in contrast to 12.5 days for all causes) at an average direct cost of US $308.55 per patient (Ramirez 1971). Moreover, in Uruguay, which has one of the highest levels of hydatid endemicity of any fairly developed country, it has been found that 60 per cent of hydatid surgical patients are unable to resume a normal working life 4 months after leaving hospital and 40 per cent are still unable to after 6 months (Schantz 1972a). Other Australian data summarised by Kumaratilake and Thompson (1982) indicate that the surgical fees for abdominal or thoracic operations in Australia are A$194–320 and hospitalisation charges per hydatid patient average an additional A$1105–1955 in different parts of the country. These most direct costs of the disease do not include other services such as radiology or repeat surgery.

Geographical considerations

The known geographical distributions of *Echinococcus* spp. have been discussed in Chapter 2 and tabulations of published human surgical case rate data for the world have been made by Gemmell (1960), Simitch (1964), Schantz and Schwabe (1969) and Williams *et al.* (1971). Matossian *et al.* (1977) and Schantz (1982) have supplemented these compilations with more recent occurrence and incidence information. Many such statistics represent only officially reported cases, often only from government hospitals, or result from incomplete hospital surveys. Further, they infrequently differentiate first diagnoses from readmissions. These facts render many such statistics of dubious accuracy (Schwabe, 1968). For this reason, Schantz (1982) felt that 'comparing data on the prevalence of echinococcosis, particularly in humans, is a frustrating exercise'.

However, in some instances, even quite cursory hospital surveys have yielded evidence of human infections never officially recorded. For example, a mailed questionnaire to eight medical colleges in Bangladesh disclosed a substantial number of cases in a country from which human infection was previously regarded as non-existent or very rare (Islam & Rahman 1975). This is likely to occur on the periphery of the known geographical range of *E. granulosus* and other species of the genus. Human cases may also be suspected in countries or parts of countries where echinococcal infections have been recorded for any period of time in domestic animals raised within the country. Such has been true in Korea, for example, where the first two known cases of human hydatidosis were isolated ones reported in 1938 and 1962 respectively (cited by Moon 1976), though infections in animals had long been known. A similar situation has existed also in Indonesia and countries of the Indo-Chinese peninsula. Thus, *E. granulosus* has been known from animals in Indo-China since 1905 (including infection in a wild canid *Cyon primaerus*), but the first human case was one reported from Laos only in 1975 (Fontan *et al.* 1975).

Moreover, for individual countries even very incomplete statistics can constitute starting points for reaching initial decisions as to what national public health priority to assign hydatidosis. Such decisions, in turn, may provide justification for more adequate baseline or pre-control surveillance (Schwabe 1984). Even with poorly recorded data, marked differences in frequency of diagnoses within different segments of national populations may sometimes be apparent (Schwabe 1979). Kenya provides an excellent example. There, human hydatid disease occurs with very high frequency in only one of several pastoral tribes, the Turkana. It is rarely seen among other peoples like the Masai who have superficially similar customs (Eugster 1978), although their animals may have comparable rates of infection to those owned by Turkana. Furthermore, even among the

Turkana, who numbered about 143 000 in 1979 and range with their approximately 2.7 million sheep and goats, 0.5 million cattle and more than 10 000 camels over some 6.2×10^6 ha (24 000 square miles) of northwestern Kenya, annual surgical incidence rates vary markedly from 18 per 100 000 people in the south of their territory to an estimated 220 per 100 000 people in the north (French & Nelson 1982, Macpherson 1983).

Some of the human factors which have been identified as possibly influencing such variations in human risk, and factors associated with introductions of the parasites into new areas, will be discussed below. Other factors which pertain more to distribution of the parasites themselves are only now beginning to be explored. For instance, relatively few data are yet available on the effects of climatic variables upon risk of infection in domestic animals (or man) within countries in which infection is endemic. Pappaioanou (1982) has demonstrated, however, that the prevalence of *E. granulosus* in sheep in Cyprus varies from village to village in indirect relation to local rainfall, confirming earlier experimental findings of Sweatman and Williams (1963) on viable egg availability in two areas of New Zealand.

Changes in hydatid disease frequency over time

Complete data for hydatid disease cases treated surgically, from all hospitals for extended periods of time, does not exist for any country. One of the more extensive was compiled by Burridge *et al.* (1977a,b) for New Zealand government hospitals. However, during the period 1891–1972 only 53.9 per cent of New Zealanders dying from hydatid disease did so in government hospitals, suggesting the incomplete nature even of these data. Moreover, until 1951, hospital case records were not systematically collected in New Zealand and, prior to 1945, first admissions were not differentiated from readmissions. Even so, it is possible to conclude from this compilation that the total hydatid case rate for the country increased quite steadily from 1878 to 1954. This was probably true, for most of that period, also for the incidence of new cases. The availability of actual incidence rates for new cases was more or less coincident with the beginning of their steady decline. This change reflected a control programme which was implemented in 1959 (Laing 1961, Burridge & Schwabe 1977a,b), following a period of less organised educational efforts.

Perceived public health priorities may change particularly rapidly under circumstances where new national, regional or community development efforts are accompanied by the institution of improved primary care services where few or none previously existed. For example, in the Turkana District of Kenya, where there were no medical facilities at all in 1961 and tribesmen had to walk a very long distance to the closest Kenyan hospital at Kitale, Schwabe (1964) was able to estimate from the records of that hospital alone, a *minimum* yearly surgical incidence rate of 40 cases per

100 000 Turkana; a rate higher than that then recorded for any country. With the subsequent introduction of a Flying Doctor Service by the African Medical and Research Foundation and establishment of six primary care stations within the Turkana territory, even this high incidence estimate could immediately be revised very substantially upward (Irwin 1974, O'Leary 1976 and see above).

VETERINARY-ECONOMIC IMPORTANCE OF HYDATID DISEASE

Beyond the social and economic tolls human hydatid infection exacts, are the poorly estimated costs of infection among domestic animals. Almost no clinical cases of hydatid disease are diagnosed in most domestic animal species, except *post mortem*, and even these are generally only in individually valuable draught or multipurpose species (see above). Though prevalence of hydatid infections has been better estimated in domestic food animals in most countries than in man as the result of routine veterinary diagnoses at slaughter, and of special surveys, their economic consequences have been poorly ascertained. Data cited by Thompson (1977) and Thompson and Smyth (1975) suggest that annual losses solely from condemnation of offal from cattle, sheep, swine and horses in Great Britain, where hydatidosis is regarded as a minor disease, were about £70 000. In more highly endemic situations such losses may be much more. In Australia, for example, they were estimated as A$1.2 million per year (Kumaratilake & Thompson 1982) and for Chile US$5 million (Neghme & Silva 1970). Beyond a few examples such as these, data are almost completely lacking. Estimates of effects of hydatid infection on animal production are rare and almost all from the Soviet Union (see Rausch 1975, Kumaratilake & Thompson 1982). Most of this literature examined by the author reports few details of the study design or its results. Badly needed from many countries, therefore, are follow-ups to such suggestions as that of Ramazanov *et al.* (1978) that a 7 per cent loss in milk production in ewes, as compared to controls, results from infection with 3000 *E. granulosus* eggs. Determination of the effects of often heavy echinococcal infections in common domestic animals upon growth, meat quality and quantity, milk, wool and other product production and quality, is an urgent research requirement if proper priorities are to be assigned to hydatid control. Demonstrated interference by hydatidosis into its extensive lamb and mutton export trade provided an important impetus to hydatid control in New Zealand.

SPREAD OF INFECTION

Rausch (1967) has conjectured interestingly on the early evolution and spread of *E. granulosus* infections in the Northern Hemisphere before the domestication of mammals. He considers that extensions of the parasite's range in historic times to Iceland, South America, Australasia and into the domestic animal populations of North America, resulted largely from European colonisation, accompanied by importation of infected domestic species. He cites several specific instances of known movements of infected animals in more modern times.

Some other apparent instances of the spread of infection probably represent recent recognition or reporting of infections that actually existed previously. Probable examples include some comparatively recent reports from the subsaharan sudanic zone of Africa (Graber *et al.* 1969, Dada *et al.* 1979), from Kuwait (Hassounah & Behbehani 1976) and from Bangladesh (Shamsul Islam 1979, Islam & Rahman 1975). Kuwait represents an instance, however, of an area in which infection has, no doubt, intensified considerably in recent years. This has been the result of a significant economic transformation accompanied by the wholesale importation of domestic livestock from abroad. Australia alone exported 1.8 million live sheep in 1976 (Kumaratilake & Thompson 1982), many to the Middle East, and Yamashita *et al.* (1956) have reported that Australian sheep imported live to Japan harbour hydatid cysts.

The only major area of the globe from which *E. granulosus* is apparently absent at the present time is most of the insular Pacific. Relatively recent spread and intensification of infection appears to be occurring, however, on the southwestern fringe of the Pacific basin, especially in the Indo-Chinese peninsula (Le Van Hoa 1967, Fontan *et al.* 1975) and extending beyond into the islands of the Indonesian archipelago. Areas of Central Africa are still an unknown, but there has been some evidence for recent spread of the parasite into new areas, such as in parts of Uganda with movements of refugee populations and their livestock (Owor & Bitakaramire 1975). Within only a few countries has it been possible to document in any detail the spread of unilocular hydatid infection into previously uninfected areas. The United States is, perhaps, the best case in point (Pappaioanou *et al.* 1977). There, infection was apparently introduced into the southeastern part of the country in imported swine in the late 19th century. Infection established itself with local transmission to swine and man taking place on tenant and other smallholdings where a few pigs were raised and slaughtered for home consumption. Poor farmers of that area, many of whom were black, usually kept one or more dogs, often hounds, for hunting raccoons and opposums. Hydatid infection in that initially infected area has since declined in importance with general improvements in the standard of living and, specifically, a marked decline in home slaughter of swine. Rare hydatid cysts also were detected in cattle slaughtered elsewhere in the United States during that early period, as evidenced by specimens in the US National Museum. It seems probable that these were in cattle originating in the south-east and shipped to other areas for fattening or slaughter (see Schwabe 1984 for data on similar US cattle movements in that period in connection with the better known spread in the US of contagious bovine pleuropneumonia). Early reports of hydatid cysts in American sheep from meat inspection statistics of the US Department of Agriculture almost certainly represent misdiagnoses of *Taenia hydatigena* cysts, since Curtice (1890) and Hall (1915, 1920) reported that *E. granulosus* was absent or very rare in that species and no museum specimens exist. The first proven spread of *E. granulosus* into the sheep population of the United States occurred in the western United States, first in California, and was coincident with movements of large numbers of impoverished farm families (and their dogs) from the south-east (the 'Grapes of Wrath' migration) during the great economic depression of the 1930s and continuing into the World War II years (Pappaioanou *et al.* 1977). A number of transmission sites in California were located beginning in the 1960s through a programme of slaughterhouse surveillance (Sawyer *et al.* 1969), which resulted also in traceback of infected sheep to Utah and Idaho. Subsequent epidemiological follow-up investigations in California, Utah, New Mexico and Arizona (Schantz *et al.* 1970, Kahn *et al.* 1972, Andersen *et al.* 1973, Schantz *et al.* 1977) indicate that *E. granulosus* is being transmitted currently over a large area of the western United States in which transhumant systems of sheep husbandry still prevail. Although focally distributed, the potential exists for hydatidosis to become a problem of sizeable public health importance in these parts of the American West.

Another very serious problem from the standpoint of potential control concerns the spread of infections into wildlife where this may not have occurred previously. Few instances are known with certainty because wildlife reservoirs have been little investigated. Possible examples, however, are infections in wolves and jackals in parts of Iran (Sadighian, 1969, Modebi *et al.* 1973) and coyotes and deer in California (Liu *et al.* 1970, Romano *et al.* 1974). In most areas the epidemiological significance of wildlife infections with *E. granulosus* remains completely unknown. There is the enigma, for example, of infection in 60 per cent of zebras in one area of South Africa, with experimental demonstration of the transmissibility of this parasite to lions (Young 1975a,b). There is further evidence for naturally occurring lion infections in Kenya, Uganda and Tanzania, with existence of a possible lion–wart-hog cycle in the Central African Republic (Graber & Thal 1980).

Evidence is somewhat more clear cut that *E. multilocularis* continues to spread geographically and that it could become of public health importance in several countries where it had not been known until recently. In the Eastern Hemisphere there appears to be a steady extension southward of the range of the parasite, but this has been relatively little investigated with respect to the zoogeography of its natural reservoir hosts. In northwestern Iran, however, infection has been found in the red fox, *Vulpes vulpes* (Mobedi & Sadighian 1971). Recent identification of *E. multilocularis* in cats in Jordan (Morsy *et al.* 1980), probably indicates the southernmost point of this extension. Other evidence of spread, reflecting a potential public health problem, has been forthcoming from diagnosis of the first human cases of alveolar infection in such new areas as northern

India, including Kashmir (Aikat *et al.* 1978, Khuroo *et al.* 1980) and northwestern China (Cipeng 1981). Within Europe, the western range of the parasite has also extended fairly recently from Switzerland into northeastern France, where infections occur in the red fox (Coudert *et al.* 1970) and a quite large number of human cases have been diagnosed (Miguet *et al.* 1976, Thierry *et al.* 1978). In North America, conclusive evidence exists for comparatively recent introduction of the parasite into the red fox, coyote, vole and deer mouse populations of north-central United States (Minnesota, Iowa, Illinois, Nebraska, North and South Dakota, Montana and Wyoming) (Leiby *et al.* 1970, Ballard & Vande Vusse 1984, Schantz 1983) and contiguous areas of central Canada (Manitoba, Saskatchewan and Alberta) (Schantz 1982). There is as yet no evidence that this large pocket of infection in wildlife, which has resulted so far in only two diagnosed human infections, one in a Manitoba resident in 1928 (James & Boyd 1937) and the second in a rural Minnesota housewife in 1977 (Gamble *et al.* 1979), is continuous with the extensive boreal range of this parasite in the northern tundra. Rapidly increasing prevalence of *E. multilocularis* infection in red foxes from this middle western and now largely agricultural, grain-producing area – that was until comparatively recently virgin grassland – suggests that the accompanying build-up of small rodent populations and their predators may be responsible for a potentially dangerous public health problem (Schantz 1983). One infected animal has been found within 24 km (15 miles) of the city of Chicago, heightening possibilities for transmission to sizeable dog and cat populations. Infection rates in farm cats in North Dakota have varied in recent years from 1 to 5 per cent (Kritsky & Leiby, as cited in Gamble *et al.* 1979).

HUMAN FACTORS ASSOCIATED WITH THE DISTRIBUTION AND IMPORTANCE OF HYDATID DISEASE

Ethnic/cultural factors

Among differences in ethnic risk to hydatid disease that have been demonstrated within countries, are a preponderantly greater risk of 1340 times among Californians of Basque origin or extraction than among other California residents (Araujo *et al.* 1975); a 6.4 times greater risk among New Zealand Maoris than among New Zealanders of other ethnic origins (Burridge & Schwabe 1977a,b, Burridge *et al.* 1977a,b); and a greater risk among Greek than among Turkish Cypriots (Pappaioanou 1982). Some culturally related differences in risk of infection among different populations in the same area may be ones associated with their religious beliefs (see below). Thus, in both Lebanon (Schwabe & Abou Daoud 1961) and Cyprus (Pappaioanou 1982), Christians are operated on for hydatidosis more frequently than are Moslems, and in the former country at least, this does not reflect differences in accessibility to or use of medical facilities.

An obviously important but little investigated aspect of such differences in human risk of *E. granulosus* infection is the extent and nature of different people's associations with dogs, particularly in the keeping of dogs as pets. The much higher infection rate among the Polynesian Maori of New Zealand than among New Zealanders of European extraction is associated with their different customs regarding sheep-dogs (Burridge & Schwabe 1977a,b), especially their dogs' additional function as house pets. The dog was a traditional Maori animal which in former times was highly valued both as a pet and as a source of food. Thus while hydatid disease in the Maori was not mentioned in the early New Zealand medical literature, their dogs eventually became infected at a much higher rate than those owned by other New Zealanders. None of this heightened Maori risk is associated, however, with peculiarities of their sheep husbandry practices *per se* (Burridge *et al.* 1977a,b). This is not surprising since sheep were introduced into New Zealand by Europeans, from whom Maori have learned sheep husbandry methods only in the last generation or so.

The higher surgical incidence rate in Lebanese Christians than in Lebanese Moslems also seems to parallel closely their respective associations with the dog (Schwabe & Abou Daoud 1961). In the Moslem *Hadith* (sayings of the Prophet), the following are among several recorded statements about the undesirability of close contact with dogs: 'If a dog drinks from your vessel, you must wash the vessel seven times'; 'Angels do not enter a house where there is a dog'. Nonetheless, even non-nomadic Moslem families in some countries may commonly keep dogs. This is true, for example, in parts of Afghanistan where Buck *et al.* (1972) reported dog ownership rates for households ranging from 7.8 to 64.3 per cent, depending upon village, with 5.5 per cent of households in one village owning three or more dogs. In Beirut, Lebanon, Abou Daoud and Schwabe (1964) showed that hydatid disease patients were 21.5 times more likely to have owned a dog than were their uninfected neighbours matched for sex and age. More detailed knowledge may be necessary to explain several well documented familial outbreaks of hydatidosis. For example, in one family of six persons in Tasmania, the father had lung cysts removed in 1959 and 1961; the mother was operated on for a subcutaneous cyst and a 10-year-old son for a liver cyst both in 1963; while in 1965 the 22-year-old daughter had two cysts of the liver removed (Schwabe 1984). This family kept three dogs, one of which was a household pet. In a similar episode in Israel, Romanoff and Krausz (1975) reported diagnosis of lung infection in a 6-year-old boy in 1960; in one of his brothers (age 14) the same year; in the father in 1963; liver cysts in his 25-year-old sister at about the same time; liver and lung cysts in another 21-year-old brother in 1972 and a brain cyst in the boy's mother in 1975. In all, six of the eight members of this family acquired the disease. Though they had had a house dog for some years, there was no indication in this report that the dog was ever examined by the arecoline hydrobromide test, or disposed of, during the 15 years this particular family's tragedy had unfolded.

The Turkana of Kenya maintain a large number of dogs and sleep with them to keep warm on the desert (Schwabe 1964). Women of child-bearing age also keep dogs as 'nurses' to lick infants clean after they defecate or vomit (O'Leary 1976, French *et al.* 1982, Macpherson 1983). Turkana eat the intestines of animals with little cooking, and Macpherson *et al.* (1983) indicate that they will readily eat jackals and hyaenas, though they deny eating dogs. In addition, human Turkana dead, except for the important and elderly, are laid out in the desert for dogs and wild carnivores to eat (O'Leary 1976, Macpherson 1983), so man too may fill a biological role in perpetuating the hydatid cycle. This latter custom of Turkana is shared by some but not all other Nilotic tribes (Schwabe 1978).

Occupational factors

A presumed high risk of hydatid infection among sheep raisers generally has been documented in very few areas. In California, an increased risk has been shown to be associated virtually entirely with one system of sheep raising practised largely by sheepmen of Basque extraction (Araujo *et al.* 1975 and see below). Other less expected occupational risks have rarely been identified. A high level of hydatid infection among Lebanese shoemakers (14.3 per cent of patients for whom occupation was known) led, however, to disclosure of the formerly common practice there of bating hides in a mixture of dog faeces and water; a method of preparing leather which was once in use in many parts of the world and has not disappeared altogether even today (Schwabe & Abou-Daoud 1961).

Sex differences in risk of infection may simply reflect the respective occupational exposures of men and women. Thus, in the transhumant sheep-raising area of California, autochthonous cases of hydatidosis were over five times more common in men than in women (Miller *et al.* 1971). In Turkanaland, in contrast, females are about 2.5 times as likely to be operated on for hydatidosis than men (Macpherson 1983). However, very little sex discrepancy apparently exists among Turkana less than 10 years of age; it becomes marked only from young adulthood, suggesting it reflects the decreased risk in young men who are out herding the livestock and removed from the homestead where large numbers of dogs are concentrated.

Economic variables

Hydatid transmission, especially non-occupational transmission, is probably favoured by poor sanitary conditions and practices usually associated with poverty and lack of education. In few instances, however, has economic status been considered in relation to risk of hydatidosis either in individuals or among populations of different geographical areas of the same country. Even in such cases, indirect indicators of economic levels have had to be resorted to, rather than direct measures, because all studies to date have been undertaken retrospectively and proper data collection could not be incorporated in the study design. Thus, in New Zealand, Burridge *et al.* (1977a,b) found no clear-cut effect of economics (as measured by percentage of employed rural males earning less than the national median income for that group) upon district to district prevalence of *E. granulosus* in dogs. However, in Greek villages in Cyprus, Pappaioanou (1982) found that the poorer the village, as measured by the average number of rooms per house, the higher the prevalence of *E. granulosus* infection in the village's dogs.

Husbandry practices and beliefs

Specific livestock husbandry practices have also been little studied with reference to hydatidosis risk. In California, it was found that a peculiar geographical restriction of the disease, almost entirely to about one-third of the sheep-raising region of that state, was accounted for by a particular form of husbandry practised by sheepmen of Basque descent (Sawyer *et al.* 1969, Schantz *et al.* 1970, Schwabe *et al.* 1972, Araujo *et al.* 1975). These Americans of Basque origin were shown to follow a transhumant system of 'ranching without ranches' in which sheep were grazed successively on leased pastures, cropped-over lands and government-owned deserts and forests. This system, in which sheep-dogs play a prominent and necessary role, contrasts with an alternative system in other parts of California of raising sheep on rancher-owned, permanent fenced pastureland, a system in which dogs are not employed. The transhumant system is restricted almost exclusively to the Central Valley of California south of Sacramento and is 87 per cent Basque-operated, while almost no Basques operate permanent pasture systems in other parts of the state. A similar transhumant system is associated with transmission of *E. granulosus* to Indians living on the Navajo and Zuni reservations of New Mexico and Arizona (Schantz *et al.* 1977). In Utah, on the other hand, Crellin *et al.* (1982) have noted that a transhumant system of sheep husbandry has been the predominant system followed by largely Mormon herders in most areas of that state since the 19th century, but that infection is endemic only in one county. They attribute this endemic hydatid situation in Sanpete County to an initial introduction of *E. granulosus* from outside Utah into an area of transhumance where trucking sheep from grazing site to grazing site has not replaced a formerly universal practice of trailing sheep overland with the help of groups of dogs. Many sheepherders and their dogs still use the same trails in Sanpete County, thereby exposing multiple bands of sheep to parasite eggs deposited by even a few infected dogs. Moreover, herders in that county commonly rotate dogs between the trail and the home and family members still accompany some herders on the trail, thereby offering opportunities for wider human exposure.

Locally held beliefs about hydatid cysts in animals may not coincide with scientific knowledge and, if not ascertained and possibly corrected, may result in lack of interest in the disease or lack of co-operation in its control. One known instance was a commonly held belief among both Turkana pastoralists and some Cypriot sheepherders that hydatid cysts in their animals were a physiological storage device for water in times of drought and, therefore, were desirable (Schwabe 1984). Such beliefs may change, however, or not be uniformally held. For example, while the author found that no Turkana interviewed in 1961 understood that these well recognised 'water sacks' in sheep were the same as the cause of the big-belly disease in themselves, O'Leary (1976) reported that some patients treated by her during 1971–5 had by then made that association. In contrast, several Turkana stated their belief in 1961 that the human disease was a visitation upon them by their traditional enemies, the Murle (Marile; Dassanetch), who range from the adjacent areas of Ethiopia into the southeastern Sudan (Schwabe 1964). In fact, some cases operated upon in Turkanaland are in ethnic Murle, and they are known also to be infected in Ethiopia (Fuller & Fuller 1981).

PROGNOSTICATION

It is impossible to know whether hydatid infection will continue to spread and intensify or whether wide application of well organised and pursued control programmes, as in New Zealand, Tasmania and Cyprus, will reverse this trend. Much will depend upon priorities assigned to this problem by governments, which in turn will be dependent upon research to disclose the actual hydatid situation in most countries. As for other zoonoses, the total importance of hydatid disease tends to be underestimated and research goes unsupported because interest in and responsibility for different aspects of the disease reside with different ministries of the government. These authorities may, in turn, be unaccustomed to considering both the public health and veterinary economic costs of zoonoses in arriving at overall programme priorities. In too many instances, in consequence, concern for hydatidosis and other important zoonoses 'falls between administrative chairs', with the public the clear loser (Schwabe 1981). One certain way to reduce this prospect is to establish a small veterinary public health unit within each ministry of health as a complement to and for liaison with the main veterinary services, which usually are based within ministries of agriculture (Schwabe 1984).

REFERENCES

Abou-Daoud, K. and C. W. Schwabe 1964. Epidemiology of echinococcosis in the Middle East. III. A study of hydatid disease patients from the city of Beirut. *Am. J. Trop. Med. Hyg.* **13**, 681–5.

Afshar, A., I. Nazarian and B. Baghban-Baseer 1971. A survey of the incidence of hydatid cyst in camels in south Iran. *Br. Vet. J.* **127**, 544–6.

Aikat, B. K., S. R. Bhusnurmath, M. Cadersa, P. N. Chhuttani and S. K. Mitra 1978. *Echinococcus multilocularis* infections in India: first case report proved at autopsy. *Trans. R. Soc. Trop. Med. Hyg.* **72**, 619–21.

Ali-Khan, Z. 1978. *Echinococcus multilocularis*: cell-mediated immune response in early and chronic alveolar murine hydatidosis. *Exp. Parasitol.* **46**, 157–65.

Amir-Jahed, A. K., R. Fardin, A. Farzad and K. Bakshandeh 1975. Clinical echinococcosis. *Ann. Surg.* **182**, 541–6.

Andersen, F. L., P. D. Wright and C. Mortenson 1973. Prevalence of *Echinococcus granulosus* infection in dogs and sheep in central Utah. *J. Am. Vet. Med. Ass.* **163**, 1168–71.

Araujo, F. P., C. W. Schwabe, J. C. Sawyer and W. G. Davis 1975. Hydatid disease transmission in California: a study of the Basque connection. *Am. J. Epidemiol.* **102**, 291–302.

Arora, R. G. and S. N. Dixit 1970. Generalised hydatidosis in a bullock. *Punjab Vet.* **9**, 33–6.

Arseni, C. and V. Marinescu 1974. Epilepsy in cerebral hydatidosis. *Epilepsia* **15**, 45–54.

Awachat, K. G. and G. R. Iyer 1971. Rumeno-reticular dysfunction due to hydatid cyst of spleen in a bullock. *Indian Vet. J.* **48**, 967–9.

Bähr, R. 1981. *Die Echiookokkose des Menschen.* Stuttgart: Enke Verlag.

Baldellii, B. 1947. Contributo allo studio della echinococci ossea nei bovini. *Atti Soc. Ital. Sci. Vet.* **1**, 81–9.

Bali, H. S. and R. C. Chhabra 1978. A study of secondary hydatids from a buffalo and their experimental infection in pups. *Indian J. Anim. Sci.* **48**, 432–5.

Bali, H. S., S. C. Dutt, S. S. Rathor and P. P. Gupta 1978. A note on subcutaneous hydatidosis in a bullock. *Indian Vet. J.* **55**, 735–6.

Balikian, J. P. and F. F. Mudarris 1974. Hydatid disease of the lungs – a roentgenological study of 50 cases. *Am. J. Roentgen. Rad. Ther. Nucl. Med.* **122**, 692–707.

Ballard, N. B. and F. J. Vande Vusse 1984. *Echinococcus multilocularis* in Illinois and Nebraska. *J. Parasitol.* **69**, 790–1.

Barnett, L. 1939. Hydatid disease: errors in teaching and practice. *Br. Med. J.* **2**, 593–9.

Baron, R. W. and C. E. Tanner 1977. *Echinococcus multilocularis* in the mouse: the *in vitro* protoscolicidal activity of peritoneal macrophages. *Int. J. Parasitol.* **7**, 489–95.

Barros, J. L. 1978. Hydatid disease of the liver. *Am. J. Surg.* **135**, 597–600.

Barvaux and E. Derzelle 1947. L'échinococcose equine. *Ann. Med. Vet.* **91**, 241–3.

Beard, T. C. 1978. Evidence that a hydatid cyst is seldom 'as old as the patient'. *Lancet ii*, 30–2.

Begg, N. C., A. C. Begg and R. G. Robinson 1957. Primary hydatid disease of the brain – its diagnosis, radiological investigation, treatment and prevention. *N.Z. Med. J.* **56**, 84–98.

Berenson, M. M., J. W. Freston, P. R. Koehler and F. Chang 1974. Traumatic intrahepatic rupture of an echinococcal cyst. *J. Trauma* **14**, 798–804.

Bickers, M. M. 1970. Hydatid disease of the female pelvis. *Am. J. Obstet. Gynec.* **107**, 477-83.

Boko, F. and S. Barušić 1963. *Echinococcus cysticus* in the endocardium and the calcified hydatid cysts in the liver and lungs of cattle. *Veterinaria, Serajevo* **12**, 89–91.

Buck, A. A., R. I. Anderson, K. Kawata, I. W. Abrahams, R. A. Ward and T. T. Sasaki 1972. *Health and disease in rural Afghanistan.* Baltimore: York.

Burridge, M. J. and C. W. Schwabe 1977a. Hydatid disease in New Zealand: an epidemiological study of transmission among Maoris. *Am. J. Trop. Med. Hyg.* **26**, 258–65.

Burridge, M. J. and C. W. Schwabe 1977b. Epidemiological analysis of factors influencing rate of progress in *Echinococcus granulosus* control in New Zealand. *J. Hyg.* **78**, 151–63.

Burridge, M. J., C. W. Schwabe and J. Fraser 1977a. Hydatid disease in New Zealand: changing patterns in human infection, 1878–1972. *N.Z. Med. J.* **85**, 173–7.

Burridge, M. J., C. W. Schwabe and T. W. Pullum 1977b. Path analysis: application in an epidemiological study of echinococcosis in New Zealand. *J. Hyg.* **78**, 135–49.

Čaklovisa, F., F. Sudarit and A. Milanovic 1981. Nalaz ciste *Echinococcus granulosus* u srčanom mišiću goveda. *Veterinaria, Serajevo* **30**, 473–7 [*Helminthol. Abstr. A* **52**, 64 (1983)].

Calamai, G., Am. Perna and A. Venturini 1974. Hydatid disease of the heart – report of five cases and review of the literature. *Thorax* **29**, 451–8.

Cameron, T. W. M. 1927. Some modern biological conceptions of hydatid. *Proc. R. Soc. Med.* **20**, 272–83.

Chin, D. D. 1981. Hydatid cyst of the heart presenting as cerebral and cerebellar infarctions. *Med. J. Aust.* **2**, 556–7.

Cipeng, J. 1981. Liver alveolar echinococcosis in the northwest. Report of 15 patients and a collective analysis of 90 cases. *China Med. J.* **94**, 771–8.

Coudert, J. and P. Goinard 1967. *Le kyste hydatique du foie.* Lyon: Simep Editions.

Coudert, J., J. Euzeby and J. P. Garin 1970. Frequence d'*Echinococcus multilocularis* chez le renard (*Vulpes vulpes*) dans le secteur nord-est de la France. *Lyon Med.* **224**, 293–8.

Crellin, J. R., F. L. Andersen, P. M. Schantz and S. J. Condie 1982. Possible factors influencing distribution and prevalence of *Echinococcus granulosus* in Utah. *Am. J. Epidem.* **116**, 463–74.

Curtice, C. 1890. *The animal parasites of sheep.* Washington: US Department of Agriculture.

Cuthbert, R. 1975. Sylvatic pulmonary hydatid disease: a radiological survey. *J. Ass. Can. Radiol.* **26**, 132–8.

Dada, J. O. and E. D. Belino 1978. Prevalence of hydatidosis and cysticercosis in slaughtered livestock in Nigeria. *Vet. Rec.* **103**, 311–2.

Dada, J. O., D. S. Adegboye and A. N. Mohammed 1979. The epidemiology of *Echinococcus* infection in Kaduna State, Nigeria. *Vet. Rec.* **104**, 312–3.

Dailey, M. D. and G. K. Sweatman 1965. The taxonomy of *Echinococcus granulosus* in the donkey and dromedary in Lebanon and Syria. *Ann. Trop. Med. Parasitol.* **4**, 463–77.

D'Alessandro, A., R. L. Rausch, C. Cuello and N. Aristizabal 1979. *Echinococcus vogeli* in man, with a review of polycystic hydatid disease in Colombia and neighboring countries. *Am. J. Trop. Med. Hyg.* **28**, 303–17.

Deineka, I. Ia. 1968. *Ekhinokokkoz cheloveka.* Moscow: Meditsina.

Deklotz, R. J. 1976. Echinococcal cyst involving the prostate and seminal vesicles: a case report. *J. Urol.* **115**, 116–7.

Dent, C. H. R. 1960. Cerebral hydatids in a cow. *Aust. Vet. J.* **42**, 28.

Dévé, F. 1946. *L'echinococcose secondaire.* Paris: Masson.

Dévé, F. 1949. *L'echinococcose primitive.* Paris: Masson.

Dew, H. R. 1925. The histogenesis of the hydatid parasite (*Taenia echinococcus*) in the pig. *Med. J. Aust.* (12th year) **1**, 101–10.

Dew, H. R. 1928. *Hydatid disease – its pathology, diagnosis and treatment.* Sydney: Australasian Medical Publishing.

Dew, H. R. 1953. Pleomorphism in hydatid disease. *Arch. Int. Hidat.* **13**, 284–95.

Dew, H. R. 1958. Morphological variation in hydatid disease. *Br. J. Surg.* **45**, 447–53.

Dixon, J. B., J. K. Baker-Smith and J. C. Greatorex 1973. Incidence of hydatid cysts in old cattle. *Vet. Rec.* **93**, 470.

Duran, H., L. Ferrandez, F. Gomez-Castesana, L. Lopez-Duran, P. Mata, D. Brandau and A. Sanchez-Barba 1978. Osseous hydatidosis. *J. Bone Joint Surg.* 60–*A* **60**, 685–90.

Editorial 1976. The invisible worm. *Lancet ii*, 552–3.

Eugster, R. O. 1978. *A contribution to the epidemiology of echinococcosis/hydatidosis in Kenya (East Africa) with special reference to the Kajiado district.* DVM thesis, University of Zurich.

Euzéby, J. 1971. *Les échinococcoses animales et leur relations avec les échinococcoses de l'homme.* Paris: Vigot Freres.

Fairley, W. H. and R. J. Wright-Smith 1929. Hydatid infestation (*Echinococcus granulosus*) in sheep, oxen and pigs, with special reference to daughter cyst formation. *J. Path. Bact.* **32**, 309–35.

Fontan, R., F. Beauchamp and P. C. Beaver 1975. Sur quelques helminthiases nouvelles au Laos. II. Platyhelminthes. *Bull. Soc. Path. Exot.* **6**, 566–73.

Freedman, A. N. 1974. Muscular hydatid disease: report of a case and a review of the literature. *Can. J. Surg.* **17**, 232–4.

French, C. M. and G. S. Nelson 1982. Hydatid disease in the Turkana District of Kenya. II. A study in medical geography. *Ann. Trop. Med. Parasitol.* **76**, 439–57.

French, C. M., G. S. Nelson and A. M. Wood 1982. Hydatid disease in the Turkana District of Kenya. I. The background to the problem with hypotheses to account for the remarkably high prevalence of the disease in man. *Ann. Trop. Med. Parasitol.* **76**, 425–37.

Front, D. and O. Israel 1981. Hydatid disease: the value of whole-body screening by scintigraphy with technetium-99m-labelled red blood cells. *Br. J. Radiol.* **54**, 241–4.

Fuller, G. K. and D. C. Fuller 1981. Hydatid disease in Ethiopia: clinical survey with some immunodiagnostic test results. *Am. J. Trop. Med. Hyg.* **30**, 645–52.

Gamble, W. G., M. Segal, P. M. Schantz and R. L. Rausch 1979. Alveolar hydatid disease in Minnesota. First human case acquired in the contiguous United States. *J. Am. Med. Ass.* **241**, 904–7.

Gemmell, M. A. 1960. Advances in knowledge on the distribution and importance of hydatid disease as world health and economic problems during the decade 1950–1959. *Helminthol. Abstr.* **29**, 355–69.

Gemmell, M. A. 1979. Hydatidosis – a global view. *Aust. Vet. J.* **55**, 118–25.

Gill, H. S. 1968. Secondary echinococcosis in an Indian water buffalo (*Bos bubalis*). *J. Parasitol.* **54**, 949.

Gluhovschi, N., E. Simionescu and D. Orbulescu 1970. Cas rare d'echinococcose prénatale chez le veau. *Rec. Med. Vet.* **146**, 1457–63.

Goel, V. P., T. N. Mehrotra, P. R. Bhatia and S. N. Gupta 1974. Hydatid cyst of the tongue. *J. Indian Med. Assoc.* **63**, 28–30.

Golematis, B. 1983. Hydatid cyst of the pancreas: case report. *Mt Sinai J. Med.* **50**, 76–80.

Grabbe, E., P. Kern and M. Heller 1981. Human echinococcosis: diagnostic value of computerized tomography. *Tropenmed. Parasitol.* **32**, 35–8.

Graber, M., P. Troncy, R. Tabo, J. Service and O. Oumatie 1969. L'echinococcose-hydatidose en Afrique centrale. I. Echinococcose des animaux domestiques et sauvages. *Rev. Elev. Méd. Vét. Pays Trop.* **22**, 55–67.

Graber, M. and J. Thal 1980. L'echinococcose des artiodactyles sauvages de la République Centrafricaine: existence probable d'un cycle lion-phacochere. *Rev. Elev. Méd. Vét. Pays Trop.* **33**, 51–9.

Graham, J. 1891. *Hydatid disease in its clinical aspects.* London: Young J. Pentland.

Gupta, P. P. and B. Singh 1975. A note on an unusual case of echinococcosis in a buffalo (*Bos bubalis*) *Zbl. Veterinärmed. B* **22**, 793–5.

Hall, M. C. 1915. The dog as a carrier of parasites and disease. *U.S. Dept Agric. Bull.* no. 260.

Hall, M. C. 1920. Parasites and parasitic diseases of sheep. *U.S. Dept Agric. Bull.* no. 1150.

Harris, L. S. 1976. Lateral chest wall cyst in a woman with disseminated echinococcal disease. *Mt Sinai J. Med.* **43**, 182–8.

Hassounah, O. and K. Behbehani 1976. The epidemiology of *Echinococcus* infection in Kuwait. *J. Helminthol.* **50**, 65–73.

Heath, D. D. 1971. The migration of oncospheres of *Taenia pisiformis, T. serialis* and *Echinococcus granulosus* within the intermediate host. *Int. J. Parasitol.* **1**, 145–52.

Hoeppli, R. 1959. *Parasites and parasitic infections in early medicine and science*, p. 32. Singapore: University of Malaya Press.

Holgado Rivas, D. E. 1969. Sobre un notable caso do hidatidosis testicular bilateral en un porcino. *Gac. Vet., Buenos Aires* **31**, 263–5.

Hosemann, G., E. Schwarz, J. C. Lehmann and A. Posselt 1928. *Die Echinokokkenkrankheiten.* Stuttgart: F. Enke.

Irwin, A. D. 1974. Hydatidosis in human patients from Turkana. *Trop. Geogr. Med.* **26**, 157–9.

Islam, N. and M. Rahman 1975. Echinococcosis in Bangladesh. *Trop. Geogr. Med.* **27**, 305–6.

Jakubowski, M. S. and D. E. Barnard 1971. Anaphylactic shock during operation for hydatid disease. *Anesthesiology* **34**, 197–9.

James, E. and W. Boyd 1937. *Echinococcus alveolaris. Can. Med. Ass. J.* **36**, 354–6.

Jones, W. H. S. (transl.) 1948–53. *Hippocrates*, Vol. 4, *Aphorisms*, section 7, no. 55. Cambridge: Harvard University Press.

Kahn, J. B., S. L. Spruance, J. Harbottle, P. Cannon and M. G. Schultz 1972. Echinococcosis in Utah. *Am. J. Trop. Med. Hyg.* **21**, 185–8.

Khuroo, M. S., D. V. Datta, A. Khoshy, S. K. Mitra and P. N. Chhuttani 1980. Alveolar hydatid disease of the liver with Budd–Chiari syndrome. *Postgrad. Med. J.* **56**, 197–201.

Kirkland, K. 1966. Urological aspects of hydatid disease. *Br. J. Urol.* **38**, 241–54.

Kirkman, J. 1863. Chronic disease of the bones of the cranium of the horse, associated with the existence of hydatids within a cyst at the interior part of the eye. *Veterinarian, London* **36**, 77–80.

Kumaratilake, L. M. and R. C. A. Thompson 1982. Hydatidosis/echinococcosis in Australia. *Helminthol. Abstr. A* **51**, 233–52.

Laclainche, E. 1936. *Histoire de la médicine vétérinaire.* Toulouse: Office du Livre.

Laing, A. D. M. G. 1961. The implementation of hydatid eradication measures in New Zealand. *Bull. Off. Int. Epizoot.* **56**, 1030–9.

Larsson, S., A. K. Soe and K. Zahoory 1983. Hydatidcysta på ovanlig plats hos får. *Svensk Vet.* **35**, 229–30 [*Helminthol. Abstr. A* **52**, 2874 (1983)].

Le Van Hoa 1967. Sur la presence des cestodes *Echinococcus granulosus* chez le chien sauvage au Sud Viet-Nam. *Bull. Soc. Path. Exot.* **60**, 64–71.

Leiby, P. L., W. P. Carney and C. E. Woods 1970. Studies on sylvatic echinococcosis. III. Host occurrence and geographic distribution of *Echinococus multilocularis* in the north central United States. *J. Parasitol.* **56**, 1141–50.

LeRiche, P. D. and R. J. Jorgensen 1971. *Echinococcosis (hydatidosis) and its control*, Near East Animal Health Institutes, Handbook no. 6. Rome: United Nations Food and Agricultural Organization.

Little, J. M. 1976. Hydatid disease at Royal Prince Alfred Hospital, 1964 to 1974. *Med. J. Aust.* **1**, 903–8.

Littré, E. 1962 (1851). *Oeuvres completes d'Hippocrate,* VII. Amsterdam: Halckert, pp. 224–5.

Liu, I. K. M., C. W. Schwabe, P. M. Schantz and M. N. Allison 1970. The occurrence of *Echinococcus granulosus* in coyotes (*Canis latrans*) in the central valley of California. *J. Parasitol.* **56**, 1135–7.

Lukashenko, N. P. 1975. [*Alveococcus.*] Moscow: Medicine.

Lupascu, Gh. and D. Panaitescu 1968. *Hidatidoza.* Bucharest: Editura Academiei Republicii Socialiste Romania.

Macpherson, C. N. L. 1983. An active intermediate host role for man in the life cycle of *Echinococcus granulosus* in Turkana, Kenya. *Am. J. Trop. Med. Hyg.* **32**, 397–404.

Macpherson, C. N. L., L. Karstad, P. Stevenson and J. H. Arundel 1983. Hydatid disease in the Turkana District of Kenya. III. The significance of wild animals in the transmission of *Echinococcus granulosus*, with particular reference to Turkana and Masailand in Kenya. *Ann. Trop. Med. Parasitol.* **77**, 61–73.

Mandal, P. C. 1977. Fatal hydatid disease with involvement of the cerebrum in buffaloes (*Bos bubalis*). *Zbl. Vet. Med. B.* **24**, 678–9.

Matossian, R. M., M. D. Rickard and J. D. Smyth 1977. Hydatidosis: a global problem of increasing importance. *Bull. Wld Hlth Org.* **55**, 499–507.

Meldrum, G. K. and J. D. McConnell 1968. The control of hydatid disease in Tasmania. *Aust. Vet. J.* **44**, 2121–7.

Miguet, J.-P., C. Monange, J.-P. Ricatte, F. Weill, G. Camelot, M. Gillet, P. Carayon and H. Gisselbrecht 1976. L'échinococcose alvéolaire du foie. A propos de 20 cas observés en Franche Comté. I. Etude épidemiologique, biologigue, radiologique et échorgraphique. *Archs Er. Mal. App. Dig.* **65**, 9–21.

Miller, C. W., R. Ruppanner and C. W. Schwabe 1971. Hydatid disease in California: study of hospital records, 1960 through 1969. *Am. J. Trop. Med. Hyg.* **20**, 904–13.

Mobedi, I., R. A. Bray, F. Arfaa and K. Movafag 1973. A study of the cestodes of carnivores in the northwest of Iran. *J. Helminthol.* **47**, 277–81.

Mobedi, I. and A. Sadighian 1971. *Echinococcus multilocularis* in red foxes, *Vulpes vulpes*, in Moghan, Azerbaijen Province, northwest of Iran. *J. Parasitol.* **57**, 493.

Moon, J. R. 1976. Public health significance of zoonotic tapeworms in Korea. *J. Zoonoses* **3**, 1–18.

Morsy, T. A., S. A. Michael and A. M. E. Disi 1980. Cats as reservoir hosts of human parasites in Amman, Jordan. *J. Egypt. Soc. Parasitol.* **10**, 5–18.

Nasseh, G. A. and B. Khadivi 1975. Epidemiological and clinical aspects of echinococcosis in East Iran. *J. Trop. Med. Hyg.* **78**, 120–2.

Neghme, E. and R. Silva 1970. A hidatidose como problema médico, sanitário e social e esbôço básico para sua profilaxia. *Rev. Ass. Med. Brasil* **16**, 279–86.

Nelson, G. S. and R. L. Rausch 1963. *Echinococcus* infections in man and animals in Kenya. *Ann. Trop. Med. Parasitol.* **57**, 136–49.

Niron, E. A. and H. Özer 1981. Ultrasound appearance of liver hydatid disease. *Br. J. Radiol.* **54**, 335–8.

Odend'hal, S. 1972. Energetics of Indian cattle in their environment. *Human Ecology* **1**, 3–22.

OIE 1979. The OIE Working Group on Echinococcosis–Hydatidosis. No. VIII of Reports by the Permanent Commissions and Working Groups, Paris, 21–26 May 1979. *Bull. Off. Int. Epizoot.* **91** (numéro spécial), 64–7.

O'Leary, P. 1976. A five-year review of human hydatid cyst disease in Turkana District, Kenya. *E. Afr. Med. J.* **53**, 540–4.

Owor, R. and P. K. Bitakaramire 1975. Hydatid disease in Uganda. *E. Afr. Med. J.* **52**, 700–4.

Pal, A. K. and P. K. Sinha 1970. Multilocular hydatidosis in a bullock. *Indian Vet. J.* **47**, 910-2.

Panner, B. and J. Leonard 1960. Hydatid disease with *Salmonella* infection of the echinococcal cyst. *Med. Times* **88**, 980–4.

Pappaioanou, M. 1982. *An epidemiological study of the Cyprus anti-echinococcus campaign*. PhD dissertation, University of California, Davis.

Pappaioanou, M., C. W. Schwabe and D. M. Sard 1977. An evolving pattern of human hydatid disease transmission in the United States. *Am. J. Trop. Med. Hyg.* **26**, 732–42.

Perez-Gomez, F., H. Duran, S. Tamames, J. L. Perrote and A. Blanes 1973. Cardiac echinococcosis: clinical picture and complications. *Br. Heart J.* **35**, 1326–31.

Pierotti, P. 1954. Echinococcosi in equino. *Atti Soc. Ital. Sci. Vet.* **8**, 692–4.

Pieters, G., A. van den Spiegel and P. Demeester 1976. Les guérisons spontanées de l'hydatidose pulmonaire. *Tunisie Méd.* **54**, 487–9.

Pinch, L. W. and J. F. Wilson 1973. Non-surgical management of cystic hydatid disease in Alaska – a review of 30 cases of *Echinococcus granulosus* infection treated without operation. *Ann. Surg.* **178**, 45–8.

Polydorou, K. 1980. The control of echinococcosis in Cyprus. *Wld. Anim. Rev.* **33**, 19–25.

Powers, L. E. and C. W. Churchill 1959. *Bibliography of echinococcosis with selected abstracts*. Beirut: American University of Beirut.

Purriel, P., P. M. Schantz, H. Beovide and G. Mendoze 1973. Human echinococcosis (hydatidosis) in Uruguay: a comparison of indices of morbidity and mortality, 1962–71. *Bull. Wld Hlth Org.* **49**, 395–402.

Ramazanov, V. T., Y. Kereev, R. G. Ismagilova and K. Kosmoldanov 1978. [Effect of hydatid disease on milk production in sheep.] *Trudў Kazakh. Nauch. Vet. Inst.* **17**, 120–3. [In Russian.]

Ramírez, R. 1971. Algunos aspectos bioestadísticos de la hidatidosis humana en Chile durante los años 1969, 1970. *Bol. Chil. Parasitol.* **26**, 84–8.

Rausch, R. L. 1967. On the ecology and distribution of *Echinococcus* spp. (Cestoda: Taeniidae), and characteristics of their development in the intermediate host. *Ann. Parasitol.* **42**, 19–63.

Rausch, R. L. 1975. Taeniidae. In *Diseases transmitted from animals to man*, W. T. Hubbert, W. F. McCulloch and P. R. Schurrenberger (eds). p. 678–707. Springfield, Ill.: Thomas.

Rausch, R. L. and J. J. Bernstein 1972. *Echinococcus vogeli* sp. In (Cestoda: Taeniidae) from the bush dog, *Speothos venaticus* (Lund). *Z. Tropenmed. Parasitol.* **23**, 25–34.

Rausch, R. L. and E. L. Schiller 1956. Studies on the helminth fauna of Alaska. XXV. The ecology and public health significance of *Echinococcus sibiricensis* Rausch and Schiller, 1954, on St Lawrence Island. *Parasitology* **46**, 395–419.

Rivera, R. and J. L. Delcan 1980. Surgical treatment of coronary insufficiency produced by cardiac echinococcosis. *Chest* **78**, 849–52.

Romano, M. N., O. A. Brunetti, C. W. Schwabe and M. N. Rosen 1974. Probable transmission of *Echinococcus granulosus* between deer and coyotes in California. *J. Wildl. Dis.* **10**, 225–7.

Romanoff, H. and M. Krausz 1975. Surgical aspects of pulmonary hydatid disease and report of a familial hydatidosis. *Int. Surg.* **60**, 361–4.

Ronéus, O., D. Christensson and N.-G. Nilsson 1982. The longevity of hydatid cysts in horses. *Vet. Parasitol.* **11**, 149–54.

Sadighian, A. 1969. Helminth parasites of stray dogs and jackals in Shahsavar area, Caspian region, Iran. *J. Parasitol.* **55**, 372–4.

Sami, M. A. 1938. Hydatid disease in the Punjab. *Indian Med. Gaz.* **73**, 90.

Sapunar, J. and E. Cancino 1974. Siembra hidatídica subcutánea. *Bol. Chil. Parasitol.* **29**, 103–6.

Sawyer, J. C., P. M. Schantz, C. W. Schwabe and M. W. Newbold 1969. Identification of transmission foci of hydatid disease in California. *Pub. Hlth Rep., Wash.* **84**, 531–41.

Schantz, P. M. 1972a. Hidatidosis: magnitud del problemay perspectivas de control. *Bol. Ofic. Sanit. Panamer.* **74**, 187–97.

Schantz, P. M. 1972b. Localizacion de la hidatidosis en el sistema nerviosa central. *Bol. Ofic. Sanit. Panamer.* **63**, 198–202.

Schantz, P. M. 1977. *Echinococcus granulosus*: acute systemic allergic reactions to hydatid cyst fluid in infected sheep. *Exp. Parasitol.* **43**, 268–85.

Schantz, P. M. 1982. Echinococcosis. In *CRC handbook series in zoonoses, Section C: Parasitic zoonoses*, J. Steele (ed.) **1**, 231–77. Baton Roca, Fla: CRC Press.

Schantz, P. M. 1983. Emergent and newly recognized parasitic zoonoses. *Comp. Contin. Educ. Pract. Vet.* **5**, 163–74.

Schantz, P. M. and C. W. Schwabe 1969. Worldwide status of hydatid disease control. *J. Am. Vet. Med. Assoc.* **155**, 2104–21.

Schantz, P. M., J. F. Williams and C. Riva Posse 1973. The epidemiology of hydatid disease in southern Argentina. Comparison of morbidity indices, evaluation of immunodiagnostic tests and factors affecting transmission in southern Rio Negro province. *Am. J. Trop. Med. Hyg.* **22**, 629–41.

Schantz, P. M., R. P. Clérou, I. K. M. Liu and C. W. Schwabe 1970. Hydatid disease in the Central Valley of California: transmission of infection among dogs, sheep, and man in Kern County. *Am. J. Trop. Med. Hyg.* **19**, 823–30.

Schantz, P. M., C. F. von Reyn, T. Welty, F. L. Andersen, M. G. Schultz and I. G. Kagan 1977. Epidemiologic investigation of echinococcosis in American Indians living in Arizona and New Mexico. *Am. J. Trop. Med. Hyg.* **26**, 121–6.

Schwabe, C. W. 1961a. *Report on veterinary public health, Cyprus. A preliminary assessment of the hydatid disease problem and the present programme for control.* World Health Organization, WHO Project EM/Zoonoses/11, Cyprus 12/TA.

Schwabe, C. W. 1961b. *Report on visits to laboratories engaged in hydatid disease research, April 14–June 26, 1961.* WHO Project Z 2/133/2(a).

Schwabe, C. W. 1964. *Veterinary medicine and human health.* Baltimore: Williams and Wilkins, pp. 211 and 395.

Schwabe, C. W. 1968. Epidemiology of echinococcosis. *Bull. Wld Hlth Org.* **39**, 131–5.

Schwabe, C. W. 1978. *Cattle, priests and progress in medicine*, 4th Spink Lectures in Comparative Medicine. Minneapolis: University of Minnesota Press.

Schwabe, C. W. 1979. Epidemiological aspects of the planning and evaluation of hydatid disease control. *Aust. Vet. J.* **55**, 109–17.

Schwabe, C. W. 1981. Animal diseases and primary health care: intersectoral challenges. *WHO Chron.* **35**, 227–32.

Schwabe, C. W. 1984. *Veterinary medicine and human health*, 3rd edn. Baltimore: Williams and Wilkins.

Schwabe, C. W. and K. Abou-Daoud 1961. Epidemiology of echinococcosis in the Middle East. I. Human infection in Lebanon, 1949 to 1959. *Am. J. Trop. Med. Hyg.* **10**, 374–81.

Schwabe, C. W., A. Kilejian and G. Lainas 1970. The propagation of secondary cysts of *Echinococcus granulosus* in the Mongolian jird, *Meriones unguiculatus*. *J. Parasitol.* **56**, 80–3.

Schwabe, C. W., L. A. Schinazi and A. Kilejian 1959. Host–parasite relationships in echinococcosis. II. Age resistance to secondary echinococcosis in the white mouse. *Am. J. Trop. Med. Hyg.* **8**, 29–36.

Schwabe, C. W., G. Luttermoser, M. Koussa and S. Ali 1964. Serial passage of fertile hydatid cysts of *Echinococcus granulosus* in absence of the definitive host. *J. Parasitol.* **50**, 260.

Schwabe, C. W., R. Ruppanner, C. W. Miller, R. E. Fontaine and I. G. Kagan 1972. Hydatid disease is endemic in California. *Calif. Med.* **117**, 13–7.

Shamsul Islam, A. W. M. 1979. Hydatid disease in sheep of Mymensingh District, Bangladesh. *J. Parasitol.* **65**, 37.

Shanbhag, A. M., L. V. Baxi and A. S. Punde 1974. Obstructed labour due to a pelvic hydatid cyst. *J. Obstet. Gynaec. Br. Commonw.* **81**, 825–6.

Simitch, T. 1964. Frequence et répartition géographique dans le monde de l'échinococcose-hydatidose due à *Echinococcus multilocularis et à Echinococcus granulosus*. *Bull. Off. Int. Epizoot.* **62**, 1031–61.

Simpson, D. A. and P. W. Verco 1976. Cerebral hydatid cysts in colonial Australia. *Surg. Neurol.* **6**, 377–80.

Slais, J. 1980. Experimental infection on sheep and pigs with *Echinococcus granulosus* (Batsch, 1786), and the origin of pouching in hydatid cysts. *Acta Vet. Acad. Sci. Hung.* **28**, 375–87.

Smyth, J. D. and M. M. Smyth 1964. Natural and experimental hosts of *Echinococcus granulosus* and *E. multilocularis*, with comments on the genetics of speciation in the genus *Echinococcus*. *Parasitology* **54**, 493–514.

Spruance, S. L. 1974. Latent period of 53 years in a case of hydatid cyst disease. *Arch. Intern. Med.* **134**, 741–2.

Suić, M. 1952. *Ehinokoza*. Zagreb: Yugoslav Akad. Znanosti i Umjetnosti.

Sweatman, G. K. and R. J. Williams 1963. Survival of *Echinococcus granulosus* and *Taenia hydatigena* eggs in two extreme climatic regions of New Zealand. *Res. Vet. Sci.* **4**, 199–216.

Tenhaeff, C. and S. F. Ferwerda 1935. Over de localisatie van de echinococcose in de organen van de slachddieren. *Tijdschr. Diergeneesk.* **62**, 79–94.

Teymoorian, G. A. and F. Bagheri 1976. Hydatid cyst of the skull: report of four cases. *Radiology* **118**, 97–100.

Thatcher, V. E. 1972. Neotropical echinococcosis in Colombia. *Ann. Trop. Med. Parasitol.* **66**, 99–105.

Thierry, A., P. Cortet, R. Michiels, C. Seigneuric, D. Binnert, M. C. Pelikan and J. L. Sautreaux 1978. Exérese chirurgicale des localisations cérébrales de l'échinococcose multiloculaire. *Neurochirurgie* **24**, 123–8.

Thomas, J. D. 1884. *Hydatid disease with special reference to its prevalence in Australia*. Adelaide: Spiller.

Thomas, J. D. 1894. *Hydatid disease*, Vol. 2 (A. A. Lendon, ed.), Sydney: Bruck.

Tomb, J. and R. Matossian 1976. Diagnosis of pulmonary hydatidosis by sputum cytology. *Johns Hopkins Med. J.* **139**, 38–40.

Thompson, R. C. A. 1977. Hydatidosis in Great Britain. *Helminthol. Abstr. A* **46**, 837–61.

Thompson, R. C. A. and J. D. Smyth 1975. Equine hydatidosis: a review of the current status in Great Britain and the results of an epidemiological survey. *Vet. Parasitol.* **1**, 107–27.

Vicary, F. R., G. Cusick, I. M. Shirley and R. J. Blackwell 1977. Ultrasound and abdominal hydatid disease. *Trans. R. Soc. Trop. Med. Hyg.* **71**, 29–31.

Vogel, H. 1957. Über den *Echinococcus multilocularis* Suddeutschlands. I. Das Bandwormstadium von Stammen menschlicher und tierischer Herkunft. *Tropenmed. Parasitol.* **8**, 404–56.

Volokh, Iu. A. 1965. *Ekhinokokkoz i Al'veokokkoz Cheloveka.* Frunze, Kyrgystan.

WHO 1968. Research needs in echinococcosis (hydatidosis). *Bull. Wld Hlth Org.* **39**, 101–13.

WHO/FAO/UNEP 1981. *Guidelines for surveillance, prevention and control of echinococcosis/hydatidosis*, WHO VPH/81.28. Geneva: WHO.

Williams, J. F., H. L. Adaros and A. Trejos 1971. Current prevalence and distribution of hydatidosis, with special reference to the Americas. *Am. J. Trop. Med. Hyg.* **20**, 224–36.

Wilson, J. F., A. C. Diddams and R. L. Rausch 1968. Cystic hydatid disease in Alaska – a review of 101 autochthonous cases of *Echinococcus granulosus* infection. *Am. Rev. Resp. Dis.* **98**, 1–15.

Wilson, J. F. and R. L. Rausch 1980. Alveolar hydatid disease: a review of clinical features of 33 indigenous cases of *Echinococcus granulosus* infection in Alaskan Eskimos. *Am. J. Trop. Med. Hyg.* **29**, 1340–55.

Yamashita, J., M. Ohbayashi and S. Konno 1956. Studies on echinococcosis. III. On experimental infection of dogs, especially on the development of *Echinococcus granulosus* (Batsch, 1786). *Japan. J. Vet. Res.* **4**, 113–22.

Young, E. 1975a. Some important parasitic and other diseases of lion, *Panthera leo*, in the Kruger National Park. *J. S. Afr. Vet. Assoc.* **46**, 181–3.

Young, E. 1975b. Echinococcosis (hydatidosis) in wild animals of the Kruger National Park. *J. S. Afr. Vet. Ass.* **46**, 285–6.

Yusuf, J. N. and G. J. Frayha 1975. *Echinococcus granulosus*: host lymphocyte transformation by parasitic antigens. *Exp. Parasitol.* **38**, 30–7.

4 Biochemistry and physiology of *Echinococcus*

D. P. McMANUS AND C. BRYANT

INTRODUCTION

Studies of the biochemistry of the Platyhelminthes lag behind similar studies of the Aschelminthes. For example, *Ascaris* figured in the classical experiments of Keilin (1925) when he rediscovered the cytochromes and wondered about their function. No tapeworm was used in a major biochemical study before the 1930s although one important piece of work on free-living Platyhelminthes (Hyman 1919) surely indicated that the group as a whole would repay interest. Hyman showed that *Planaria* were not easily killed by cyanide, but as it was yet years to the discovery of cytochromes the proper inferences could not be drawn.

It would be superfluous to comment here on the great contribution that Theodor von Brand made to parasite biochemistry; suffice to say that, in the early 1930s, he first drew attention to the fact that parasites (including cestodes) secreted succinic acid into their incubation media. This key observation was later extended in the 1940s when it was established that *Moniezia benedeni*, a tapeworm of ruminants, and the liver fluke, *Fasciola hepatica*, possessed a metabolism which differed in many important respects from the model which was at that time emerging from the laboratories of the 'mainline' biochemists. These two organisms were chosen for study for the same reason that Bueding, Saz and co-workers chose *Ascaris* for their metabolic experiments. They are large and readily obtainable in bulk, which was an important consideration given the lack of sensitivity of instruments and assays at that time (von Brand 1979).

From the 1950s onwards, there was a steady increase in interest in parasite biochemistry. In America, biochemists began amassing information about the composition of parasitic helminths and elucidating what may now be called the helminth pattern of metabolism. It is a measure of the contribution of scientists such as Theodor von Brand, Clark Read, Ernest Bueding and Howard Saz that the principles they established for parasite biochemistry are good today. There are many more pathways than they conceived of, regulation of metabolism is infinitely more subtle, and there are profound dangers in generalising from one phylum (or even genus) of helminths to another. However, the idea of an anaerobic metabolism side by side, on occasion, with a primitive but specialised version of aerobic metabolism is still true of all the helminth groups.

In 1952, Read published the first of his 'contributions to cestode enzymology', a systematic study of cytochromes, succinic dehydrogenase and metabolism generally in the rat tapeworm, *Hymenolepis diminuta*. In this, and earlier papers, Read's emphasis was on comparative biochemistry and established clearly that cestodes, too, conform to the rather odd pattern that was being worked out for the nematodes. It set the scene for a second series of papers on the role of carbohydrates in the biology of cestodes (Read & Rothman 1957). In turn, this provided the stimulus for a series of classical papers by Agosin and his colleagues (who included von Brand) on the protoscoleces of *Echinococcus granulosus* from South American sheep (Agosin *et al.* 1957).

Scientists who study the biochemistry of parasites are faced with a problem that every parasitologist is aware of, but which assumes a special significance for biochemists. A parasite with a complex life-cycle is adapted to more than one environment. The environments may be very different in their physical and chemical characteristics – temperature, pH, oxygen tension, carbon dioxide concentration, to name a few – so that the organisation and metabolic patterns appropriate in one environment may not serve for another. In the transition between environments, the adaptational programme may require a new set of enzymes to be activated, others deactivated, and new patterns of resource partitioning established.

In this account of the biochemistry of *Echinococcus* we are concerned with adaptive as well as descriptive biochemistry. For zoologists, there is a wealth of difference between the two. It is only in the attempt to view the parasite as part of a host–parasite system, rather than as a bag of independently performing biochemical molecules, that function can be discerned. The concepts of function and adaptation are irrevocably intertwined, never more so than in the intimacy of the parasitic relationship.

CHEMICAL COMPOSITION

Other than protein composition, of which a relatively substantial literature now exists (reviewed in detail, see below), there is very little recent information concerning other chemical and biochemical components of *Echinococcus*. Sanchez and Sanchez (1971) carried out a very comprehensive comparative study of the hydatid fluid (HF) from cysts of human, sheep and cattle origin. This investigation included estimations of pH, density, inorganic substances (Na, K, Mg, Cu, Fe, Cl, P), lipids, cholesterol, glucose, urea, proteins, amino acids (aspartate, glutamate, serine, glycine, glucosamine, threonine, alanine, valine, arginine), pentoses, levulose and enzymes [glutamic oxaloacetic transaminase (GOT), glutamic pyruvic transaminase (GPT), alkaline and acid phosphatases]. Many of these fluid components differed qualitatively or quantitatively, depending on the cyst location and host origin, probably relating to strain characteristics.

Na, Mg, Ca, P and Cl were also detectable in sheep HF in another study (Frayha & Haddad 1980). With the exception of Cl, these components and bicarbonate were also present in protoscoleces. RNA, DNA and ammonia, found in substantial amounts in protoscoleces, were almost totally absent from HF. The reverse was observed with urea, uric acid, creatinine and bilirubin. Cholesterol, cholesterol esters, mono-, di and triglycerides, phospholipids and fatty acids were detected mainly in protoscoleces. Glycogen, trehalose, glucose and alkali-stable carbohydrates were detected in protoscoleces and, interestingly, sucrose was present in protoscoleces and HF. The major proteins in HF were albumin and globulin and these formed one-third of the protein composition of protoscoleces. Among enzymes, lactate dehydrogenase, phosphatases, GOT and GPT exhibited high activities.

Chemical analysis (RNA, DNA, protein, lipids and polysaccharides) of protoscoleces indicated basic differences between the UK horse and sheep strains of *E. granulosus* and between these and *Echinococcus multilocularis* (McManus & Smyth 1978). A subsequent study of the biochemical composition of *E. granulosus* in Kenya (McManus 1981) revealed differences between protoscoleces of cattle, goat, camel and sheep origin but similarities between the sheep and human parasites. Differences in chemical composition were also apparent between adult worms obtained by experimental infection and those obtained from naturally infected dogs. This may have been a consequence of the original hydatid source and/or the differing stages of development of the analysed adult worms. The results of biochemical analysis from the two studies are shown in Table 4.1.

As in other larval cestodes, calcareous corpuscles are a major component of protoscoleces (14.3 per cent of dried tissue; von Brand *et al.* 1965). They consist of an organic base together with inorganic material (von Brand 1979). The composition of the inorganic constituents varies slightly in specimens of *E. granulosus* from different countries (von Brand *et al.* 1965), which again probably reflects minor strain differences. The functions of the calcareous corpuscles are not well understood but they may be antigenic or they may serve as buffer substances and/or reservoirs of phosphate for metabolic requirements (von Brand 1979). The latter is suggested by *in vitro* culture studies. The first indication of strobilar development in *E. granulosus* (Smyth 1967) and in *E. multilocularis* (Barrett 1984) is a gradual but observable reduction in the numbers of the calcareous corpuscles, which finally disappear completely. It has also been suggested that anti-complementary factors are associated with the calcareous corpuscles of *E. granulosus* and *E. multilocularis* (Kassis & Tanner 1976).

The hydatid cyst of *E. granulosus* is characterised by a pericyst (adventitial layer) and laminated layer surrounding the germinal layer from which develop the brood capsules and protoscoleces (Morseth 1967). Biochemically the laminated layer (from cattle cysts) was shown to be a periodic acid–schiff (PAS)-positive carbohydrate–protein (mucopolysaccharide) complex (Kilejian *et al.* 1961, 1962, Kilejian & Schwabe 1971). The carbohydrate component, composed of galactose, galactosamine and

Table 4.1 The biochemical composition (in micrograms per milligram dry weight ± S.E.) of protoscoleces and adults of *E. granulosus* from Kenya and the UK, and of protoscoleces of *E. multilocularis* (Data from McManus & Smyth 1978, McManus 1981).

Parasite	Host origin	Protein	Polysaccharides	Lipids	RNA	DNA
E. multilocularis	cotton rat	618 ± 11	120 ± 7	161 ± 13	73 ± 1	8 ± 0.3
E. granulosus	horse*	550 ± 10	177 ± 2	109 ± 4	60 ± 4	5 ± 0.1
	sheep*	625 ± 12	169 ± 1	88 ± 3	89 ± 4	5 ± 0.1
	sheep	592 ± 16	166 ± 4	76 ± 4	74 ± 6	7 ± 1
	cattle	547 ± 14	146 ± 3	118 ± 6	52 ± 4	6 ± 1
	goat	569 ± 16	166 ± 4	95 ± 3	54 ± 4	6 ± 1
	camel	550 ± 17	215 ± 6	113 ± 4	53 ± 4	5 ± 1
	human	668 ± 16	164 ± 4	122 ± 4	57 ± 5	4 ± 1
	dog†	712 ± 18	139 ± 5	143 ± 4	96 ± 6	6 ± 1
	dog (natural)	584 ± 16	213 ± 8	122 ± 4	203 ± 7	4 ± 1

* From the UK.

† Experimental infection with protoscoleces of human origin.

glucosamine, predominated and displayed infra-red spectral characteristics similar to chitin and to Type XIV pneumococcal polysaccharides. These early results have, in general, been confirmed histochemically by Richards (1984), working with the horse strain of *E. granulosus*, passaged into BALB/c mice. This study also showed that the carbohydrate component possessed 1,2-glycols, that the protein complex was predominantly basic with identifiable SS groups and that acid mucopolysaccharide material was present in the laminated layer. The mucopolysaccharide material is produced in and subsequently released from mucopolysaccharide bodies present in the lipid and glycogen-rich germinal layer (Richards *et al.* 1984).

Mucopolysaccharides are also present in HF, protoscoleces and adults (Kilejian *et al.* 1962). Upon electrophoresis, the mucopolysaccharide from HF and the laminated layer migrated differently to that from protoscoleces and adults suggesting differences in the number of ionised sites per polymer unit. Moreover, that in the laminated layer was destroyed by Pflüger's treatment (involving digestion in concentrated potassium hydroxide) but not that from protoscoleces and adults, indicating a major difference in biophysical properties.

RESPIRATORY METABOLISM

Metacestode

Protoscoleces of *E. granulosus* live in a complex environment within the hydatid cyst. Cyst fluid contains a range of substances – acetic, propionic, valeric, succinic and higher fatty acids, various amino acids and carbohydrates (see above) – all of which testify to the specialised metabolism of cyst tissue. Agosin *et al.* (1957), found that protoscoleces have aerobic and anaerobic components of respiration. Both modes are clearly dependent on glycolysis, as glycolytic inhibitors are effective against each of them. At least four hexokinases are present, and there was some evidence for their modulation by adenine nucleotides. Many other enzymes of glycolysis, as well as myokinase, mannose isomerase and phosphatases, were detected. Pentose phosphate pathway enzyme activities suggest that the pathway may operate *in vivo* (Agosin & Aravena 1959, 1960a,b). Further evidence to support this view was obtained using glucose labelled with radiocarbon in the 1 or 6 positions (Agosin & Repetto 1961).

Although aerobic respiration is cyanide and fluoracetate sensitive, implying the involvement of cytochromes and the tricarboxylic acid cycle (citrate synthase), malonate is without effect. Malonate is a potent inhibitor of succinic dehydrogenase, so it seems likely that the tricarboxylic acid cycle is incomplete. The major respiratory substrate appears to be glycogen (Agosin 1957) under both aerobic and anaerobic conditions, and it is probable that greater amounts of glycogen are used when oxygen is absent. The most important respiratory end products are lactic and succinic acids, but acetic and pyruvic acids and ethanol are also produced in small quantities.

Agosin and Repetto (1963) found that intact scoleces and whole homogenates oxidise a range of tricarboxylic acid intermediates as well as glutamate, glyoxylate, glycollate, acetate and lactate. All the enzymes of the tricarboxylic acid cycle were found either in whole homogenates or acetone powders. However, malate synthase and isocitrate lyase were not detected, providing circumstantial but not definitive evidence for the absence of the glyoxylate cycle. Glutamate uptake was presumed to be mediated by glutamate dehydrogenase or transaminase, yielding 2-oxoglutarate which enters the tricarboxylic acid cycle. Acetate is activated by an acetyl coenzyme A (acetyl CoA) kinase, and used for polysaccharide synthesis, although radiocarbon from acetate appears in respiratory end products also. Radiocarbon from $^{14}CO_2$ is incorporated – as is commonly observed – into a wide range of cell components, probably via phosphoenolpyruvate carboxykinase and malic enzyme activities. The former enzyme is an important component in the path to succinic acid (Agosin & Repetto 1965).

Fumarate reductase is another key enzyme on the path to succinic acid. It is an important component of anaerobic metabolism, because it transfers electrons from reduced nicotinamide adenine dinucleotide to fumarate, which thus becomes reduced to succinate. A molecule of ATP is generated in the process. Fumarate reductase activity is present in protoscoleces and is evidenced by the presence of a *b*-type cytochrome which is reduced by NADH and which, in turn, reduces fumarate. This also provides support for the idea that *E. granulosus* possesses a cytochrome system similar to that observed in *Moniezia expansa* and the Taeniid tapeworms (Bryant 1970).

Adult

Remarkably little work has been carried out on the adult stage. Bryant and Morseth (1968), using 33 day old adult worms from artificially infected dogs, showed that fumarate is rapidly taken up under aerobic conditions and converted to succinate and malate. Alanine was also formed. Uptake of radiocarbon from a range of substrates produced incorporation patterns consistent with the view that adults, like the larvae, possess an incomplete tricarboxylic acid cycle and emphasise succinic acid production via a fumarate reductase.

In summary, therefore, it appears that *E. granulosus* possesses the usual glycolytic sequence to the level of phosphoenolpyruvate. A variety of compounds, glycogen and six-carbon sugars can be used as respiratory substrates. As in other helminths there are several options for the further metabolism of phosphoenolpyruvate: formation of pyruvate and lactic acid, or acetyl CoA and partial oxidation via an incomplete tricarboxylic acid cycle, or conversion to oxaloacetate, malate, fumarate and succinate.

Regulation of respiratory pathways

In recent years, the emphasis in studies of parasite biochemistry has drifted away from the elucidation of pathways and has moved towards attempting to understand how the pathways are regulated. Although there are numerous instances of such parasitological studies in the literature, only one has been carried out with *E. granulosus*: that of McManus and Smyth (1982).

McManus and Smyth (1982) measured the activities of glycolytic and associated enzymes and the concentrations of their substrates in the protoscoleces of two strains of *E. granulosus* and one of *E. multilocularis*. They were able to demonstrate, by assays of each of the enzymes, a complete glycolytic pathway. By comparing the observed mass action ratios of these enzymes with their theoretical equilibrium constants, they determined that phosphorylase, hexokinase, phosphofructokinase and pyruvate kinase were regulators of carbon flow in glycolysis. This observation is similar to those made with other organisms.

Pyruvate kinase from the two species of *Echinococcus* was stimulated by fructose bisphosphate but was not inhibited by alanine, a common invertebrate allosteric effector. However, in cestodes it has been observed that malate is inhibitory to pyruvate kinase (Bryant 1972), and it is possible that it has the same role in *E. granulosus*. Phosphoenolpyruvate carboxykinase is more specific for IDP than ADP but is activated to a greater extent by Mg^{2+} than Mn^{2+}. This conflicts with observations made by Agosin and Repetto (1965) on protoscoleces from their South American sheep strain, and with those of other workers on other parasites (Bryant 1975). In each of these cases the enzyme is more sensitive to Mn^{2+}.

The three parasites investigated by McManus and Smyth (1982) possess complete tricarboxylic acid cycles with relatively high activities. On the other hand fumarate reductase, which catalyses the reverse reaction to succinic dehydrogenase, had a low activity (Table 4.2). However, the authors consider that their assay method would have seriously underestimated fumarate reductase activity, because of its instability and because it is notoriously difficult to measure.

The precise role of the tricarboxylic acid cycle is difficult to assess in parasitic helminths because a respiratory end product is also an intermediate in the cycle. However, McManus and Smyth (1978) showed that there were marked differences in oxygen uptake between the sheep and horse strains of *E. granulosus*. This may imply that there exist biochemical 'morphs' with greater or lesser dependence of tricarboxylic acid cycle activity. If this is so, the phenomenon may be similar to that observed in *Haemonchus contortus* by Bennet and Bryant (1984).

It is clear from end product analysis that, while the tricarboxylic acid cycle is functional at least in part in *E. granulosus*, fermentative pathways yielding acetic, succinic and lactic acid occur even under aerobic conditions. Presumably, as in other helminths, the formation of succinic

Table 4.2 The activities of the tricarboxylic acid cycle enzymes in protoscoleces of *E. granulosus* (horse and sheep strains) and *E. multilocularis* (from McManus and Smyth 1982); activities, expressed as nanomoles per minute per milligram of protein at 30°C, are means ± S.E.M.; for malate dehydrogenase (OXO–MAL), n = 8; for all other enzymes, n = 3.

Enzyme	*E. g.* horse	*E. g.* sheep	*E. m.*
citrate synthase	60 ± 8	36 ± 5	23 ± 4
aconitase	25 ± 5	62 ± 7	43 ± 6
isocitrate dehydrogenase			
NADP; Mn^{2+}	25 ± 3	73 ± 6	193 ± 24
NADP; Mg^{2+}	17 ± 2	44 ± 3	86 ± 10
NAD; Mn^{2+}	35 ± 4	29 ± 3	16 ± 2
NAD; Mg^{2+}	29 ± 2	18 ± 2	12 ± 1
2-oxoglutarate dehydrogenase	60 ± 10	20 ± 4	46 ± 6
succinate dehydrogenase	13 ± 3	7 ± 2	11 ± 3
fumarate reductase	1 ± 0.3	2 ± 1	1 ± 0.4
fumarase	36 ± 9	39 ± 6	39 ± 7
malate dehydrogenase			
OXO–MAL	4769 ± 389	6809 ± 542	7023 ± 623
MAL–OXO	20 ± 4	14 ± 3	13 ± 2

and acetic acids occur in the mitochondria. Whether this occurs in the same mitochondria which house the tricarboxylic acid cycle is unknown.

In the pathway illustrated in Figure 4.1, NAD(P)H produced from the glyceraldehyde-3-phosphate dehydrogenase step in glycolysis and by the activity of cytoplasmic malic enzyme can be reoxidised by the reduction of pyruvate to lactate or ethanol and of oxaloacetate to malate. It is possible, however, that the cytoplasmic malic enzyme is an artefact of preparation, and results from mitochondrial disruption. In *Ascaris*, what appears to be a soluble malic enzyme is located in the intercristal space of the mitochondria (Köhler *et al.* 1983). In the mitochondrion, reducing equivalents generated on the acetate arm are used to drive the fumarate reductase reaction in the generation of succinate.

The adenine nucleotide contents of the protoscoleces of *E. granulosus* and *E. multilocularis* are comparable with those of other parasites; the adenylate energy charges ([ATP] + [ADP])/([ATP] + [ADP] + [AMP]), at 0.86–0.92 are, however, the highest recorded for a parasite (McManus & Smyth 1982). ATP:AMP ratios are also very high and probably reflect the low demand for ATP in a fully developed protoscolex in a hydatid cyst.

PROTEINS AND AMINO ACIDS

Composition

Other than some information on the composition of the scolex hooks, little is known of the structural proteins in *E. granulosus*. As in a number

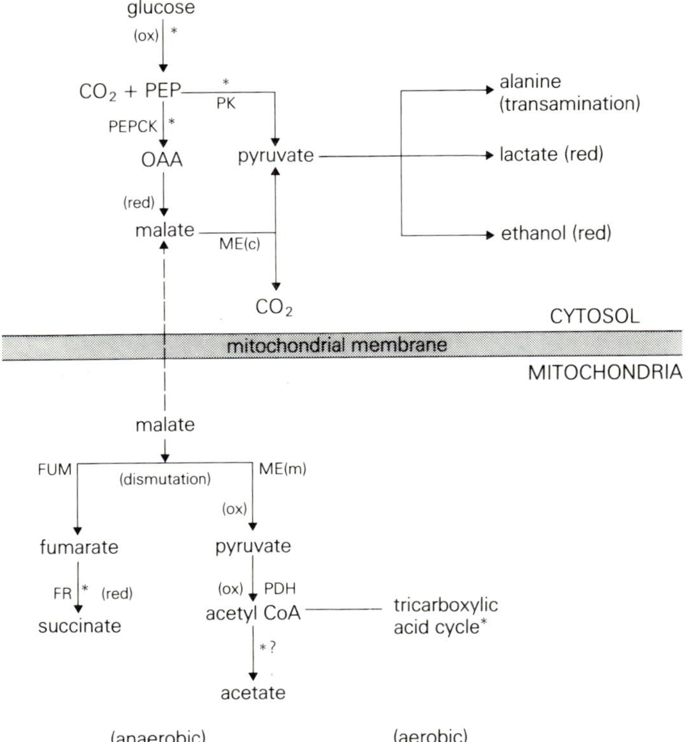

Figure 4.1 Respiratory metabolism in *E. granulosus*. ★, sites of ATP synthesis; ox, red, oxidative and reductive processes; PK, pyruvate kinase; PEPCK, phosphoenolpyruvate carboxykinase; ME(c), ME(m), malic enzyme (cytosolic) or (mitochondrial); FR, fumarate reductase; PDH, pyruvate dehydrogenase complex. When cytosol or mitochondria are in redox equilibrium, the number of oxidative reactions equals the number of reductive ones. This is achieved by regulating the carbon flow.

of other cyclophyllidean species, the hooks give histochemical reactions and have chemical and physical properties consistent with those of a keratin-type protein (Gallagher 1964).

In contrast, soluble proteins have received special attention mainly because their study facilitates the identification and characterisation of specific antigens for use in serological diagnosis, and for study of the immune response in hydatid disease. These aspects will be covered in detail elsewhere (Ch. 6 & 8). However, it is appropriate to outline here some of the methods used in attempts to characterise *E. granulosus* proteins. Despite a large number of studies, information concerning the precise nature of these proteins is very limited. Moreover, it is restricted to the cystic stage as almost nothing is known of the adult proteins.

The complexity of the proteins of *E. granulosus* has been appreciated only since immunoelectrophoresis (IEP), immunodiffusion, isoelectric focusing (IEF), polyacrylamide gel electrophoresis (PAGE) and sodium dodecylsulphate polyacrylamide gel electrophoresis (SDS-PAGE) have been introduced. Most attention has been paid to the protein composition of hydatid fluid (HF), particularly that of sheep cyst origin. IEP has revealed at least 19 components, of which 10 are distinct antigens of parasite origin (Biguet *et al.* 1962, Chordi & Kagan 1965, Capron *et al.* 1967, Castagnari & Pozzuoli 1969). PAGE separated sheep HF into 17 protein fractions (Muntyan 1973) and preliminary analysis, by SDS-PAGE (D. P. McManus, unpublished), has revealed at least 20 components. Currently only two of the parasite proteins in HF have been purified and their chemical and immunological characteristics studied, namely the thermolabile lipoprotein, Antigen A (also referred to as Antigen 5) (Capron *et al.* 1967) and the thermostable lipoprotein, Antigen B (Oriol *et al.* 1971). Both antigens also occur in *E. multilocularis* (Varela-Diaz *et al.* 1977, Rickard *et al.* 1977, Davies *et al.* 1978). (For a full discussion of antigen characterisation and terminology, see Ch. 8.)

The host serum components demonstrated in HF of *E. granulosus* include albumin and several different classes of immunoglobulin (IgG, IgG_1, IgG_2 and IgM, but not IgA) (Kagan & Agosin 1968, Coltorti & Varela-Diaz 1974, 1975, Hustead & Williams 1977, Edwards 1982). Similarly, host serum proteins (IgG and IgM) are present within the layers of the cyst and on the surface of protoscoleces of *E. multilocularis* (Kassis & Tanner 1977). IgG_1, IgG_{2a}, IgG_{2b} were also detectable on the laminated layer of intact cysts but not on the germinal layer; in contrast albumin was found on the laminated layer, germinal layer and within the intact cyst (Ali-Khan & Siboo 1981).

In vitro permeability studies on hydatid cysts of *E. granulosus*, obtained from rodents by experimental secondary infection, have shown protein uptake to be irregular; only a small percentage (20 per cent) of cysts took up ^{125}I–labelled proteins (Coltorti & Varela-Diaz 1975, Hustead & Williams 1977 and see Ch. 9). It was suggested (Coltorti & Varela-Diaz 1975) that, as the germinal layer regulates protein entry, the germinal layer had been fissured in these particular cysts. An alternative explanation was put forward by Hustead and Williams (1977) who speculated on the occurrence of intermittent or cyclic uptake activity combined with rapid degradation of internalised proteins. It is clear that much more information is required in this important area and, in particular, future emphasis might be placed on understanding protein uptake mechanisms in cysts obtained by the primary infection route, i.e. cysts originating from eggs fed *per os*.

In *E. granulosus* 15 and 19 protein fractions were identified by PAGE in soluble extracts of the germinal (+ laminated?) layer and protoscoleces respectively (Muntyan 1973). IEF separated extracts, both of protoscoleces of *E. granulosus* and total larval tissue of *E. multilocularis*, into a larger number (*c.* 60) of protein components (Kumaratilake & Thompson 1979, Kumaratilake *et al.* 1979). Similarly, as depicted in Figure 4.2a, the SDS-PAGE protein profile for protoscoleces of *E. granulosus* (horse strain) is

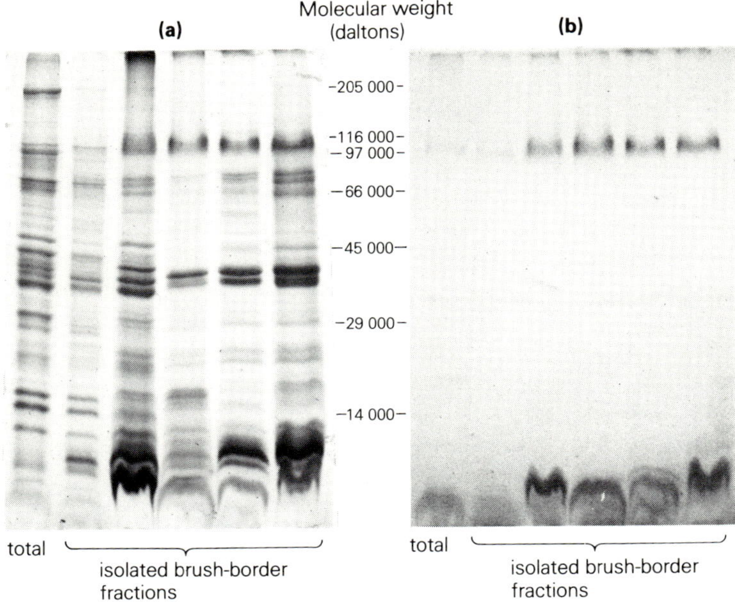

Figure 4.2 SDS-PAGE (5–15 per cent linear gradient gel) separated proteins of the total worm homogenate and isolated brush border fractions from protoscoleces of *E. granulosus* (horse strain). (a) Coomassie blue staining; (b) Periodic acid-Schiff (PAS) staining. *Note*: in (b) the two major staining glycoproteins (arrowed) and the pronounced PAS staining material running close to, or with, the tracking dye at the end of the gel. [Reproduced by kind permission of Cambridge University Press.]

equally complex and at least 50 polypeptides, ranging in approximate molecular weight greater than 200 000 daltons to less than 14 000 daltons, can be identified (McManus & Barrett 1985). The protein profiles for isolated brush-border fractions (enriched with microtriches and external plasma membrane) are also illustrated in Figure 4.2a. Two major PAS-staining bands, representing glycopeptides and/or glycoproteins of 110 000 daltons and >200 000 daltons, and PAS-positive material running close to or with the tracking dye (probably glycolipid) are detectable in all preparations (Fig. 4.2b). It is probable that these PAS-positive components originate principally from the glycocalyx. This polyionic covering, rich in carbohydrates, is particularly dense in the posterior region of the protoscolex where it covers the developing microtriches (Smyth 1969a). The glycocalyx is also present in protoscoleces of *E. multilocularis* (Sakamoto & Sugimura 1969) and it seems likely that in both parasites this layer acts as a protective covering against host proteolytic enzymes and/or immunoglobulin action.

According to Kagan (1963), the protoscolex is composed mainly of parasitic antigenic components but, as discussed above, HF in which brood capsules and protoscoleces are bathed contains a number of host proteins. Moreover, albumins and globulins formed one-third of the protein composition of protoscoleces obtained from sheep cysts (Frayha & Haddad 1980). An immunochemical approach for identifying the origin of the polypeptides depicted in Figure 4.2 has, therefore, been developed (McManus & Macpherson 1984). It involves a modification of techniques developed for the molecular analysis of the nematode surface and subsequently used to characterise surface antigens of *Schistosoma mansoni* (reviewed by Philipp & Rumjanek 1984). In short, proteins on the parasite surface are labelled with $Na^{125}I$ by the iodogen method (Fraker & Speck 1978) and/or Bolton–Hunter reagent (Bolton & Hunter 1973). In the former method, radiolabel is coupled to tyrosine and, in the latter, lysine residues. Radiolabelled proteins are then solubilised in deoxycholate and separated into lentil–lectin adherent (glycoprotein) or non-adherent fractions prior to further fractionation by SDS-PAGE and autoradiography. Proteins which are of host origin can be immune precipitated by incubation of labelled extracts in antiserum raised in rabbits against the serum components of the host animal (sheep, horse, man, etc.), followed by precipitation of antigen–antibody complexes with an excess of the appropriate anti-Ig serum. Precipitated host antigens can then be analysed by electrophoresis and autoradiography. Using these methods, a pilot programme (D. P. McManus & R. M. E. Parkhouse unpublished) showed that the external surface of protoscoleces of the horse and sheep strains of *E. granulosus* could be labelled, both with iodogen and with the Bolton–Hunter reagent. These results are illustrated in Figure 4.3 and they indicate that different proteins are labelled by the two techniques and that significant qualitative differences exist between the surface proteins of the two strains.

An interesting protein, probably a lipoprotein, with a relatively large amount of cystine, has been demonstrated histochemically in rostellar gland secretions of *E. granulosus* (Smyth 1964, Smyth *et al.* 1969, Thompson *et al.* 1979). Various functions have been suggested for these secretions, including association with hook formation, nutrition, adhesion, regulation of mitochondrial biogenesis, maturation of ova, release of gravid proglottids, and protection by inhibiting the ability of the host to detect the worm's presence or blocking the action of the host's immune response (see also Ch. 1). These secretions thus represent an especially fascinating aspect of the host–parasite relationship. Their characterisation, and particularly that of the lipoprotein component, using biochemical fractionation techniques, would clearly be rewarding.

Metabolism

Acid and alkaline phosphatases, 5'-nucleotidase and maltase have recently been shown, by enzyme analysis, to be present in the surface of protoscoleces of *E. granulosus* (McManus & Barrett 1985). This finding supports previous evidence from *in vitro* studies (Smyth 1972) that the

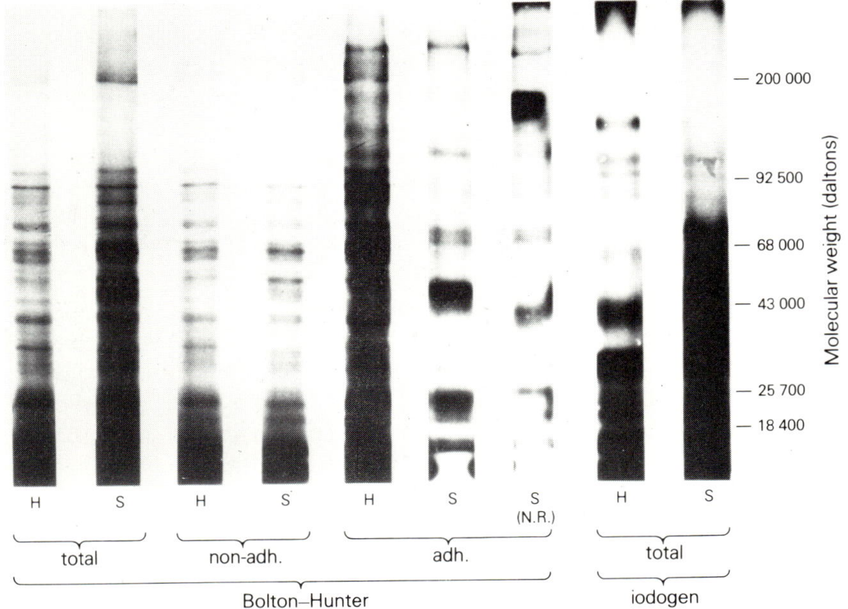

Figure 4.3 Iodination of protoscoleces of the horse (H) and sheep (S) strains of *E. granulosus*. Tot., total soluble protein fractions; Adh., lentil–lectin adherent fractions; Non-adh., non-adherent fractions; N.R., separation under non-reducing conditions, i.e. without β-mercaptoethanol.

scolex of *E. granulosus* can digest proteins at the host/parasite interface by membrane (contact) digestion. Whether proteins are, additionally, taken up by pinocytosis is, as yet, not known; early attempts to demonstrate this process in *E. granulosus* using ferritin proved unsuccessful (Smyth 1969a). Only recently, with the use of horseradish peroxidase, ruthenium red and lanthanum nitrate, has it been shown unequivocally that macromolecular uptake occurs in cestodes (Hopkins *et al.* 1978, Threadgold & Hopkins 1981). Clearly, it would be of particular interest to use these more appropriate tracers to assess the role and extent of pinocytosis occurring both in the larval and adult stages of *E. granulosus*.

With regard to amino acids, no unusual information has emerged from limited, early studies restricted to the cystic stage of *E. granulosus* (Pozzi & Pirosky 1953, Krvavica *et al.* 1959, Mastrandrea *et al.* 1962, Sanchez & Sanchez 1971). Amino acid content (both bound and free pool) shows no major departure from that found in other organisms, although the uncommon β-alanine has been reported in the cyst fluid and germinal layer of sterile pig cysts (Krvavica *et al.* 1959). No information is available for the precise amino acid requirements of *E. granulosus* but successful culture *in vitro* (see Ch. 5) can only be obtained with the use of tissue culture media (e.g. NCTC 135) containing a complex mixture of amino acids (Smyth & Davies 1974). Similarly, there are no data on amino acid uptake mechanisms in *E. granulosus* and knowledge of biosynthetic pathways is scanty. Transamination reactions, involving aminotransferases, for the interconversion of amino acids probably occur, GOT and GPT having been detected in cyst fluid and protoscoleces (Sanchez & Sanchez 1971, Frayha & Haddad 1980).

Amino acids (Krvavica *et al.* 1959), urea, uric acid, creatinine and betaine (Codounis & Polydoridès 1936) have long been considered as end products of protein metabolism in *E. granulosus* but the metabolic pathways whereby these components are produced are almost unknown. An ornithine–urea cycle does not appear to function despite the presence of ornithine transcarbamylase, arginino-succinate lyase and arginase (Janssens & Bryant 1969). Urea must, therefore, be formed by some as yet undetermined pathway, such as that of purine degradation.

LIPIDS

Knowledge of lipid metabolism in *E. granulosus* is limited. Studies have been confined mainly to quantitative and qualitative examination of the lipid content and its distribution in the larval stage of *E. granulosus*. Some data also exist on the total lipid content of the adults of *E. granulosus* and protoscoleces of *E. multilocularis* (Table 4.1). Much of the available information has been comprehensively reviewed recently by Frayha and Smyth (1983).

Coutelen (1931b) performed an early histochemical investigation of the germinal layer and found some cells charged with neutral lipids. Vercelli-Retta *et al.* (1975) showed that these lipids were especially accumulated in the differentiated metabolic zones related to brood capsule insertions. In other zones, esterase, lipase and dehydrogenase enzymes, involved in energy metabolism, were very active. They concluded that a metabolic cellular cycle was operating in the germinal layer and that esterified lipids of host origin could be hydrolysed for use by the germinal layer and/or by the brood capsules and protoscoleces.

Early biochemical investigations (Flössner 1924, 1925, Coutelen 1931a) identified acetic, propionic, valeric and higher fatty acids in HF. Acetate and, to a lesser extent, propionate were subsequently detected as metabolic end products of protoscoleces of *E. granulosus* and *E. multilocularis*; acetate was also secreted by adults of *E. granulosus* (Agosin 1957, Dicowsky *et al.* 1968, McManus & Smyth 1978, McManus 1981). Isotope studies (Frayha 1971) showed that acetate could also be used as a substrate by larvae of *E. granulosus* and *E. multilocularis*, being oxidised to CO_2 and incorporated into saponifiable and non-saponifiable lipids.

Digenis *et al.* (1970) identified 17 fatty acids in protoscoleces of *E. granulosus* ranging in chain length from 12 to 20 carbon atoms. Vessal *et al.* (1972) identified an additional major saturated fatty acid category with 22 carbon atoms and found that more than 50 per cent of the total fatty acids were composed of C_{18} fatty acids. There is no information on long chain fatty acid synthesis in *Echinococcus* species, but platyhelminths generally appear unable to synthesise long chain fatty acids *de novo* or desaturate preformed long chain fatty acids (Barrett 1981).

Vessal *et al.* (1972) also fractionated the polar lipids of protoscoleces into lysolecithin, sphingomyelin, lecithin, phosphatidylinositol, sulfatides, cerebrosides, cephalins and cholesterol. These findings were substantiated by Frayha's group (Frayha *et al.* 1980), which also identified the presence of seven major classes of lipids (phospholipids, fatty acids, cholesterol, cholesterol esters, mono-, di- and triglycerides) both in HF and protoscoleces (Frayha *et al.* 1980, Frayha & Haddad 1980). Lecithin and cholesterol in *E. granulosus* (Kilejian *et al.* 1962) and triglycerides in *E. multilocularis* (Wasylishen & Novak 1983) have also been detected by infra-red and ^{13}C-nuclear magnetic resonance (NMR) spectroscopy respectively.

Cholesterol is the only sterol so far identified in *Echinococcus* and is present in the layers of the hydatid cyst (Čmelik 1952) and in protoscoleces of *E. granulosus* and *E. multilocularis* (Frayha 1974, Frayha *et al.* 1980, Frayha & Haddad 1980). As is the case with other helminths (Barrett 1981), this sterol cannot be synthesised *de novo* from acetate or mevalonate by the *Echinococcus* organisms. Instead, it is obtained either directly from the host (Frayha 1968) or in an esterified form which is subsequently hydrolysed by an esterase (Digenis *et al.* 1970). A study of the mechanisms for cholesterol absorption by hydatid cysts of *E. granulosus* (Bahr *et al.* 1979) indicated that simple diffusion and possibly exchange diffusion operate, at least *in vitro*.

NUCLEIC ACIDS

Only limited work has been carried out on nucleic acids and nucleic acid metabolism in *Echinococcus*. In early investigations, Čmelik and Briski (1953) were unable to demonstrate DNA in the hydatid cyst wall of *E. granulosus* but, Kilejian *et al.* (1961) found variable amounts in the germinal but not laminated layer. In regard to protoscoleces, DNA and RNA represented 0.8 and 7.3 per cent of the dry weight respectively in *E. multilocularis* (Table 4.1; McManus & Smyth 1978). The values for *E. granulosus* depended on the strain analysed and varied between 0.4 and 0.8 per cent of the dry weight for DNA and between 5.2 and 8.9 per cent of the dry weight for RNA (Table 4.1; McManus & Smyth 1978, McManus 1981). In adults of *E. granulosus*, DNA constituted about 0.5 per cent of the dry weight but RNA varied between 10 and 20 per cent, depending on the stage of development of analysed worms. As might be expected, the RNA content was greater in mature egg-producing worms undergoing rapid protein synthesis (McManus 1981).

The base composition of nuclear DNA is characteristic of an organism and is usually expressed as the percentage of guanosine + cytosine (G+C) bases. Thus, the G+C value for the DNA of *E. multilocularis* was found to be 44 per cent (Kilejian & MacInnis 1976), a value similar to that of invertebrates generally. Similar data are not yet available for the DNA of *E. granulosus*, although Zekavat and Khayat (1971) found that DNA, isolated from protoscoleces of sheep origin, had a melting point of 78°C and an adenine:thymine ratio of 0.87. In addition, these workers obtained a melting point of 56°C for the parasite amino-acyl soluble RNA (sRNA) and found the ratios of RNA phosphorus and DNA phosphorus in protoscoleces and in cat, sheep and human liver to be very similar. Their main conclusion was that the sRNA and DNA of protoscoleces had similar structural and biochemical features to those of the host.

There are three different types of RNA in cells, namely, ribosomal RNA (rRNA), transfer RNA (tRNA) and messenger RNA (mRNA). The RNA species from protoscoleces of *E. granulosus* of sheep origin have been very comprehensively characterised in terms of nucleotide composition, sedimentation properties, template activity and with regard to biosynthetic kinetics (Agosin *et al.* 1971). The rRNAs had sedimentation coefficients of 29.4 and 19.6, were rich in guanosine-5'-monosphosphate and did not show 1:1 base pairing with regard to adenosine–uracil and guanosine–cytosine. In addition, a light RNA fraction (sedimentation coefficient = 6.3) was isolated which corresponded with tRNA, and two additional, heavier RNA fractions (sedimentation coefficients of 35 and 40–42.5) were apparent when labelled nuclear or total RNA was analysed. Biosynthesis of RNA followed the pattern established for eukaryotic cells and involved the synthesis of low molecular weight RNA species in the first instance and the synthesis of heavier RNAs subsequently. The 35 and 40–42.5 s RNAs were shown to be precursors of rRNA as these were the first species to disappear when protoscoleces were incubated with actinomycin D. A rapidly labelled RNA fraction (corresponding to a sedimentation coefficient of 13–14 s) had substantial template (i.e. stimulated protein synthesis *in vitro*) activity and it was suggested that this fraction contained mRNA.

OSMOTIC AND IONIC RELATIONSHIPS

This is an important but again little explored area with regard to *Echinococcus*. The permeability of secondary *E. granulosus* hydatid cysts to water, sodium and chloride ions has been determined *in vitro* under steady-state conditions by Rotunno *et al.* (1974) (see also Ch. 9). Water diffused rapidly across the layers of the cyst (diffusional permeability, 1.88×10^{-4} $cm^2\ s^{-1}$) and this rate increased after preincubation of cysts with antidiuretic hormone; permeability to sodium and chloride was, in contrast, relatively slow (0.13 and 0.035 $\mu mol\ h^{-1}\ cm^{-1}$ respectively).

Studies of water and electrolyte balance in protoscoleces of *E. granulosus* from sheep have been carried out *in vitro* by Reisin and his co-workers (Reisin & Rotunno 1981, Reisin *et al.* 1981). Their data imply the existence of an active transport mechanism for Na^+ and K^+ and they suggested that the energy required to maintain the Na–K balance within protoscoleces is largely provided by anaerobic pathways, with oxidative metabolism being only accessory to the energy balance.

The relationship between osmotic pressure and protoscolex evagination was studied by De Rycke and his group using various media including Ringer's solution, sodium glycocholate, sodium taurocholate (De Rycke 1968), sodium chloride and sucrose (De Rycke & van Grembergen 1969). In general, evagination occurred in hyposmotic media below 1.5–2.5 atm (as a result of endosmosis and hence designated 'passive evagination') or in isosmotic media, i.e. 5–7 atm (due to muscular activity leading to 'active evagination'). Evagination was inhibited in hyperosomotic media and complete incubation occurred at 10–13 atm. Pretreatment of protoscoleces in artificial gastric juice minimised these effects and it was concluded that gastric juice, and not osmotic pressure, probably provides the essential influence for rapid evagination *in vivo*. In fact, it is now generally recognised that bile salts provide the major trigger for evagination of the scolex, both in *Echinococcus* and other cestodes (Smyth 1969a, and see Chs 1 & 5).

STRAIN VARIATION

Biochemical composition

An interesting problem in parasite biochemistry, illustrated well by the *Echinococcus* complex, is that of strain variation. The biological and physiological variation which occurs between different isolates of *E. granulosus* is dealt with elsewhere in this book (Ch. 1). Biochemical differences between strains are just as marked and provide a striking example of a phenomenon which is now also apparent in other helminths, for example *Hymenlopis diminuta* and *Haemonchus contortus* (Bryant 1983). McManus and Smyth (1978) found significant differences in the biochemical compositions of horse and sheep strains of *E. granulosus* protoscoleces. The horse strain contained less protein and RNA and more lipid than the sheep strain. *E. multilocularis* had more lipid and DNA than either; otherwise it occupied an intermediate position. Of much greater interest were the differences in respiratory parameters. Under aerobic conditions, the sheep strain used more oxygen and glycogen and produced more succinic and acetic acids but less lactic acid than the horse strain. Anaerobically, there was little difference in glycogen utilisation, but the sheep strain produced less succinic and lactic acids, and more acetic acid and ethanol. In other words, both aerobically and anaerobically, the major end products of the sheep strain were mainly acetic acid with some succinic acid, whereas those of the horse strain were mainly lactic acid with some succinic acid. *E. multilocularis* showed an entirely different pattern in each case which is not surprising in view of its separate status as a species.

A much wider ranging study of *E. granulosus* from Kenya involving protoscoleces from five different host species and adults confirmed this variability (McManus 1981). Lactic acid production varied from about 5 per cent (goat, anaerobic) to about 45 per cent (man, aerobic), acetate from about 13 per cent (camel, aerobic) to about 55 per cent (sheep, anaerobic), and succinic acid from 15 per cent (sheep, aerobic) to about 55 per cent (cattle, aerobic). Similar variations occur in Australian strains of *E. granulosus*. For example, protoscoleces from sheep in New South Wales produced, on incubation, 41 per cent succinic acid and 25 per cent lactic acid, whereas those from Tasmanian sheep produced 29 and 35 per cent respectively. The differences are significant at the level $P<0.025$. Further, protoscoleces isolated from a wallaby in Queensland excreted almost no succinic acid, 61 per cent lactic acid and 35 per cent acetic acid (C. A. Behm, C. Bryant & R. C. A. Thompson unpublished).

Metabolism

The significance of the above variation is not clear and neither is its full extent known. However, it is important to distinguish between adaptation and regulation. The changes which take place when protoscoleces of a given strain are incubated first aerobically and then anaerobically are regulatory. That is, the changed environment imposes constraints on metabolism, pool sizes of metabolites adjust and a new pattern of carbon flow is achieved which presumably optimises energy production for that organism under those particular conditions. This is because the activities of enzymes are modulated by the changes in concentrations of intermediates in the metabolic pathways. The proportion of end products thus change as an indirect result of environmental change.

Adaptation is a condition of permanency, in which one organism differs from another because it has been 'tuned' to a different environment. Tuning may be the result of modifications in the genome or in the control of genomic expression. Theoretically, it is not reversible, but regulation within the boundaries of that adaptation is still possible. Thus, the differences observed in the formation of respiratory end products between the strains from various sources when incubated anaerobically are adaptive; the changes which take place when their environments are changed are regulatory.

This idea has a considerable impact on our understanding of metabolism, and it becomes important to distinguish between the terms 'optimal' and 'maximal' when applied to energy metabolism in parasites. In an optimal energy-producing system, production of ATP is not maximised, but held at the highest possible level consistent with other constraints on the organisms. In a maximal system, the theoretical yield of ATP from a given amount of substrate is achieved. If different strains of *E. granulosus* vary in the relative amounts of end products that they produce, then they may be optimising energy production, but they are not necessarily maximising it. This idea has been developed more fully by

Hochachka (1980) in his book *Living without oxygen*. In the evolution of metabolic systems, he sees two needs, the first is the capacity to compete successfully for substrates on the one hand (kinetic efficiency) and the need to maximise energy production on the other (energetics). Although he is discussing glycolysis, his concluding observation is worth repeating. Hochachka writes that '. . . neither ATP yield nor competitive capacity was maximised. Rather both were compromised. And in the compromise between energetics and kinetic efficiency (undoubtedly set in primeval time) the overall biological function was optimised.' If such a compromise is necessary for the evolution of a metabolic pathway, it is even more necessary for the subsequent evolution of organisms. Variation is symptomatic of adaptation and adaptation is the stuff of speciation. The biochemical compromises made by *E. granulosus* in adapting to new hosts can only be conjectured. However, they provide a marvellous opportunity for the biologist to observe speciation in action.

To illustrate this point, Table 4.3 shows the result of calculations of ATP yield of the various strains studied by McManus (1981) in Kenya and the UK. It is assumed that the conversion of one molecule of phosphoenolpyruvate to lactic acid yields one molecule of ATP at the pyruvate kinase step; that the conversion of one molecule of phosphoenolpyruvate to acetic acid yields two molecules of ATP, at the phosphoenolpyruvate carboxykinase and pyruvate decarboxylase steps and that the conversion of one molecule of phosphoenolpyruvate to succinic acid yields two molecules of ATP at the phosphoenolpyruvate carboxykinase and fumarate reductase steps. The maximum yield of ATP,

Table 4.3 Optimisation or maximisation? ATP production by anaerobic processes in *E. granulosus*: number of moles of ATP generated per 50 mol of end products formed, calculated from observed end-product formation by parasites from the UK and Kenya; calculated from data in McManus (1981).

	Incubation condition	
	O_2 absent	O_2 present
maximum theoretical yield	100	100
larvae		
sheep (UK)	92	89
sheep	92	90
cattle	–	85
goat	97	88
camel	–	80
man	92	78
adults		
dog (experimentally infected)	93	92
dog (natural infection)	91	85

from phosphoenolpyruvate with mitochondria in redox balance giving 33.3 per cent acetic and 66.6 per cent succinic acids, is 100 moles for each 50 moles of end products. The average observed yield aerobically is about 87, increasing to about 93 anaerobically. This increase (significant at the level $P<.05$) is generally achieved by shifting emphasis away from lactic acid production to the production of acetic and succinic acids. The results are surprisingly consistent; however, when reducing equivalents are calculated for mitochondria alone, in almost all cases there is an apparent imbalance. Acetic acid is usually produced in the largest amounts, and that means that there is an apparent excess of reducing equivalents. It implies the existence of other, unknown, metabolic pathways in mitochondria.

Of course, although in other helminths there is strong circumstantial evidence for the existence of the phosphorylation steps discussed here, there is as yet no definitive proof for their presence in *E. granulosus*. The one for which there is the greatest uncertainty is that associated with pyruvate decarboxylation to acetic acid; however, the evidence suggests that acetic acid formation is accompanied by ATP formation in *F. hepatica* at least (Tielens *et al.* 1982).

The cause of variation in metabolism remains a puzzle. In *Hymenolepis diminuta* two strains which show marked variation in end product formation have markedly different enzyme profiles, especially of fumarase (Kohlhagen *et al.* 1985). If this is also true for *E. granulosus* then strain variation may arise either from the regulation of protein synthesis, or the regulation of the expression of the DNA, or from a change in the genome itself. In *H. diminuta* there is evidence that both intermediate and definitive host have a selecting effect on strain formation (Mettrick & Rahman 1984). This view is certainly supported by experiments on isoelectric focusing of proteins from *E. granulosus*. Kumaratilake *et al.* (1979) were able to distinguish between two strains (horse and sheep) on the basis of total protein separations. A more detailed study was carried out by Macpherson and McManus (1982), in which electrophoretic distributions of glucose-phosphate isomerase and phosphoglucose mutase from protoscoleces, derived from cysts from different tissues, and different geographical localities were examined. Uniformly consistent and identical isoenzyme patterns for *E. granulosus* from sheep and humans suggested that they represented a single Kenyan strain. The camel material was distinct from the sheep–human strain but that from goats suggested the presence of at least two variants, one of which was similar to the sheep–human strain and one, possibly, to a camel strain.

Differences in isozyme patterns are, of course, indicative of differences in gene expression, but it is not clear whether the differences are constitutive or regulatory. Neither is it known whether these differences are adaptive, nor whether true 'zymodemes' (populations whose individuals carry the same isoenzyme pattern) correlated with the other characteristics of the strain, actually exist. Sample sizes reported in published work are too small to resolve this question, and too small to make even an estimate of the extent of variation.

CHEMOTHERAPY OF *ECHINOCOCCUS*
(see also Ch. 9 for full discussion)

Although the title of this very short section appears to offer grounds for optimism, the facts are that chemotherapeutic treatment of hydatid disease meets with variable success. The benzimidazole anthelmintics, mebendazole and flubendazole, are the only ones that offer any chance of recovery without surgical intervention and even these may best be restricted to presurgical use to decrease turgor within the cyst and to reduce the chances of secondary infection. Both the compounds are poorly absorbed – less than 10 per cent of an oral dose – necessitating the administration of large quantities at frequent intervals. Fortunately the compounds have very low toxicity with few side effects.

The benzimidazole anthelmintics exert a number of deleterious effects on cestode metabolism: these include interference with energy metabolism, impairment of nutrient uptake and specific enzyme inhibition. Ultrastructural studies have shown that microtubule formation is modified and that the tegument is damaged. All this leads to a failure of homeostasis and to autolysis. Finally, the damage may render the cysts vulnerable to attack from the immune system. The general problem has been well reviewed by Schantz *et al.* (1982).

It has been suggested that the resistance of hydatid cysts to chemotherapy is due to their capacity to detoxify drugs. A recent study has shown the presence of a highly active glutathione *S*-transferase, an enzyme which conjugates organic molecules with glutathione in protoscoleces (Morella, Repetto & Atias 1982). However, while this enzyme may have a role, there are many other pharmacokinetic parameters which have yet to be taken into account.

The adult cestodes in the dog are readily removed by any of the standard modern anthelmintics, although praziquantel is the drug of choice because of its low dose rate and its low toxicity for the host. Praziquantel appears to act by interfering with calcium flux across membranes.

PROSPECTS

In 1969, Desmond Smyth (1969b) wrote a paper entitled 'Parasites as biological models'. In it he argued that *E. granulosus* would make an excellent organism for the study of genetics, differentiation, immunology, pathology, biochemistry and biophysics. It is easy to dismiss this paper as the special pleading of an enthusiast; but modern technology makes the sort of studies that he envisaged far more accessible to the ordinary parasitologist. Perhaps Smyth's vision is focused on a point too distant for us even now, in the middle 1980s; a more myopic view, however, suggests that *E. granulosus* can be an extraordinarily useful parasitological model for biochemists and physiologists. Its advantages are many: it can be maintained for much of its life-cycle in axenic culture in defined media; it is often relatively easy to produce in gram quantities; it can be triggered to develop in two distinct directions, strobilar or cystic; and the raw material is easily acquired.

A possible role for *E. granulosus* is implied in an excellent review by Rickard and Williams (1982) on the immunology of hydatidosis: new techniques of immunology and genetic engineering can clearly take advantage of the opportunities afforded by axenic culture. But so, too, can biochemistry.

The recent rapid development of recombinant DNA and bacterial cloning technology in a wide range of biological problems of gene structure and function (Gilbert & Villa-Komaroff 1980, Williamson 1982), opens up new avenues for the identification and synthesis of parasite gene products. There is every reason to believe that these powerful techniques of molecular biology, if applied to the *Echinococcus* organisms, will provide fundamental information regarding our understanding of their biology and particularly their relationship with their various hosts.

For example, techniques are available for the extraction of undegraded RNA, containing messenger sequences which code for and direct the synthesis *in vitro* of important proteins. Such proteins might include antigens for use in immunodiagnosis and/or vaccination, or polypeptides which might prove particularly susceptible to chemotherapy, including structural proteins and proteins involved in growth, development, differentiation, metabolism or transport. A cell-free system capable of synthesising proteins has already been prepared and characterised from protoscoleces of *E. granulosus* (Agosin & Repetto 1967). It is the first protein synthesising system to be developed from a parasitic helminth.

The isolation of the relevant mRNA coding for a specific protein of importance and the synthesis *in vitro* of the complementary DNA (cDNA) by reverse transcriptase is another possibility. The production of double-stranded cDNA, its introduction into a plasmid vector and its cloning into a suitable recipient bacterium such as *Escherischia coli* should follow, allowing proteins of interest to be synthesised in almost unlimited quantities. A particular advantage of this approach is that a protein subsequently may be characterised in total isolation from other contaminating proteins, either of parasite or host origin.

Restriction enzyme and Southern blot analyses of DNA will provide information about the nature and size of the major repetitive sequences. Such studies will form the basis for future applications of recombinant DNA technology to the study of *Echinococcus* and hydatid disease. Already Simpson and his co-workers (Simpson *et al.* 1982, McGutchan *et al.* 1984) have detected species, strain and sex-specific genetic markers for the genus *Schistosoma* by Southern blot analysis of its isolated DNA using cloned DNA segments of the *S. mansoni* ribosomal gene as probes. Experiments along similar lines with *E. granulosus* (and *E. multilocularis*) will help to clarify the complex picture of strains currently emerging from different areas of the world. In addition, the use of cloned DNA markers offers significant potential for the development of a sensitive method for differentiation of taeniid eggs.

Another approach is suggested by nuclear magnetic resonance. NMR is a standard analytical technique for chemists, has been adopted by many mainstream biochemists and is now beginning to find application in parasite biochemistry. Although as an analytical tool it lacks the sensitivity of modern biochemical techniques, its great advantage is that it is non-invasive. It permits the detection of, for example, ^{31}P- or ^{13}C-containing compounds *in vivo* and allows the organisms to be recovered unharmed at the end of the data-gathering period. The technique and its applications have been extensively reviewed (see, for example, Iles *et al.* 1982), so further details are redundant here. The value of this technique in the study of *E. granulosus* is immediately apparent. With the judicious use of labelled substrates it will enable the continuous monitoring, in axenic cultures, of the biochemistry of whole developmental sequences, and perhaps permit an analysis of the regulatory changes involved in the shift from the strobilar to the cystic mode.

Like any other discipline, that of biochemical parasitology was the art of the possible before the 1950s. The difficulties of obtaining large quantities of parasitic material to compensate for the lack of sensitivity of analytical techniques impeded progress. In the 1960s and 1970s the development and availability of enzymes for assay procedures and the refinement of analytical tools with microprocessor control and data reduction has led to an exponential increase in interest in the biochemical aspects of parasitism. Today, technology has at last caught up with the opportunities afforded by many years of painstaking research and the future holds promise of many new insights.

REFERENCES

Agosin, M. 1957. Studies on the metabolism of *Echinococcus granulosus*. II. Some observations on the carbohydrate metabolism of hydatid cyst scolices. *Exp. Parasitol.* **6**, 586–93.

Agosin, M. and L. Aravena 1959. Studies on the metabolism of *Echinococcus granulosus*. III. Glycolysis, with special reference to hexokinases and related glycolytic enzymes. *Biochim. Biophys. Acta* **34**, 90–102.

Agosin, M. and L. Aravena 1960a. Studies on the metabolism of *Echinococcus granulosus*. IV. Enzymes of the pentose phosphate pathway. *Exp. Parasitol.* **10**, 28–38.

Agosin, M. and L. Aravena 1960b. Studies on the metabolism of *Echinococcus granulosus*. V. The phosphopentose isomerase of hydatid cyst scolices. *Enzymologia* **22**, 281–94.

Agosin, M. and Y. Repetto 1961. Studies on the metabolism of *Echinococcus granulosus*. VI. Pathways of glucose C^{14} metabolism in *E. granulosus* scolices. *Biologica* **23**, 33–8.

Agosin, M. and Y. Repetto 1963. Studies on the metabolism of *Echinococcus granulosus*. VII. Reactions of the tricarboxylic acid cycle in *E. granulosus* scolices. *Comp. Biochem. Physiol.* **8**, 245–61.

Agosin, M. and Y. Repetto 1965. Studies on the metabolism of *Echinococcus granulosus*. VIII. The pathway to succinate in *E. granulosus* scolices. *Comp. Biochem. Physiol.* **14**, 299–309.

Agosin, M. and Y. Repetto 1967. Studies on the metabolism of *Echinococcus granulosus*. XI. Protein synthesis in scolices. *Exp. Parasitol.* **21**, 195–208.

Agosin, M., Y. Repetto and L. Dicowsky 1971. RNA of *Echinococcus granulosus* protoscolices. *Exp. Parasitol.* **30**, 233–43.

Agosin, M., T. von Brand, G. F. Rivera and P. McMahon 1957. Studies on the metabolism of *Echinococcus granulosus*. I. General chemical composition and respiratory reactions. *Exp. Parasitol.* **6**, 37–51.

Ali-Khan, A. and R. Siboo 1981. *Echinococcus multilocularis*: distribution and persistence of specific host immunoglobulins on cyst membranes. *Exp. Parasitol.* **51**, 159–68.

Bahr, J. M., G. J. Frayha and J. J. Hajjar 1979. Mechanisms of cholesterol absorption by the hydatid cysts of *Echinococcus granulosus* (Cestoda). *Comp. Biochem. Physiol.* **62A**, 485–90.

Barrett, J. 1981. *Biochemistry of parasitic helminths*. London: Macmillan.

Barrett, N. J. 1984. Developmental biology of *Echinococcus multilocularis in vivo* and *in vitro*. PhD thesis, University of London.

Bennet, E.-M and C. Bryant 1984. Energy metabolism of adult *Haemonchus contortus in vitro*: a comparison of benzimidazole susceptible and resistant strains. *Molec. Biochem. Parasitol.* **10**, 335–46.

Biguet, J., A. Capron, P. Tran Van Ky and R. D'Haussy 1962. Étude immunoélectrophorétique comparée des antigénes de divers helminthes. *C. R. Hebd. Séanc. Acad. Sci., Paris* **254**, 3600–2.

Bolton, A. E. and W. M. Hunter 1973. The labelling of proteins to high specific radioactivities by conjugation to a ^{125}I-containing acylating agent. *Biochem. J.* **133**, 529–39.

Brand, T. von 1979. *Biochemistry and physiology of endoparasites*. Amsterdam: Elsevier.

Brand, T. von, M. U. Nylen, D. B. Scott and G. N. Martin 1965. Observations on calcareous corpuscles of larval *Echinococcus granulosus* of various geographic origins. *Proc. Soc. Exp. Biol. Med.* **120**, 383–5.

Bryant, C. 1970. Electron transport in parasitic helminths and protozoa. *Adv. Parasitol.* **8**, 139–72.

Bryant, C. 1972. Metabolic regulation in *Moniezia expansa:* the role of pyruvate kinase. *Int. J. Parasitol.* **2**, 333–40.

Bryant, C. 1975. Carbon dioxide utilisation and the regulation of respiratory metabolic pathways in parasitic helminths. *Adv. Parasitol.* **13**, 35–69.

Bryant, C. 1983. Intraspecies variation of energy metabolism in parasitic helminths. *Int. J. Parasitol.* **13**, 327–32.

Bryant, C. and D. J. Morseth 1968. The metabolism of radioactive fumaric acid and some other substrates by whole adult *Echinococcus granulosus* (Cestoda). *Comp. Biochem. Physiol.* **25**, 541–6.

Capron, A., A. Vernes and J. Biguet 1967. Le diagnostic immunoélectrophorétique de l'hydatidose. In *Le kyste hydatique du foie*, J. Coudert (ed.), 27–40. Lyon: Journées Lyonnaises d'Hydatidologie SIMEP.

Castagnari, L. and R. Pozzuoli 1969. Studio electroforetico e immunoelectroforetico del liquido idatideo. *Ann. Sclavo* **11**, 99-107.

Chordi, A. and I. G. Kagan 1965. Identification and characterisation of antigenic components of sheep hydatid fluid by immunoelectrophoresis. *J. Parasitol.* **51**, 63–71.

Čmelik, S. 1952. Zur kenntnis der lipoide aus den cystenmembranen von *Taenia echinococcus*. *Z. Physiol. Chem.* **289**, 78–9.

Čmelik, S. and B. Briski 1953. Untersuchungen uber Eiweissfraktionen von *Taenia echinococcus*. *Biochem. Z.* **324**, 104–14.

Codounis, A. and. J. Polydoridès 1936. Sur les constituants du liquide deskystes hydatiques. *Proc. 3rd Int. Congr. Comp. Path., Athens* **2**, 195–202.

Coltorti, E. A. and V. M. Varela-Diaz 1974. *Echinococcus granulosus*: penetration of macromolecules and their localization on the parasite membranes of cysts. *Exp. Parasitol.* **35**, 225–31.

Coltorti, E. A. and V. M. Varela-Diaz 1975. Penetration of host IgG molecules into hydatid cysts. *Z. ParasitKde* **48**, 47–51.

Coutelen, F. R. 1931a. Présence chez les hydatides echinococciques de cellules libres a glycogene et a graisses. *Annls Parasitol. Hum. Comp.* **9**, 97–100.

Coutelen, F. R. 1931b. Histogénesè des cellules libres à glycogenè et à graisses, des hydatides echinococciques. *Annls Parasitol. Hum. Comp.* **9**, 101–3.

Davies, C., M. D. Rickard, T. D. Bout and J. D. Smyth 1978. Ultrastructural immunocytochemical localisation of two hydatid fluid antigens (antigen 5 and antigen B) in the brood capsules and protoscoleces of ovine and equine *Echinococcus granulosus* and *E. multilocularis*. *Parasitology* **77**, 143–57.

De Rycke, P. H. 1968. The evagination of *Echinococcus granulosus* in media with different osmotic pressures. *Z. ParasitKde* **30**, 192–8.

De Rycke, P. H. and G. van Grembergen 1969. Study on the relation between the osmotic pressure and the evagination of *Echinococcus granulosus*. *Z. ParasitKde* **32**, 128–34.

Dicowsky, L., Y. Repetto and M. Agosin 1968. Studies of the metabolism of *Echinococcus granulosus*. X. The mechanism of production of volatile fatty acids. *Comp. Biochem. Physiol.* **24**, 763–72.

Digenis, G. A., R. E. Thorson and A. Konyalian 1970. Cholesterol biosynthesis and lipid biochemistry in the scolex of *Echinococcus granulosus*. *J. Pharm. Sci.* **59**, 676–9.

Edwards, G. T. 1982. Host immunoglobulin G in equine cyst fluid. *Ann. Trop. Med. Parasitol.* **76**, 485–8.

Flössner, O. N. 1924. Neue untersuchungen ueber die Echinokokkusfluessigkeit. *Z. Biol.* **80**, 225–60.

Flössner, O. N. 1925. Neue untersuchungen ueber die Echinokokkusfluessigkeit. *Z. Biol.* **82**, 297–301.

Fraker, P. J. and J. C. R. Speck 1978. Protein and cell membrane iodinations with a sparingly soluble chloramide, 1,3,4,6-tetrachloro-3,6-diphenylglycoluril. *Biochem. Biophys. Res. Commun.* **80**, 849-57.

Frayha, G. J. 1968. A study on the synthesis and absorption of cholesterol in hydatid cysts (*Echinococcus granulosus*). *Comp. Biochem. Physiol.* **27**, 875–8.

Frayha, G. J. 1971. Comparative metabolism of acetate in the taeniid tapeworms *Echinococcus granulosus, Echinococcus multilocularis* and *Taenia hydatigena*. *Comp. Biochem. Physiol.* **39B**, 167–70.

Frayha, G. J. 1974. Synthesis of certain cholesterol precursors by hydatid protoscoleces of *Echinococcus granulosus* and cysticerci of *Taenia hydatigena*. *Comp. Biochem. Physiol.* **49B**, 93–8.

Frayha, G. J. and R. Haddad 1980. Comparative chemical composition of protoscoleces and hydatid cyst fluid of *Echinococcus granulosus* (Cestoda). *Int. J. Parasitol.* **10**, 359–64.

Frayha, G. J. and J. D. Smyth 1983. Lipid metabolism in parasitic helminths. *Adv. Parasitol.* **22**, 310–87.

Frayha, G. J., G. M. Bahr and R. Haddad 1980. The lipids and phospholipids of hydatid protoscoleces of *Echinococcus granulosus* (Cestoda). *Int. J. Parasitol.* **10**, 213–6.

Gallagher, I. H. C. 1964. Chemical composition of hooks isolated from hydatid scolices. *Exp. Parasitol.* **15**, 110–17.

Gilbert, W. and L. Villa-Komaroff 1980. Useful proteins from recombinant bacteria. *Scient. Am.* **242**, 68–84.

Hochachka, P. W. 1980. *Living without oxygen.* Cambridge, Mass.: Harvard University Press.

Hopkins, C. A., L. M. Law and L. T. Threadgold 1978. *Schistocephalus solidus*: pinocytosis by the plerocercoid tegument. *Exp. Parasitol.* **44**, 161–72.

Hustead, S. T. and J. F. Williams 1977. Permeability studies on taeniid metacestodes. Part I. Uptake of proteins by larval stages of *Taenia taeniaeformis, Taenia crassiceps* and *Echinococcus granulosus*. *J. Parasitol.* **63**, 314–21.

Hyman, L. H. 1919. On the action of certain substances on oxygen consumption. II. Action of potassium cyanide on *Planaria*. *Am. J. Physiol.* **48**, 340–71.

Iles, R. A., A. N. Stevens and J. R. Griffith 1982. NMR studies of metabolites in living tissue. *Progr. NMR Spectr.* **15**, 49–200.

Janssens, P. A. and C. Bryant 1969. The ornithine–urea cycle in some parasitic helminths. *Comp. Biochem. Physiol.* **30**, 261–72.

Kagan, I. G. 1963. Seminar on immunity to parasitic helminths. IV. Hydatid disease. *Exp. Parasitol.* **13**, 57–71.

Kagan, I. G. and M. Agosin 1968. *Echinococcus* antigens. *Bull. Wld Hlth Org.* **39**, 13–20.

Kassis, A. I. and C. E. Tanner 1976. The role of complement in hydatid disease: *in vitro* studies. *Int. J. Parasitol.* **6**, 25–35.

Kassis, A. I. and C. E. Tanner 1977. Host serum proteins in *Echinococcus multilocularis*: complement activation via the classical pathway. *Immunology* **33**, 1–10.

Keilin, D. 1925. On cytochrome, a respiratory pigment common to animals, yeast and higher plants. *Proc. R. Soc. B.* **98**, 312–39.

Kilejian, A. and A. J. MacInnis 1976. Density distribution of DNA from parasitic helminths with special reference to *Ascaris lumbricoides*. *Rice Univ. Studies* **62**, 161–74.

Kilejian, A. and C. W. Schwabe, 1971. Studies on the polysaccharides of the *Echinococcus granulosus* cyst, with observations on a possible mechanism for laminated membrane formation. *Comp. Biochem. Physiol.* **40B**, 25–36.

Kilejian, A., K. Sauer and C. W. Schwabe 1962. Host–parasite relationships in echinococcosis. VIII. Infra-red spectra and chemical composition of the hydatid cyst. *Exp. Parasitol.* **12**, 377–9.

Kilejian, A., L. A. Schinazi and C. W. Schwabe 1961. Host–parasite relationships in echinococcosis. V. Histochemical observation on *Echinococcus granulosus*. *J. Parasitol.* **47**, 181–8.

Köhler, P., J. Gisler, R. Bachmann and P. Wild 1983. The localisation of fumarase and malic enzyme in muscle mitochondria of *Ascaris suum*. *Molec. Biochem. Parasitol.* **9**, 329–36.

Kohlhagen, S., C. A. Behm and C. Bryant 1985. Strain variation in *Hymenolepis diminuta*: enzyme profiles. *Int. J. Parasitol.* (in press).

Krvavica, S., T. Martinčič and R. Asaj 1959. [Metabolism of amino acids in some parasites. II. Amino acids in the hydatid fluid and germinal layer of *Echinococcus*.] *Vet. Arh.* **29**, 314–21.

Kumaratilake, L. M. and R. C. A. Thompson 1979. A standardised technique for the comparison of tapeworm soluble proteins by thin-layer iso-electric focusing in polyacrylamide gels, with particular reference to *Echinococcus granulosus*. *Science Tools* **26**, 21–4.

Kumaratilake, L. M., R. C. A. Thompson and J. D. Dunsmore 1979. Intraspecific variation in *Echinococcus*: a biochemical approach. *Z. ParasitKde* **60**, 291–4.

McGutchan, T. F., A. J. G. Simpson, J. A. Mullins, A. Sher, T. E. Nash, F. Lewis and C. Richards 1984. Differentiation of schistosomes by species, strain, and sex by using cloned DNA markers. *Proc. Natn. Acad. Sci. U.S.A.* **81**, 889–93.

McManus, D. P. 1981. A biochemical study of adult and cystic stages of *Echinococcus granulosus* of human and animal origin from Kenya. *J. Helminthol.* **55**, 21–7.

McManus, D. P. and N. J. Barrett 1985. Isolation, fractionation and partial characterisation of the tegumental surface from protoscoleces of the hydatid organism, *Echinococcus granulosus*. *Parasitology* **90**, 111–29.

McManus, D. P. and C. N. L. Macpherson 1984. Strain characterisation in the hydatid organism, *Echinococcus granulosus*: current status and new perspectives. *Ann. Trop. Med. Parasitol.* **78**, 193–8.

McManus, D. P. and J. D. Smyth 1978. Differences in the chemical composition and carbohydrate metabolism of *Echinococcus granulosus* (horse and sheep strains) and *E. multilocularis*. *Parasitology* **77**, 103–9.

McManus, D. P. and J. D. Smyth 1982. Intermediary carbohydrate metabolism in protoscoleces of *Echinococcus granulosus* (horse and sheep strains) and *E. multilocularis*. *Parasitology* **84**, 351–66.

Macpherson, C. N. L. and D. P. McManus 1982. A comparative study of *Echinococcus granulosus* from human and animal hosts in Kenya using isoelectric focusing and isoenzyme analysis. *Int. J. Parasitol.* **12**, 515–21.

Mastrandrea, G., M. Mazzett and G. Mele 1962. Studio cromatografico sul contenuto in aminoacidi del liquido idatideo. *Rass. Ital. Gastroenterol.* **8**, 556–61.

Mettrick, D. F. and M. S. Rahman 1984. Effect of strain of parasite and species of intermediate host on carbohydrate intermediary metabolism in the rat tapeworm, *Hymenolepis diminuta*. *Can. J. Zool.* **62**, 355–61.

Morello, A., Y. Repetto and A. Atias 1982. Glutathione *S*-transferase activity in *Echinococcus granulosus*. *Comp. Biochem. Physiol.* **72B**, 449–52.

Morseth, D. J. 1967. Fine structure of the hydatid cyst and protoscolex of *Echinococcus granulosus*. *J. Parasitol.* **53**, 312–25.

Muntyan, N. A. 1973. [Disc electrophoretic analysis of echinococcal fluid and extracts from scolices and germinative membranes of the larval cyst of *Echinococcus granulosus*.] *Medskaya Parazit.* **42**, 544–8.

Oriol, R., J. F. Williams, M. V. Perez Esandi and C. Oriol 1971. Purification of lipoprotein antigens of *Echinococcus granulosus* from sheep hydatid fluid. *Am. J. Trop. Med. Hyg.* **20**, 569–74.

Philipp, M. and F. D. Rumjanek 1984. Antigenic and dynamic properties of helminth surface structures. *Molec. Biochem. Parasitol.* **10**, 245–68.

Pozzi, G. and I. Pirosky 1953. Contribución al estudio de la proteina de la hidátide de *Tenia equinococcus*. Análisis cromatografico en papel. *Archos Int. Hidatid.* **13**, 232.

Read, C. P. 1952. Contributions to cestode enzymology. I. The cytochrome system and succinic dehydrogenase in *Hymenolepis diminuta*. *Exp. Parasitol.* **1**, 353–62.

Read, C. P. and A. Rothman 1957. The role of carbohydrates in the biology of cestodes. I. The effect of dietary carbohydrate quality on the size of *Hymenolepis diminuta*. *Exp. Parasitol.* **6**, 1–7.

Reisin, I. L. and C. A. Rotunno 1981. Water and electrolyte balance in protoscoleces of *Echinococcus granulosus* incubated *in vitro*: general procedures for the determination of water, sodium, potassium and chloride in protoscoleces. *Int. J. Parasitol.* **11**, 399–404.

Reisin, I. L., C. A. Rabito and H. F. Cantiello 1981. Water and electrolyte balance in protoscoleces of *Echinococcus granulosus* incubated *in vitro*: effect of metabolic inhibitors. *Int. J. Parasitol.* **11**, 405–10.

Richards, K. S. 1984. *Echinococcus granulosus equinus*: the histochemistry of the laminated layer of the hydatid cyst. *Folia Histochem. Cytobiol.* **22**, 21–3.

Richards, K. S., C. Arme and J. F. Bridges 1984. *Echinococcus granulosus equinus*: variation in the germinal layer of murine hydatids and evidence of autophagy. *Parasitology* **89**, 35–47.

Rickard, M. D. and J. F. Williams 1982. Hydatidosis/cysticercosis: immune mechanisms and immunisation against infection. *Adv. Parasitol.* **21**, 230–96.

Rickard, M. D., C. Davies, D. T. Bout and J. D. Smyth 1977. Immunohistological localisation of two hydatid antigens (antigen 5 and antigen B) in the cyst wall, brood capsules and protoscoleces of *Echinococcus granulosus* (ovine and equine) and *E. multilocularis* using immunoperoxidase methods. *J. Helminthol.* **51**, 359–64.

Rotunno, C. A., W. S. Kammerer, M. V. Perez Esandi and M. Cereijido 1974. Studies on the permeability to water, sodium and chloride of the hydatid cyst of *Echinococcus granulosus*. *J. Parasitol.* **60**, 613–20.

Sakamoto, T. and M. Sugimura 1969. Studies on echinococcosis. XXI. Electron microscopical observations on general structure of larval tissue of multilocular *Echinococcus*. *Jap. J. Vet. Res.* **17**, 67–80.

Sanchez, F. A. and A. C. Sanchez 1971. Estudio de algunas propiedades fisicas y componentes quimicos del liquido y pared germinativa de quistes hidatidicos de diversas especies y de diferente localizacion. *Revta Iber. Parasitol.* **31**, 347–66.

Schantz, P. M., H. Van den Bossche and J. Eckert 1982. Chemotherapy for larval echinococcosis in animals and humans: report of a workshop. *Z. ParasitKde* **67**, 5–26.

Simpson, A. J. G., A. Sher and T. F. McGutchan 1982. The genome of *Schistosoma mansoni*: isolation of DNA, its size, bases and repetitive sequences. *Molec. Biochem. Parasitol.* **6**, 125–37.

Smyth, J. D. 1964. Observations on the scolex of *Echinococcus granulosus*, with special reference to the occurrence of secretory cells in the rostellum. *Parasitology* **54**, 515–26.

Smyth, J. D. 1967. Studies on tapeworm physiology. XI. *In vitro* cultivation of *Echinococcus granulosus* from the protoscolex to the strobilate stage. *Parasitology* **57**, 111–33.

Smyth, J. D. 1969a. *The physiology of cestodes.* Edinburgh: Oliver & Boyd.

Smyth, J. D. 1969b. Parasites as biological models. *Parasitology* **59**, 73–91.

Smyth, J. D. 1972. Changes in the digestive-absorptive surface of cestodes during larval/adult differentiation. *Symp. Br. Soc. Parasitol.* **10**, 41–70.

Smyth, J. D. and Z. Davies, 1974. *In vitro* culture of the strobilar stage of *Echinococcus granulosus* (sheep strain): a review of basic problems and results. *Int. J. Parasitol.* **4**, 631–44.

Smyth, J. D., D. J. Morseth and M. M. Smyth 1969. Observations on nuclear secretions in the rostellar gland cells of *Echinococcus granulosus* (Cestoda). *The Nucleus* **12**, 47–56.

Tielens, A. G. M., J. M. van den Heuvel and S. G. van den Bergh 1982. Changes in energy metabolism of the juvenile *Fasciola hepatica* during its development in liver parenchyma. *Molec. Biochem. Parasitol.* **6**, 277–86.

Thompson, R. C. A., J. D. Dunsmore and A. R. Hayton 1979. *Echinococcus granulosus*: secretory activity of the rostellum of the adult cestode *in situ* in the dog. *Exp. Parasitol.* **48**, 144–63.

Threadgold, L. T. and C. A. Hopkins 1981. *Schistocephalus solidus* and *Ligula intestinalis*: pinocytosis by the tegument. *Exp. Parasitol.* **51**, 444–56.

Varela-Diaz, V. M., J. Eckert, R. L. Rausch, E. A. Coltorti and U. Hess 1977. Detection of the *Echinococcus granulosus* diagnostic arc 5 in sera from patients with surgically confirmed *E. multilocularis* infection. *Z. ParasitKde* **53**, 183–8.

Vercelli-Retta, J., N. J. Reissenweber, W. Lozano and A. M. Siri 1975. Histochemistry and histoenzymology of the hydatid cyst of *Echinococcus granulosus*. Part I. The germinal membrane. *Z. ParasitKde* **48**, 15–23.

Vessal, M., S. Y. Zekavat and A. A. Mohammadzadeh-k 1972. Lipids of *Echinococcus granulosus* protoscoleces. *Lipids* **7**, 289–96.

Wasylishen, R. E. and M. Novak 1983. Natural abundance of ^{13}C nuclear magnetic resonance studies of live cestodes. *Comp. Biochem. Physiol.* **74B**, 303–6.

Williamson, R. (ed.) 1982. *Genetic engineering*, vol. 3. London: Academic Press.

Zekavat, S. Y. and A. A. M. Khayat 1971. *Echinococcus granulosus*. Isolation and partial characterization of sRNA and DNA. *Isr. J. Med. Sci.* **7**, 1292–4.

5 Cultivation of *Echinococcus* species *in vitro*

M. J. HOWELL

INTRODUCTION

The cultivation of metazoan parasites *in vitro* is a more difficult proposition than cell culture and has a shorter history. Its successes are more modest but nevertheless quite outstanding technical feats. The problems confronting attempts to grow a highly specialised organism *in vitro* in ignorance of the factors which regulate its development are formidable ones demanding inordinate amounts of flair, ingenuity and patience for their resolution. They are compounded by the fact that metazoan parasites have complex life-cycles often involving development in different hosts. Because progress in this area tends to proceed in a largely empirical way, *in vitro* cultivation of parasites can be regarded more as an art-form than a science! It is, however, in investigating secondary problems that are suggested by *in vitro* observations that the scientific skills of the investigator are brought to the forefront. This is amply demonstrated with respect to cestodes, as this review will attempt to show.

What are the objectives of *in vitro* cultivation of metazoan parasites? Simply stated, to be able to observe parasitological phenomena unfettered by the complexities of the host environment. It can be argued that if a life-cycle can be duplicated *in vitro* a complete description of a parasite's morphogenesis, nutrition, physiology and biochemistry is within reach, and details of the complex interactions between host and parasite, particularly those of an immunological nature, are more readily unravelled. In a practical sense there are great benefits; the need to maintain infected animals is obviated and a source of antigenic material is always available. But there are also benefits that extend beyond the realm of parasitology. For example, metazoan parasites exhibit profound and abrupt changes in gene expression at several stages of their life-cycles. *In vitro* techniques that can initiate and sustain these changes provide a means of studying the most fundamental of all biological problems, namely that of differentiation.

Attempts to cultivate cestodes *in vitro* are marked by many outstanding achievements and the contributions of Desmond Smyth have dominated the field for almost 40 years. Studies on *Echinococcus granulosus* in particular, as well as *E. multilocularis*, have occupied him for 20 years, both in Australia and the United Kingdom. *E. granulosus* proved to be a more difficult proposition than some of his other much-admired parasites –

Schistocephalus, Ligula and *Diphyllobothrium* – on which he commenced his investigations in this field. And the refractoriness of protoscoleces of this parasite to develop in a strobilate direction *in vitro* would have daunted a much less dedicated individual. The conceptual advances made by Desmond Smyth in solving this and many other questions have led to a clearer understanding of a variety of aspects of the host–parasite relationship, not only in respect of *Echinococcus* spp., but of parasites in general. The review of the literature dealing with the cultivation of *Echinococcus* spp. *in vitro* which follows will, it is hoped, bear out this contention.

The chapter is divided essentially into two main sections: the methods and results obtained with *E. granulosus* and *E. multilocularis* with respect to their growth and development *in vitro*, and the implications this has had for a clearer understanding of the biology of these parasites. More general biological questions to which the work has relevance will also be briefly addressed.

DEVELOPMENT OF *ECHINOCOCCUS* SPP. *IN VITRO*

Major developmental sequences in the life-cycles of both *E. granulosus* and *E. multilocularis* have been duplicated *in vitro*. A few studies were made prior to the 1960s but detailed investigations were commenced by Smyth (1962a) and his contributions have dominated this field of research since then. The situation at present is that only a few gaps remain in completing the entire life-cycle of each species *in vitro*. However, these have proved to be rather intractable problems. Diagrammatic summaries of the results for *E. granulosus* and *E. multilocularis* are shown in Figures 5.1 and 5.2. The details will be elaborated upon in the following discussion and the problems that remain will be referred to where relevant. This work has been reviewed extensively (Smyth & Davies 1974b, Voge 1978, Heath 1982, Smyth 1968, 1979a, 1982). Because of this and space limitations only brief descriptions of techniques will be reported here.

There are two obvious starting points for the *in vitro* culture of these parasites – either cysts or eggs. The former are accessible, provide sterile material in the form of protoscoleces or germinal layer and are relatively safe to handle. In contrast eggs (containing the infective oncosphere) pose a serious health hazard for the worker, special facilities are essential to maintain infected dogs, and collection of eggs or gravid worms from this source raises problems of contamination by the microflora of the dog gut. Consequently, the protoscolex has been the material of choice with the added advantage that successful cultivation of this stage would obviate the need to maintain infected dogs as a source of eggs.

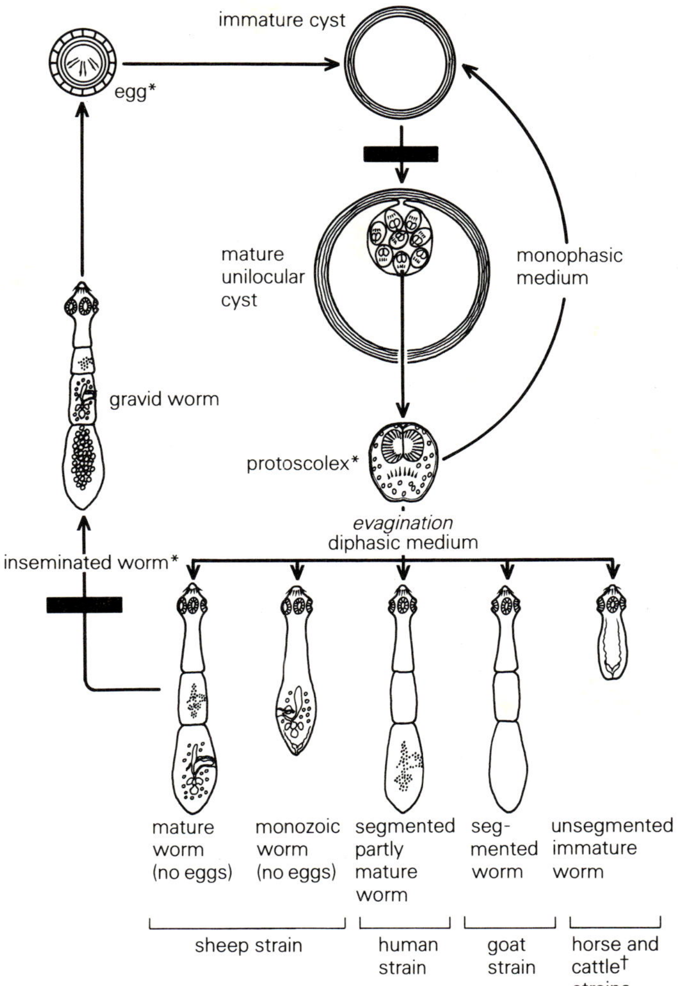

Figure 5.1 *Echinococcus granulosus*: development *in vitro*. ▬, barrier encountered; *stages used for culture; †variable, see text.

Echinococcus granulosus

PROTOSCOLEX

The protoscolex of *E. granulosus* (Fig. 5.3a,b) has the ability to differentiate in either of two directions depending on the environmental circumstances: (a) into a hydatid cyst if one should escape from an existing fertile cyst, or (b) into sexually mature segmented worms if eaten by a dog. These *in vivo* patterns of development have been replicated *in vitro*.

Cystic development Protoscoleces (Fig. 5.3a) have been cultured under a variety of conditions *in vitro* and cyst development has often been

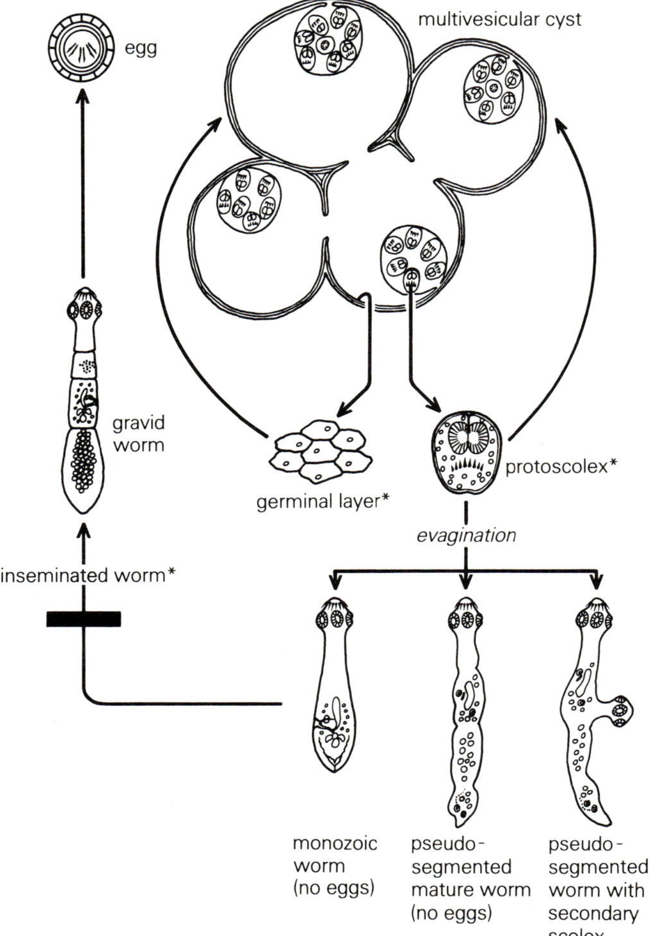

Figure 5.2 *Echinococcus multilocularis*: development *in vitro*. ▬, barrier encountered; *stages used for culture.

observed (Devé 1926, Coutelen 1927a,b, Smyth 1962a, Paulluzzi *et al.* 1965, Benex 1968, Brudnjak *et al.* 1970, Heath & Osborn 1976). In the procedure developed by Smyth (1962a), brood capsules from cysts were pretreated with pepsin to free protoscoleces and digest dead material. Trypsin digestion followed pepsin pretreatment to free protoscoleces entirely from the germinal layer (Benex 1968); in order to obtain evaginated protoscoleces (Fig. 5.3b), bile salts, particularly sodium taurocholate, have been used (Smyth 1967, 1979a, Smyth & Davies 1974b). Culture media have contained natural (commonly hydatid fluid from cysts, animal sera, yeast extract and dog bile or bile salts) and synthetic components (such as Parker 199 or 858 and NCTC-135 together with additional glucose). The most important factors to bear in mind in

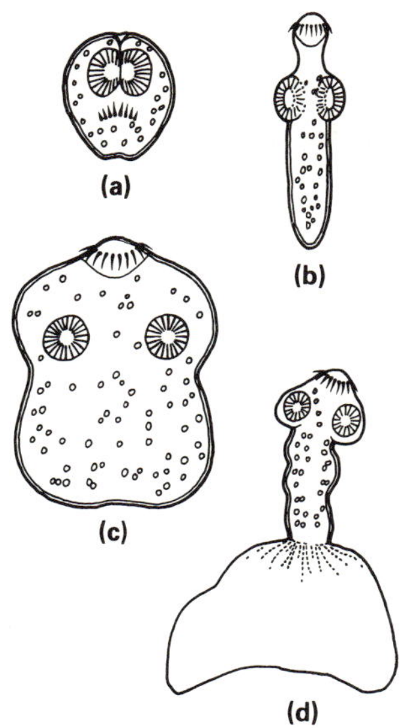

Figure 5.3 *Echinococcus* protoscoleces and developmental forms assumed *in vitro*: (a) invaginated protoscolex; (b) evaginated protoscolex; (c) vesicular protoscolex; (d) protoscolex with posterior bladder.

setting up cultures appear to be the sterility of the material, the need to use material from cysts which contain >60 per cent viable protoscoleces, the necessity to ensure that if bile salts are used for evagination they do not contain sodium deoxycholate which lyses protoscoleces, and standardisation of the sample of pepsin for its ability to free the protoscoleces and digest dead material. A variety of media support cystic development, including one which is chemically defined (Heath & Osborn 1976). Thus, the nutritional requirements for cystic development are amenable to investigation.

Two patterns of cystic development *in vitro* were described by Smyth (1962a, 1967). In the first, some protoscoleces became swollen or vesicular (Fig. 5.3c) within a few days of culture and grew into thin walled cysts. After 5–7 weeks a laminated layer, consisting of a hyaline mucopolysaccharide material laid down in concentric lamellae, developed around each cyst. Cysts increased in size over the next 4–6 weeks, by which time they were about three times the size of protoscoleces.

In the non-vesicular pattern of development, the protoscoleces each developed a posterior bladder (Fig. 5.3d) which increased substantially in size; eventually a spherical cyst formed and this became enveloped by a laminated layer. Such cysts were morphologically indistinguishable from cysts that developed from vesicular protoscoleces.

Cysts were maintained for up to 4 months, but beyond the appearance of small groups of cells on the interior of the cyst wall which may have represented the anlagen of the protoscoleces further development was not obtained. Evagination of the protoscolex with trypsin or bile treatment did not appear to influence the pattern of development Vesicular development was accelerated by very high (95 per cent) and low (0 per cent) oxygen tensions, by low (6.5) and high (8.0) pH values, and by high levels of bile. It was concluded therefore that vesicularisation was elicited by abnormal *in vitro* conditions and that it may serve a protective function. But vesicularisation could also have a detrimental effect on the parasite's survival and continued differentiation because the eventual development of the laminated layer may prevent nutrients from reaching the enclosed tissues.

Similar patterns of development have been observed by other workers but some differences have been reported regarding the competency of certain morphological types assumed by the protoscolex to undergo cystic development. For example Benex (1968) and Heath and Osborn (1976) found that only vesicular protoscoleces with associated remnants of the brood capsule wall (germinal layer) formed cysts; posterior bladder development was associated with the complete loss of the germinal layer from the protoscolex and an apparent inability to develop in a cystic direction.

The reasons for this discrepancy with Smyth's observations are unknown; they may derive from different pretreatments with enzymes or to undefined differences in the physico-chemical conditions of culture. It seems possible that those protoscoleces with posterior bladders that formed cysts in Smyth's experiments may have retained vestiges of the germinal layer. Although a number of questions have yet to be resolved, the results suggest that the germinal layer has a very influential determining potential, perhaps analagous with the dorsal lip of the blastopore in a vertebrate embryo. It would be of interest to culture germinal layer alone to see if it had the capacity to undergo cystic development in the absence of protoscolex tissue. Such has been demonstrated for *E. multilocularis* (see below).

Gurri (1963), in contrast with others, obtained cystic development but laminated layers did not form. Protoscoleces from the same source formed laminated layers *in vivo* so an explanation for this unusual result is not readily apparent. Smyth (1968) has suggested that the medium used may have lacked some factor necessary for laminated layer formation *in vitro*.

Heath and Osborn (1976) made some additional interesting observations on cystic development *in vitro*. Since the culture medium they used (NCTC-135) contained no macromolecules, they established unequivocally that the laminated layer was of parasite rather than host origin, a question that had been debated previously (Smyth 1962a and see Ch. 1). They also observed that the posterior bladders of several protoscoleces often coalesced to form a cyst-like structure with the bodies of the protoscoleces arranged peripherally; when 10–40 protoscoleces were involved, laminated layers formed.

While the development of small cysts has been achieved *in vitro*, these have not differentiated into fertile cysts containing brood capsules and protoscoleces. There would appear to be several possible reasons for this: (a) the presence of the laminated layer may prevent cells in the germinal layer from obtaining adequate nutrients for their continued differentiation; (b) some 'trigger' stimulus which initiates protoscolex differentiation may be lacking; (c) cysts may fail to reach the critical levels of water content (about 95 per cent) and size ($\simeq$ 6 mm) that are apparently required before fertility is achieved (Heath 1970); (d) cystic development *in vitro* may be an abnormal and terminal pattern of differentiation, brought on in response to abnormal or unfavourable cultural conditions such as high pH and extremely low or high O_2 tension which Smyth (1967) considered to be important factors in inducing vesicularisation of protoscoleces; (e) other physico-chemical properties of the cultures may be lacking in some way.

Clearly the area of cyst differentiation is worthy of further investigation. Initially it would be of interest to see if *in vitro* derived cysts can continue their development and become fertile if implanted into a suitable host. Indeed, such an experiment impinges on all the possibilities considered above. In particular, it would clarify whether (d) has any validity. It would also be worthwhile considering whether the so-called 'abnormal' conditions that encourage cystic development *in vitro* can be equated with any of the physico-chemical conditions of the *in vivo* environment.

Strobilate development Attempts to induce the protoscolex to differentiate into an adult tapeworm were frustrated by the ease with which this stage developed in a cystic direction. Varying a variety of physico-chemical conditions in culture such as E_h, pO_2, pH, pCO_2 and nutritional constituents had no obvious effect on the cystic pattern of development (Smyth *et al.* 1966). This led to the suggestion that some unusual stimulus or nutritional factor was lacking from the cultures which was essential for development in a strobilate direction to be initiated. An hypothesis was developed to explain the nature of the missing factor(s) based on a close examination of the relationship between the adult worm and the dog gut (Smyth 1964, Smyth *et al.* 1966, 1967, Smyth & Smyth 1969). It was suggested that because worms penetrated deeply into the crypts of Lieberkühn they could be regarded more as tissue parasites than lumen dwellers and the apposition of the scolex to the host was so intimate that the scolex could be regarded as analagous to a placenta. Ultrastructural evidence of long microtriches on the scolex and the presence of a rostellar gland reinforced this view. Thus, if development was to proceed in a strobilate direction *in vitro* it was reasoned that a solid supporting substrate providing nutrients and/or a contact stimulus would be required. The classic studies using diphasic media, consisting of a solid base with a liquid phase above, were therefore initiated (Smyth *et al.* 1966, Smyth 1967) and the results of this work have amply borne out the conclusions arrived at regarding the requirements for strobilate development. Since that time the methods have been modified to optimise development in a strobilate direction (Smyth & Davies 1974b, Smyth 1979a) and these can be summarised as follows: as the solid phase, calf serum which has been coagulated in the base of a milk dilution bottle by heating to 78–80°C is used; the liquid phase consists of 20 ml of Medium S10; 0.1 ml of packed evaginated protoscoleces (10 000) of sheep origin are added and incubated at 38.5°C with a gas phase of 5 per cent CO_2, 10 per cent O_2, 85 per cent N_2.

Under these conditions sexually mature worms with three segments developed in about twice the time required in the dog. Only a proportion of protoscoleces developed to this extent; a whole range of developmental stages could be found in any one culture, but this also characterises development *in vivo*. Two other striking observations were made. Firstly, the degree of development attained *in vitro* was dependent on the origin of the protoscoleces: those from sheep develop as described above; those from human and goats segmented and the former developed testes; those from cattle and horses failed to segment (Smyth 1982). Secondly, monozoic forms – sexually mature but unsegmented worms – appeared in some cultures (Smyth 1971), leading to the conclusion that somatic and germinal differentiation can, under certain physico-chemical conditions which are as yet undefined, take place independently of each other (see Ch. 1). Alternatively, the monozoic forms could have arisen from mutant protoscoleces in which somatic differentiation was suppressed.

The major difference between sexually mature cultured worms and dog worms was the failure of insemination to occur in the former. The uterus of the terminal proglottid became filled with ova but these were not fertilised and shells did not form. It was noted that the receptaculum seminis was empty, an indication that insemination had not occurred. Despite the fact that nearly 18 years have elapsed since strobilate worms were obtained *in vitro*, this problem has not yet been overcome.

Some important factors to consider when establishing cultures were stressed by Smyth and Davies (1974b) and Smyth (1979a), particularly (a) the need to evaginate protoscoleces prior to culture by incubation in medium 858 containing 0.002 per cent sodium taurocholate or 0.05 per cent dog bile for 18–24 h at 38°C; (b) if sodium taurocholate rather than dog bile is used care must be exercised to choose a brand which does not contain other bile salts as impurities which are lytic to protoscoleces. Variable results were a feature both within and between experiments and a particularly variable component of the culture medium was foetal calf serum. Some of the variation was also ascribed to factors such as micro-organismal contaminants, type of culture vessel, different batches of other media components, mechanical failure of equipment, unevenness in seeding cultures with protoscoleces and the nature of the protoscoleces themselves – their age, physiological condition and host of origin.

Similar results were also obtained in a 'lift' culture system in which medium slowly circulated through cellulose tubing without disturbing worms developing in the diphasic medium comprising a solid bovine serum base with liquid phase above (Smyth 1969a, Smyth & Davies 1974b). It has not been demonstrated, however, that this modification to the culture procedure significantly altered the physico-chemical conditions to which the worms were exposed.

It is of interest to note that the protoscoleces of another cyclophyllidean, *Taenia serialis*, responded in a similar way to *E. granulosus* when cultured under comparable conditions (Smyth 1969b). Thus, in monophasic media the protoscoleces became 'cystic', but in the diphasic system some worms underwent strobilisation and genitalia appeared. In a limited series of experiments, Brandt and Sewell (1980) found that metacestodes (≡ protoscoleces) of *T. saginata* underwent strobilisation in a diphasic medium in which a solid phase consisting of disrupted coagulated calf serum rather than a solid base was more effective. However strobilisation also occurred in a monophasic medium and therefore much more work needs to be carried out in an attempt to define the conditions under which it can be reproducibly achieved.

Some comments are warranted on why strobilisation of *E. granulosus* protoscoleces only occurs in diphasic media and why insemination fails to take place *in vitro*. The nature of the factors governing strobilar development are not known but two conditions need to be satisfied for it to occur: (a) the protoscoleces must be evaginated and (b) a nutritive substrate must be provided with which the protoscolex can establish intimate contact; non-nutritive substrates such as agar fail to initiate strobilisation. The type of nutritive substrate is itself critical. Coagulated bovine serum is superior to horse or dog serum and other protein bases such as gelatine or collagen do not induce strobilisation. The possible nature of the stimulus involved has been discussed in detail by Smyth (1967, 1969a, 1972) so only a brief resumé will be given here. It is believed that a contact or 'strobilisation' stimulus is provided to the scolex by the substrate and strobilar development is thereby initiated. The stimulus is either a nutritional factor derived from the substrate either directly, or indirectly by some digestive process; or a physical interaction between the substrate and microtriches on the tegument of the protoscolex which initiates neurophysiological changes. It is also worth considering that the discontinuity between solid and liquid phases in cultures may generate optimum gradients of small molecules that facilitate their uptake through the parasite's tegument. Relevant to this possibility is that strobilisation is only achieved in cultures in which the medium is undisturbed.

The failure to achieve insemination *in vitro* may be a physical rather than nutritional inadequacy of the culture system (Smyth & Davies 1974b), since self-insemination is known to occur *in vivo* (Smyth & Smyth 1969). Given that the worms are small, some special kind of compression may be required *in vitro*, in order for the cirrus to bend back on itself and enter the vagina on the same segment. In cultured worms the cirrus has certainly been observed to protrude from the genital pore. Of course some as yet unrecognised developmental abnormality of the reproductive system may prevent insemination, and even when and if the problem is solved there is no guarantee that sperm formed *in vitro* will be normal. It would be useful to implant cultured worms into dogs to see if the latter stages of sexual maturation took place. Dogs could be fed gelatine capsules containing sexually mature worms grown *in vitro* in an attempt to answer this question.

MATURATION OF PARTLY DEVELOPED WORMS

Cultivation of adult *E. granulosus in vitro* is an important objective because it would eliminate the difficulties and dangers of maintaining this highly infective stage in dogs. Because of the apparent barrier to insemination in otherwise sexually mature worms cultured in diphasic media, Smyth and Howkins (1966) sought to circumvent it by culturing partly mature worms from dogs to the ovigerous stage. They found that 28–35 d old worms from dogs (without shelled eggs in the uterus and therefore safe to handle) became ovigerous after a period of 7–22 d in culture. These worms were presumably inseminated when the cultures were initiated because this occurs between 25 and 30 d *in vivo* (Smyth & Davies 1974b).

The rate of maturation of these partly developed worms *in vitro* was slightly slower than *in vivo* and it took place in both monophasic and diphasic media. Oncospheres within eggs appeared to be normal. However, it was not until some time later that worms cultured by this method produced eggs from which oncospheres were hatched and activated (Thompson & Smyth 1976) and gave rise to fertile cysts containing apparently normal protoscoleces in mice (Kumaratilake & Thompson 1981). As a result of these studies it is now possible to maintain the life-cycle of *E. granulosus* in the laboratory in relative safety.

The physico-chemical conditions under which worms that have partly developed *in vivo* will mature *in vitro* have yet to be defined. Maturation will occur in hydatid fluid alone (although not as well as in diphasic media) so the nutritional and/or physical requirements may not be particularly demanding. A solid serum base is clearly not essential.

CYSTIC DEVELOPMENT FROM ONCOSPHERES

There have been few attempts to initiate cultures with *E. granulosus* oncospheres because of the inherent danger to the operator in handling eggs. Heath and Smyth (1970) hatched and activated oncospheres by sequential treatments with artificial gastric and intestinal solutions and cultured the parasites in medium 858 containing 20 per cent sheep serum with a gas phase of 10 per cent O_2, 5 per cent CO_2, 85 per cent N_2, pH 7.2. They obtained small cysts, up to about five times the diameter of the oncosphere, after 10 d *in vitro*; cultures were not continued beyond that point.

The development of facilities for the relatively safe handling of eggs derived from patent infections of dogs enabled Heath and Lawrence (1976) to investigate further the development of *E. granulosus* oncospheres *in vitro*. Using a medium consisting of NCTC-135, 20 per cent foetal calf or 10 week old rabbit serum (together with 1 per cent v/v rabbit red blood cells for the first 30 d), hatched and activated oncospheres developed into small cysts up to 2 cm in diameter (which represented an approximately 700-fold increase in size) at a rate comparable with, or even faster than, that observed *in vivo*. The cysts developed clearly defined laminated layers, so in many respects they resembled cysts which developed from protoscoleces. Cysts were not fertile after 120 d although they were still growing; they may not have achieved their critical mass after that time and a more prolonged period of culture may have been required for protoscoleces to develop from what appeared to be a clearly defined germinal layer within the cyst.

Echinococcus multilocularis

PROTOSCOLEX AND GERMINAL LAYER

The protoscoleces of *E. multilocularis*, like those of *E. granulosus*, exhibit a dual developmental potential – into adult worms if eaten by a carnivore such as a fox, dog or cat, or in a cystic direction if injected into an appropriate intermediate host. These patterns of development have been achieved *in vitro*; in addition, proliferation of the germinal layer into cysts has been demonstrated.

Cystic development The development of viable cysts (cysts containing protoscoleces) of *E. multilocularis in vitro* from fragments of undifferentiated germinal layer (Rausch & Jentoft 1957) and dissociated cyst tissue or protoscoleces (Lukashenko 1964) has been achieved. In both cases cultured material was infective to intermediate hosts (voles and cotton rats) and protoscoleces were also infective to a dog. The proliferation of vesicles by exogenous budding, which was thought to occur *in vivo*, was confirmed and growth rates attained *in vitro* approached those observed *in vivo*. Laminated layers formed around vesicles in some experiments (Lukashenko 1964) but apparently not in others (Rausch & Jentoft 1957). The best results in terms of rate and degree of development were obtained when intermediate host embryo extract was present in the culture media.

Yamashita *et al.* (1962) found that protoscoleces developed in a cystic direction in a manner almost exactly as described by Smyth (1962a) for *E. granulosus*. Either a protoscolex became vesicular and a laminated layer formed as cyst differentiation proceeded, or the protoscolex developed a posterior bladder which expanded as the hooks and suckers degenerated and an essentially spherical cystic form resulted. Although cultures were maintained for 60 d, protoscoleces did not develop within the cysts. This may reflect an insufficient period of culture or possibly that intermediate host embryo extract was not present; this was a component of culture media where protoscolex differentiation was achieved. However, from the little work that has been done, it is difficult to draw any definitive conclusions about the factors governing differentiation of cysts and protoscoleces of this species *in vitro*.

Strobilate development Both Lukashenko (1964) and Webster and Cameron (1963) found that a few protoscoleces in their cultures developed in a strobilate rather than a cystic direction. Although two or three segments formed, the reproductive system failed to develop. Since these events took place side by side with cystic development the conditions under which strobilisation were induced were not defined.

Smyth and Davies (1975) cultured protoscoleces of *E. multilocularis* through to sexual maturity although eggs were not produced. Further studies were reported by Smyth (1979a) and Smyth and Barret (1979) and the procedure for setting up cultures and the pattern of development obtained were as follows: protoscoleces were separated from host tissue (which tends to be spongy and calcified) by homogenisation and pepsin treatment followed by repeated sedimentation in Hank's saline to remove suspended material. They were then evaginated and cultured in monophasic and diphasic media, essentially as described above for *E. granulosus*.

Two distinct patterns of differentiation occurred irrespective of the type of culture medium (either monophasic or diphasic) used. Firstly, about 70–80 per cent of the protoscoleces developed into unsegmented worms (monozoic forms), each with a complete set of mature male and female genitalia. After about a month *in vitro* a uterus cavity containing ova and vitelline cells could be identified in the most advanced worms, but fertile eggs were not obtained, probably due to the failure of insemination to occur. The rate of development *in vitro* was not appreciably slower than *in vivo*.

The second pattern of differentiation was, in itself, multi-faceted, but generally involved (a) elongation of the worms, (b) the appearance and maturation of genitalia, (c) constrictions separating anterior and posterior portions of the worms – a phenomenon referred to as pseudosegmentation since no interproglottidal membrane was formed, (d) further pseudosegmentation into three proglottids and in long-term cultures the appearance of a fourth proglottid and supernumerary scoleces with apparently normal suckers. A considerable degree of variation was observed, especially in regard to the way in which (b), (c) and (d) were temporally related. Smyth (1979a) and Smyth and Barrett (1979) should be consulted for further details. Sexual maturity was also attained by worms that underwent pseudosegmentation but again fertile eggs were not produced.

The reasons for this highly variable pattern of development together with some abnormal features such as extra suckers and pseudosegments are not known. It would seem that varying degrees of suppression or acceleration of somatic cell differentiation can explain most of the results (Smyth & Davies 1975). That the variation can be observed in any one culture suggests that the protoscoleces are genetically heterogeneous. This would be, perhaps, expected if the protoscoleces were derived from different cysts, but if they were not, it is difficult to explain the differential effects of the same culture conditions on what are, in all probability, genetically identical organisms (Smyth 1977). This point could be tested by establishing replicate cultures of protoscoleces and ensuring that those in each were derived from the same cyst.

MATURATION OF PARTLY DEVELOPED WORMS

A similar barrier to the maturation of *E. granulosus* into ovigerous worms *in vitro* exists with respect to *E. multilocularis* and this is again apparently due to the failure of insemination to occur.

Thompson and Eckert (1982), by applying the same techniques as used with *E. granulosus*, were able to obtain gravid worms *in vitro* following partial development in the definitive host for 20–21 d. Maturation required a further 8 d and took place in both monophasic and diphasic media. Morphologically normal eggs were produced at the same time as in worms that developed to maturity in dogs, but these were not infective following oral administration to jirds, irrespective of whether the eggs were pretreated with pepsin. If this technique can be modified to produce infective eggs *in vitro*, a considerable barrier to research on this phase of the life-cycle of *E. multilocularis* will be overcome. The eggs of *E. multilocularis* are considered to be even more hazardous to work with than those of *E. granulosus* and there is little doubt that this has discouraged attempts to work with them. This would also explain why there have been no reported attempts to culture the cystic stages of *E. multilocularis* from oncospheres.

COMPARATIVE ASPECTS OF *IN VITRO* CULTURE OF *E. GRANULOSUS* AND *E. MULTILOCULARIS*

Two barriers prevent *Echinococcus granulosus* (particularly the sheep strain) from being cultured throughout its entire life-cycle *in vitro*. These are (a) the inability of sexually mature worms to self-inseminate and produce shelled eggs; (b) the failure of protoscoleces to differentiate within cysts derived from either protoscoleces or oncospheres. Since early attempts (Smyth & Davies 1974b), there has been no concerted effort made to solve these problems.

The first barrier has been recognised for a long time and, as noted above, it is presumably a physical defect in the culture system which is responsible, a judgment based on the relationship between the worms and the intestinal villi *in vivo* where the strobila is compressed between the villi and a protruding cirrus would be guided towards the vagina. The second barrier may be resolved merely by culturing the cysts for longer periods than has hitherto been attempted.

E. multilocularis, like *E. granulosus*, fails to undergo insemination *in vitro* and shelled eggs are not produced. However, protoscoleces and germinal tissue from the intermediate host differentiate *in vitro* into viable cysts containing protoscoleces which are infective to dogs. There are also other points of contrast between the two species: *E. multilocularis* undergoes sexual maturation in both monophasic and diphastic media and develops mainly into monozoic forms or less frequently into pseudosegmented forms in which segmentation is incomplete; *E. granulosus* will only undergo segmentation and some degree of sexual maturation in diphasic media provided that the protoscoleces are derived from sheep or human hydatid cysts. Protoscoleces from goats segment but fail to mature while those of horse and cattle origin fail to segment. An important feature common to both species is that development in a strobilate as opposed to a cystic direction will only take place if the protoscoleces are evaginated.

E. multilocularis is a considerably more invasive parasite in its intermediate host than *E. granulosus*. In fact, it behaves rather like a highly differentiated metastatic tumour (Mankau 1956, Swellengrebel & Sterman 1961). Moreover, it develops more rapidly in the definitive host than *E. granulosus*. These characteristics point to differences in the control of gene expression between the two species which are reflected in the *in vitro* results. It could well be that molecular biological investigations of the genomes of these species could be a profitable area of research. Some unusual genetic control mechanisms or genomic characteristics may be revealed that explain at a more fundamental level some of the differing biological properties of the organisms.

Another point is also worth making. In one study (Lubinsky & Desser 1963) it was found that *E. multilocularis* induced the formation of sarcomata in mice and in another (Vogel 1957) there appeared to be a relationship between *E. multilocularis* infection and human liver carcinoma. These observations raise questions as to whether there is some kind of genetic input into the host genome by this parasite, perhaps in a manner analogous to that which occurs in the induction of neoplasia by some retroviruses (Duesberg 1983). Probing the host genome for parasite genetic material could well be a fruitful area of investigation.

IN VITRO STUDIES AND THE BIOLOGY OF *ECHINOCOCCUS* SPP.

The principal objective of the work described above has been to cultivate *E. granulosus* and *E. multilocularis* throughout all of their life-cycle stages *in vitro*. During the course of this work significant progress has been made. Many problems have been encountered and solved, but others – such as obtaining ovigerous adult worms with viable eggs – remain.

To what extent has this work contributed to an understanding of the biology of these parasites? Before attempting to answer this question in detail, it is worth pointing out that there are three main ways in which *in vitro* studies have been able to contribute. Firstly, direct observation of the parasites *in vitro* has clarified certain aspects of their biology. Secondly, some of the problems encountered *in vitro* have led to a closer appraisal of certain aspects of the host–parasite relationship and important conceptual advances have resulted. Thirdly, some of the findings have fostered other kinds of experiments which have illuminated important biological characteristics of the organisms.

Host–parasite relationships

The dual developmental potential of both *E. granulosus* and *E. multilocularis* has been confirmed *in vitro*. Development in a cystic direction is readily achieved, particularly for *E. multilocularis*, and the laminated layer which surrounds the cyst is clearly of parasite origin. Development in a strobilate direction requires that protoscoleces be evaginated. Beyond that, no requirements have been defined for *E. multilocularis*, but for *E. granulosus* the need to culture the organisms on a solidified nutritive base to achieve segmentation is well established. The events leading to this discovery were characterised by a close analysis of the relationship between the worm and the dog gut together with ultrastructural observations of the protoscoleces (Smyth 1964, Smyth *et al.* 1966). These investigations highlighted the intimacy of contact between host and parasite, the presence of a rostellar gland and the likelihood that immunological contact with the host was established. It was also found that the protoscolex had microtriches only on the scolex; posterior to the suckers the body was covered by a dense polysaccharide coat beneath which were blunt protruberances (undeveloped microtriches) of the body wall. The idea that a solid substrate would be required for both support and as a nutrient source for the scolex was a brilliant and far-reaching deduction that proved to have validity when tested. The importance of evagination in order to obtain strobilate development was also brought into focus by the number of interesting properties of the scolex.

The two hypotheses that were proposed to account for the events which trigger strobilisation (Smyth *et al.* 1967) have been referred to earlier in this chapter; unfortunately there have been no published accounts of attempts to test them.

The failure to achieve insemination and complete the final stages of maturation *in vitro* has also been referred to above. Although the reasons for this are probably spatial, attempts to overcome the problem (e.g. enclosing worms in cellulose tubing to achieve compression of the strobila) have so far failed. An important observation to emerge from this work was that *E. granulosus* is a self-inseminating species (Smyth & Smyth 1969). To provide the appropriate physical conditions for the parasite to undertake this activity will tax the ingenuity of the *in vitro* culturist.

In the earliest attempts to culture *E. granulosus* protoscoleces *in vitro* (Smyth 1962a) no particular procedure was followed to induce evagination. Later, bile salts were used to effect and sustain this phenomenon because of its importance in relation to achieving strobilate development. Initially it was found that a sample of bile extract (commercially referred to as 'sodium tauroglycocholate') lysed and killed the organisms (Smyth 1962b). The investigation of the phenomenon which followed showed that bile from a number of herbivores lysed the protoscoleces but lysis did not occur with a number of carnivore biles. This led to an imaginative hypothesis to account for the host specificity of not only *E. granulosus* but parasites in general – namely that the nature and concentration of bile salts and soaps to which a parasite is exposed may be a fundamental controlling factor in helminth life-cycles. This hypothesis alone fails to account for the host specificity in *E. granulosus* and there is no doubt that other factors are involved (see Ch. 1). For example, cat bile was not lytic to protoscoleces (Smyth 1962b) but *E. granulosus* fails to become established as an adult worm in this host (Smyth & Smyth 1964, Euzéby 1974). In this case the topography of the gut may be unsuitable or some essential bile constituent that acts in a positive way by facilitating worm establishment is lacking (Smyth 1968).

Despite the attractiveness of the bile hypothesis and of its seemingly fundamental significance in host–parasite relationships, it has been little studied since the original paper by Smyth (1962b). Dixon (1966) and Howell (1970) have suggested a number of functions for bile such as stimulating muscular activity or triggering developmental changes in parasites in a hormonal-like fashion, but essentially the broad field of investigation highlighted by Smyth (1962b) is still open.

Parasite strains

The culture work leading to the development of strobilate *E. granulosus in vitro* was based on the use of protoscoleces derived from hydatid cysts in sheep (Smyth & Davies 1974b). When similar techniques were applied to protoscoleces from hydatid cysts in horses unexpected results were obtained (Smyth & Davies 1974a). The protoscoleces survived for long periods but grew only slightly; they failed to segment and showed no signs of sexual maturation. Various modifications to the culture conditions have failed to promote growth and development of protoscoleces of horse origin (Smyth 1977, 1979b, Smyth & Davies 1979). The reasons for this remain an enigma but are presumably related to nutritional, stimulatory or metabolic requirements peculiar to these parasites which are not supplied by the culture system used so successfully with protoscoleces of sheep origin (Smyth 1982). It became evident, therefore, that distinct physiological strains of the parasite existed. When protoscoleces from other intermediate hosts were cultured *in vitro* it was found that those from cattle (from Ireland and Kenya) behaved like those from horses (Smyth 1979b, Macpherson 1981) whereas those from goats grew and segmented but did not undergo sexual maturation (Macpherson 1981). Those from a human (from Saudi Arabia) followed a similar developmental pattern to sheep and goat protoscoleces in that segmentation took place; however, full maturity was not achieved although testes developed (Smyth *et al.* 1980). The evidence from these studies suggested that *E. granulosus* from sheep, goats and humans belonged to the same group whereas those from horses and cattle belonged to another (Smyth 1982). The demonstration of these strain differences by *in vitro* culture methods has stimulated much further work on the biochemical characterisation of strains (reviewed by Smyth 1979b, 1982; see also Chs 1 & 4).

There are biochemical differences between parasites derived from the various intermediate hosts which match the *in vitro* results. However, it is now recognised that the situation is more complex than the division into two groups based on the *in vitro* developmental pattern alone. This probably reflects differential selection on the *E. granulosus* gene pool imposed by varied ecological situations in geographically distinct regions. Thus, it is not possible to generalise as to the strain type of the parasite solely on the basis of host. For example Macpherson and Smyth (1985) have shown that Kenyan protoscoleces of human, cattle, sheep, camel and goat origin develop *in vitro* like the UK sheep strain (i.e. segment). These results contrast with earlier work on parasites from Kenyan cattle (see above) and with biochemical data on various enzymes in the Kenyan parasites: two groups could be differentiated on the basis of their isoenzyme patterns – type A (human, cattle and sheep) and type B (camel and goat) (Macpherson 1981). These problems are considered further in Chapters 1 & 4.

The *in vitro* culture of partly mature worms has also been used to characterise strains of the parasite from the same host in geographically separated regions (Kumaratilake *et al.* 1983). Egg production *in vitro* by worms removed from dogs 35 d post-infection took 7 d less in parasites of Tasmanian sheep origin than in those of mainland sheep origin. These results complemented observations made on the *in vivo* developmental pattern.

Strains of *E. multilocularis* have not been identified as yet but given the wide distribution of this parasite and its host range (Lukashenko 1971) it would seem highly likely that a similar degree of physiological complexity will be found.

The initial observations of Smyth and Davies (1974a) on strains of *E. granulosus* have thus stimulated much further work and alerted parasitologists to the need for more detailed investigation in order to understand fully the ecology of echinococcosis; they represent a very significant contribution to parasitology. An interesting practical benefit has also emerged in relation to the epidemiology of the parasite in humans. Smyth *et al.* (1980) showed that protoscoleces from a human hydatid cyst from a Saudi Arabian had the biochemical and *in vitro* developmental characteristics of the UK sheep strain. Thus, *in vitro* culture may be useful for distinguishing those strains of the parasite which are infective to humans and for corroborating conclusions drawn from other data regarding the epidemiology of echinococcosis.

CONCLUDING REMARKS

The preceding discussion has described the *in vitro* cultivation of *E. granulosus* and *E. multilocularis* and how the results of this work have clarified certain aspects of the biology of these parasites and suggested hypotheses about their relationships with their hosts. Immunological considerations have scarcely been referred to because these have not been a focus of the type of work reviewed. Although the culture methods described above have been aimed primarily at achieving growth and development they could be extended to examine the effects of immune mechanisms on the parasites by, for example, the addition of antibody, complement or lymphocytes to cultures in which the parasites are in a reasonably normal physiological state at the outset of the experiments. It would be of interest to compare the results of such studies with those derived from the kinds of *in vitro* investigations reviewed in the following chapter which have been directed at gaining an understanding of the immunology of echinococcosis.

Smyth (1969b) put forward a strong case based on his *in vitro* studies for the wider use of *E. granulosus* as an experimental animal in order to examine a variety of biological phenomena in areas such as neuromuscular physiology, cytology and differentiation. The same case could now be made for *E. multilocularis*. Differentiation, in particular, is well suited to investigation because the direction it takes in the protoscoleces of these species – either in a cystic or strobilate direction – can be controlled *in vitro*. Unfortunately, however, it has not attracted the attention it deserves. Both the factors that stimulate differentiation in these parasites and, at a more fundamental level, the genetic mechanisms that are involved would be fruitful areas for investigation. The rapid advances being made in recombinant DNA technology now make it possible to analyse the complexities of differential gene expression. The value of parasites for such studies is well exemplified by work on trypanosomes (Borst & Cross 1982) which is at the forefront of our present level of understanding of the phenomenon.

In addition to the question of differentiation, nuclear magnetic resonance techniques are available (see Ch. 4) which make it possible to monitor aspects of a parasite's biochemistry (e.g. intermediary metabolism) continuously throughout its development *in vitro*. Such methods enable essentially normal organisms to be examined and could be expected to provide more realistic and comprehensive data than short-term incubations.

In conclusion, the *in vitro* culture of *Echinococcus* spp. has offered much to parasitology in the past; may it prosper in the future and may it continue to improve our understanding of parasitological phenomena in particular and biological problems in general. Desmond Smyth's far-sighted and practical contributions to this field stand in bold relief. They provide a firm experimental and conceptual base for the imaginative researcher who is prepared to use these organisms in order to tackle some of the most challenging problems in biology.

REFERENCES

Benex, J. 1968. Considérations expérimentales nouvelles sur l'évolution *in vitro* en milieu liquide des larves d'*Echinococcus granulosus*. *Annls Parasitol.* **43**, 561–72.

Borst, P. and G. A. M. Cross 1982. Molecular basis for trypanosome antigenic variation. *Cell* **29**, 291–303.

Brandt, J. R. A. and M. M. H. Sewell 1980. Preliminary observations on the *in vitro* culture of metacestodes of *Taenia saginata*. *Vet. Sci. Commun.* **3**, 317–24.

Brudnjak, Z., S. Cvetnić and T. Wikerhauser 1970. Cystic development of the protoscoleces and brood capsules of *Echinococcus granulosus* in cell cultures and cell-free media. *Vet. Arhiv* **40**, 292–6.

Coutelen, F. 1927a. Essai de culture *in vitro* de scolex et hydatides échinococciques. *Annls Parasitol. Hum. Comp.* **5**, 1–19.

Coutelen, F. 1927b. Sur l'évolution vésiculaire *in vitro* des scolex échinococciques. *Annls Parasitol. Hum. Comp.* **5**, 239–42.

Dévé, F. 1926. Evolution vésiculaire du scolex échinococcique obtenue *in vitro*. La culture artificielle du kyste hydatique. *C. R. Soc. Biol. Paris* **94**, 440–1.

Dixon, K. E. 1966. The physiology of excystment of the metacercaria of *Fasciola hepatica* L. *Parasitology* **56**, 431–56.

Duesberg, P. H. 1983. Retroviral transforming genes in normal cells. *Nature, Lond.* **304**, 219–26.

Euzéby, J. A. 1974. Zoonotic cestodes. In *Parasitic zoonoses: clinical and experimental studies*, E. J. L. Soulsby (ed.), 151–78. New York: Academic Press.

Gurri, J. 1963. Vitalidad y evolutividad de los escólices hidátocos *in vivo* e *in vitro*. *Ann. Fac. Med. Univ. Montevideo* **48**, 372–81.

Heath, D. D. 1970. The development of *Echinococcus granulosus* larvae in laboratory animals. *Parasitology* **60**, 449–56.

Heath, D. D. 1982. *In vitro* culture of cysticerci: an aid to investigations of morphological development and host-parasite relationships. In *Cysticercosis: present state of knowledge and perspectives,* A. Flisser, K. Willons, J. P. Laclette, C. Larralde, C. Ridaura and F. Beltrán (eds), 477–93. New York: Academic Press.

Heath, D. D. and S. B. Lawrence 1976. *Echinococcus granulosus*: development *in vitro* from oncosphere to immature hydatid cyst. *Parasitology* **73**, 417–23.

Heath, D. D. and P. J. Osborn 1976. Formation of *Echinococcus granulosus* laminated membrane in a defined medium. *Int. J. Parasitol.* **6**, 467–71.

Heath, D. D. and J. D. Smyth 1970. *In vitro* cultivation of *Echinococcus granulosus, Taenia hydatigena, T. ovis, T. pisiformis* and *T. serialis* from oncosphere to cystic larva. *Parasitology* **61**, 329–43.

Howell, M. J. 1970. Excystment of the metacercariae of *Echinoparyphium serratum* (Trematoda: Echinostomatidae. *J. Helminthol*). **44**, 35–56.

Kumaratilake, L. M. and R. C. A. Thompson 1981. Maintenance of the life cycle of *Echinococcus granulosus* in the laboratory following *in vivo* and *in vitro* development. *Z. ParasitKde* **65**, 103–6.

Kumaratilake, L. M., R. C. A. Thompson and J. D. Dunsmore 1983. Comparative strobilar development of *Echinococcus granulosus* of sheep origin from different geographical areas of Australia *in vivo* and *in vitro*. *Int. J. Parasitol.* **13**, 151–6.

Lubinsky, G. and S. Desser 1963. Growth of the vegetatively propagated strain of larval *Echinococcus multilocularis* in C57L/J, B6AF$_1$, and A/J mice. *Can. J. Zool.* **41**, 1213–6.

Lukashenko, N. P. 1964. [Study of the development of *Alveococcus multilocularis* (Leuckart, 1863) *in vitro*.] *Med. Parazit. (Moskow)* **33**, 271–8. (In Russian).

Lukashenko, N. P. 1971. Problems of epidemiology and prophylaxis of alveococcosis (multilocular echinococcosis): a general review – with particular reference to the USSR. *Int. J. Parasitol.* **1**, 125–34.

Macpherson, C. 1981. *Epidemiology and strain differentiation of* Echinococcus granulosus *in Kenya.* PhD thesis, University of London.

Macpherson, C. N. L. and J. D. Smyth 1985. *In vitro* culture of the strobilar stage of *Echinococcus granulosus* from protoscoleces of human, camel, sheep and goat origin from Kenya and buffalo origin from India. *Int. J. Parasitol* **15**, 137–40.

Mankau, S. K. 1956. Studies on *Echinococcus alveolaris* (Klemm, 1883) from St Lawrence Island, Alaska. III. The histopathology caused by the infection of *E. alveolaris* in white mice. *Am. J. Trop. Med. Hyg.* **5**, 872–80.

Pauluzzi, S., F. Sorice, L. Castagnari and P. Serra 1965. Contributo allo studio delle colture *in vitro* degli scolici di *Echinococcus granulosus Annali Sclavo* **7**, 191–218.

Rausch, R. and V. L. Jentoft 1957. Studies on the helminth fauna of Alaska. XXXI. Observations on the propagation of the larval *Echinococcus multilocularis* Leuckart, 1863, *in vitro. J. Parasitol.* **43**, 1–8.

Smyth, J. D. 1962a. Studies on tapeworm physiology. X. Axenic cultivation of the hydatid organism, *Echinococcus granulosus*: establishment of a basic technique. *Parasitology* **52**, 441–57.

Smyth, J. D. 1962b. Lysis of *Echinococcus granulosus* by surface-active agents in bile and the role of this phenomenon in determining host specificity in helminths. *Proc. R. Soc. B* **156**, 553–72.

Smyth, J. D. 1964. Observations on the scolex of *Echinococcus granulosus*, with special reference to the occurrence and cytochemistry of cells in the rostellum. *Parasitology* **54**, 515–26.

Smyth, J. D. 1967. Studies on tapeworm physiology. XI. *In vitro* cultivation of *Echinococcus granulosus* from the protoscolex to the strobilate stage. *Parasitology* **57**, 111–33.

Smyth, J. D. 1968. *In vitro* studies and host-specificity in *Echinococcus. Bull. Wld Hlth Org.* **39**, 5–12.

Smyth, J. D. 1969a. *The physiology of cestodes.* Edinburgh: Oliver and Boyd.

Smyth, J. D. 1969b. Parasites as biological models. *Parasitology* **59**, 73–91.

Smyth, J. D. 1971. Development of monozoic forms of *Echinococcus granulosus* during *in vitro* culture. *Int. J. Parasitol.* **1**, 121–4.

Smyth, J. D. 1972. Changes in the digestive–absorptive surface of cestodes during larval/adult differentiation. *Symp. Br. Soc. Parasitol.* **10**, 41–70.

Smyth, J. D. 1977. Strain differences in *Echinococcus granulosus*, with special reference to the status of equine hydatidosis in the United Kingdom. *Trans. R. Soc. Trop. Med. Hyg.* **71**, 93–100.

Smyth, J. D. 1979a. *Echinococcus granulosus* and *E. multilocularis*: *in vitro* culture of the strobilar stages from protoscoleces. *Angew. Parasitol.* **20**, 137–47.

Smyth, J. D. 1979b. An *in vitro* approach to taxonomic problems in trematodes and cestodes, especially *Echinococcus. Symp. Br. Soc. Parasitol.* **17**, 75–101.

Smyth, J. D. 1982. Speciation in *Echinococcus*: biological and biochemical criteria. *Revta Iber. Parasitol.* Special Volume, 25–34.

Smyth, J. D. and N. J. Barrett 1979. *Echinococcus multilocularis*: further observations on strobilar differentiation *in vitro. Revta Iber. Parasitol.* **39**, 39–53.

Smyth, J. D. and C. J. Davies 1979. *In vitro* differentiation of *Echinococcus* as a taxonomic tool, with special reference to its use in strain identification. *Helminthologia* **16**, 5–12.

Smyth, J. D. and Z. Davies 1974a. Occurrence of physiological strains of *Echinococcus granulosus* demonstrated by *in vitro* culture of protoscoleces from sheep and horse hydatid cysts. *Int. J. Parasitol.* **4**, 443–5.

Smyth, J. D. and Z. Davies 1974b. *In vitro* culture of the strobilar stage of *Echinococcus granulosus* (sheep strain): a review of basic problems and results. *Int. J. Parasitol.* **4**, 631–44.

Smyth, J. D. and Z. Davies 1975. *In vitro* suppression of segmentation in *Echinococcus multilocularis* with morphological transformation of protoscoleces into monozoic adults. *Parasitology* **71**, 125–35.

Smyth, J. D. and A. B. Howkins 1966. An *in vitro* technique for the production of eggs of *Echinococcus granulosus* by maturation of partly developed strobila. *Parasitology* **56**, 763–6.

Smyth, J. D. and M. M. Smyth 1964. Natural and experimental hosts of *Echinococcus granulosus* and *E. multilocularis*, with comments on the genetics of speciation in the genus *Echinococcus*. *Parasitology* **54**, 493–514.

Smyth, J. D. and M. M. Smyth 1969. Self insemination in *Echinococcus granulosus in vivo*. *J. Helminthol.* **43**, 383–8.

Smyth, J. D., A. B. Howkins and M. Barton 1966. Factors controlling the differentiation of the hydatid organism, *Echinococcus granulosus*, into cystic or strobilar stages *in vitro*. *Nature, Lond.* **211**, 1374–7.

Smyth, J. D., H. J. Miller and A. B. Howkins 1967. Further analysis of the factors controlling strobilization, differentiation and maturation of *Echinococcus granulosus in vitro*. *Exp. Parasitol.* **21**, 31–41.

Smyth, J. D., D. McManus, N. J. Barrett, A. Bryceson and A. G. A. Cowie 1980. *In vitro* culture of human hydatid material. *Lancet i*, 202–3.

Swellengrebel, N. H. and M. M. Sterman 1961. *Animal parasites in man*. New York: Van Nostrand.

Thompson, R. C. A. and J. Eckert 1982. The production of eggs by *Echinococcus multilocularis* in the laboratory following *in vivo* and *in vitro* development. *Z. ParasitKde* **68**, 227–34.

Thompson, R. C. A. and J. D. Smyth 1976. Attempted infection of the rhesus monkey (*Macaca mulatta*) with the British horse strain of *Echinococcus granulosus*. *J. Helminthol.* **50**, 175–7.

Voge, M. 1978. Cestoda. In *Methods of cultivating parasites in vitro*, A. E. R. Taylor and J. R. Baker (eds), 193–225. New York: Academic Press.

Vogel, H. 1957. Uber den *Echinococcus multilocularis* Süddeutschlands. I. Das Bandwurmstadium von Stämmen menslicher und tierischer Herkunft. *Z. Tropenmed. Parasitol.* **8**, 404–54.

Webster, G. A. and T. W. M. Cameron 1963. Some preliminary observations on the development of *Echinococcus in vitro*. *Can. J. Zool.* **41**, 185–94.

Yamashita, J., M. Ohbayashi, T. Sakamoto and M. Orihara 1962. Studies on echinococcosis. XIII. Observation on the vesicular development of the scolex of *E. multilocularis in vitro*. *Jap. J. Vet. Res.* **10**, 85–96.

6 Immunobiology of *Echinococcus* infections

D. D. HEATH

INTRODUCTION

This chapter reviews the immunobiology of *Echinococcus* infections. The relative paucity of information on *E. multilocularis* compared to *E. granulosus* may reflect the lower prevalence of human infection with the former. The subject will be dealt with in two parts – adult worms in the gastrointestinal tract of the definitive host, and the metacestode stage in intermediate hosts.

ECHINOCOCCUS ADULT WORMS

Immunobiology

INNATE RESISTANCE

Between species of hosts The host specificity of *Echinococcus* in definitive hosts is examined in detail in Chapters 1 and 2 of this book.

Whether immunological mechanisms are involved in determining host specificity has not been resolved.

Within species of hosts Gemmell *et al.* (1985) examined the innate resistance of dogs to *E. granulosus*, and included the variables of age of dog (3 months, 6 months or >2 years), and dose-rate of protoscoleces (10, 100, 1000, 17 500, 87 500 and 175 000). Altogether, there were 221 dogs in this trial, with infections terminated after 28 d. There was no effect of age or dose rate on susceptibility. Within each experimental group there was a range of susceptibility. The distribution was overdispersed, with the majority of dogs harbouring very few worms or none at all, and a few dogs being moderately or highly susceptible. Although Lübke (1973) had observed a possible age effect, his experiment was confounded by giving the lowest dose rates to the youngest dogs.

The involvement of immunological mechanisms in variation in susceptibility has not been demonstrated. Immunosuppressive techniques could perhaps be used to determine whether susceptibility could be increased.

ACQUIRED RESISTANCE

In a search for evidence of acquired resistance to *E. granulosus* in dogs, Gemmell *et al.* (1985) fed 0.25 ml protoscoleces to 14 susceptible dogs on nine occasions over a period of 3 years. The infections were removed by repeated purgation with arecoline hydrobromide each time. Worm numbers and sizes were measured from the purges.

There was a significant decline in the number of worms purged from dogs, correlated with the number of challenge infections given. Eight dogs remained susceptible for varying periods and then became resistant. However, five dogs never became resistant (one dog died). In the eight dogs that became resistant, there was no significant reduction in worm length, or in oogenesis.

Immunological responses

ANTIBODY

There is very little information on serum antibody responses to taeniid tapeworms in the gastrointestinal tract of carnivores. Movsesijan and Mladenović (1971), using an indirect fluorescent antibody test, found that antibody in serum from dogs infected with *E. granulosus* precipitated on the scolex and genital pore of *E. granulosus* worms. Precipitates were not detected on the day of infection, but were demonstrable in serum from some dogs after 14 and 28 d and in all five dogs 42 d after infection. In contrast to this, Herd *et al.* (1975), using gel diffusion, were not able to demonstrate precipitating antibody to *E. granulosus* worm secretions collected *in vitro*. They tested antisera on day 38 after infection. However, gel diffusion is a relatively insensitive technique.

Recently, D. D. Heath and S. B. Lawrence (unpublished) have shown that antibody to *E. granulosus* worms can be detected in the serum of infected dogs within two weeks after infection, using *E. granulosus* worm secretions as antigen in the enzyme-linked immunosorbent assay (ELISA) test. Al-Khalidi (1982) found that dogs infected with *E. granulosus* had detectable antibodies when tested 35 d after infection. There was an increase in serum IgA and in antibodies to hydatid fluid protein that were haemagglutinating, 2-mercaptoethanol sensitive, and heterocytotropic.

Presumably, mucosal antibodies could be detected against *Echinococcus* spp. worms, but such a study has not been reported. However, Al-Khalidi (1982) found an increased level of IgM and IgA in faecal extracts from infected dogs. There is no evidence so far that antibody has an effector role in resistance by the carnivore to infection.

COMPLEMENT

Variations from normal complement levels in the dog are a manifestation of some diseases (Wolfe & Halliwell, 1980). For the purposes of this review, complement is considered to be an immunological effector mechanism. Lysis of protoscoleces and adult worms in serum *in vitro*, due to activation of the alternative pathway via C_3, has been reported (Kamiya *et al.* 1980b for *E. multilocularis*; Herd 1976 for *E. granulosus*). The classical pathway is also thought to be activated to some extent (Kassis 1977, Kassis & Tanner 1976, 1977a). The role of complement in the serum of animals resistant to reinfection has not been tested. It is difficult to relate *in vitro* lysis of protoscoleces to the conditions encountered by protoscoleces during establishment in the carnivore small intestine. There is no evidence so far that complement has an effector role. Al-Khalidi (1982) showed that the haemolytic activity of sera from dogs infected with *E. granulosus* for 35 days was positively correlated with the number and growth rate of the parasites, but an effector role for complement was not established.

LYMPHOID CELLS

In vitro studies by Al-Khalidi (1982) showed that infection of dogs with *E. granulosus* protoscoleces for 30–40 days resulted in depressed blastogenesis of non-stimulated lymphocytes and of lymphocytes stimulated with phytohemagglutinin, lipopolysaccharides or purified protein derivative. There was, however, increased reactivity of cells stimulated with concanavalin A. Most infected dogs exhibited immediate-type skin sensitising reactions to hydatid fluid protein, but there was no cutaneous delayed reactivity.

Possible mechanisms of immune evasion

E. granulosus worms can survive in the dog intestine for 1–2 years (Sweatman & Williams 1963, Aminzhanov 1975, Sokolov *et al.* 1975). The scolex of the tapeworms is often in intimate contact with the lamina propria at the base of the crypts of Lieberkühn (Smyth 1964, Thompson & Eckert 1983), and a rostellar gland secretion 'could be histolytic and associated with local proteolysis' (Smyth 1964).

Chappel *et al.* (1974) found that *E. granulosus* adult worms produce *in vitro* a substance with caseinolytic protease activity. Thompson *et al.* (1979) suggested that the rostellar gland secretion of *E. granulosus* might serve to protect the parasite by 'inhibiting the ability of the host to detect the worm's presence, or by blocking the action of the host's immune response in some way'.

With *Hymenolepis diminuta*, it has been shown by Elowni (1982) and Hopkins and Barr (1982) that the scolex is the source of a protective antigen in mice. Isaak (1983) found that the rejection of worms was due to sensitised cells, localised in the mesenteric lymph nodes and acting on the scolex. In rats, where worms are not rapidly rejected, Machnika and Choromanski (1983) concluded that the worms induced a state of specific cellular unresponsiveness. Responsiveness was re-established within 5–9 d of removal of worms.

Whether *Echinococcus* spp. worms survive in the carnivore intestine by induction of specific cellular unresponsiveness remains to be determined.

Immunoprophylaxis

IRRADIATED PROTOSCOLECES

Movsesijan *et al.* (1968) and Movsesijan and Mladenović (1970) found that irradiation of protoscoleces prevented strobilisation, and most existed only as elongated scoleces after 60 d in the dog. Oral immunisation of dogs with irradiated protoscoleces (1000–2500) induced a resistance to challenge infection that limited numbers establishing, and the proportion of established worms that were able to develop to the gravid stage. Aminzhanov (1980) achieved a similar result with 10 000 irradiated protoscoleces, even though no scoleces were present in unchallenged dogs at necropsy.

It is not known whether a similar result would have occurred with non-irradiated protoscoleces, i.e. whether there is resistance to superinfection (a new population being added to an existing population). Because of the variability between dogs in susceptibility (Gemmel *et al.* 1985 and see Ch. 7), such an experiment would require a large number of dogs in each group for statistical validity.

PROTOSCOLECES

Turner *et al.* (1933) prepared an immunogen from protoscoleces and cyst membrane, dried at 37°C, powdered and preserved with 1 per cent phenol. This was injected once subcutaneously, and thereafter intramuscularly five times at 3–5 d intervals. Challenge infection 6–15 d after the last injection resulted in very large numbers of worms in control uninjected dogs (1384 per square centimetre) and 0, 1, 3, 3, 5 and 6 in six injected dogs. In a further series of experiments, Turner *et al.* (1936) used more dogs per group and varied the immunisation procedure, giving two, three, four or five injections. There were 19 control and 61 immunised dogs, all obtained from dog catchers. Of the immunised dogs, 28 (46 per cent) had no worms, a further 19 (31 per cent) had less than 200, and 14 (23 per cent) had heavy infections. In the control group, one (5 per cent) had no worms, five (26 per cent) had less than 200 worms and 13 (69 per cent) had very heavy infections. It was also apparent that dogs immunised four or five times were more resistant than those given only two or three injections. When puppies 8–12 weeks of age were used, there was no significant difference in the proportions of the three categories between immunised and control groups.

Current knowledge of variable immunological thresholds within populations (Gemmel *et al.* 1985) would suggest that Turner *et al.* (1933, 1936) were working with a potent immunogen. Their results were subsequently confirmed by Gemmell (1962), who obtained similar results. He injected freeze-dried powdered protoscoleces, in saline or as a water-in-oil emulsion, intramuscularly, either as a single injection or as a series of five injections at 5 d intervals. Resistance to a challenge infection of 50 000 protoscoleces (as measured by numbers of dogs with <500 worms) was five out of five versus one out of four with mature dogs, but none of six versus none of five with young dogs. Growth of the terminal and subterminal segments was also depressed in mature, immunised dogs.

Recently, Aminzhanov (1980) injected dogs subcutaneously with 100–150 irradiated *E. granulosus* protoscoleces and obtained a mean of 651 worms in 10 immunised dogs versus a mean of 20 548 in four control dogs when a challenge of 25 000 protoscoleces was given 15–21 d later. This procedure, using living protoscoleces as antigen, confirms that protoscoleces are capable of eliciting a high degree of immunity in dogs against *E. granulosus* infection.

CYST FLUID

Aminzhanov (1980) immunised four dogs subcutaneously with 5 ml of *E. granulosus* cyst fluid each. At necropsy after challenge, four control dogs had a mean of 20 548 worms, while the immunised dog mean was 856. Two of the dogs had no worms at all. The results are comparable with those from injecting protoscoleces subcutaneously, but the small number of dogs precludes an overall generalisation regarding this antigen (Gemmell *et al.* 1985).

CYST MEMBRANES

Turner *et al.* (1936) immunised six dogs with membrane from sterile cysts. Three had no worms at necropsy after challenge and three were heavily infected, whereas 19 control dogs had 5 per cent with no worms, 25 per cent with light infections and 70 per cent with heavy infections. With the low number of dogs in the immunised group, it was not possible to state unequivocally that protection had been induced. A similar outcome resulted from a small experiment conducted by Gill (1969).

ADULT WORMS

Gemmell (1962) immunised two young dogs with five injections of freeze-dried, powdered *E. granulosus* worms and another two with one injection in oil-based adjuvant. A mean of 895 worms was found at necropsy versus a mean of 5457 worms in five young control dogs. Worm development was also suppressed in the immunised dogs. Another small experiment by Gill (1969) used a saline homogenate of 112 'cephalic ends' (scoleces) of *E. granulosus* worms injected once subcutaneously. Two immunised dogs had 44 and no worms as opposed to 897 and 274 in control dogs.

WORM SECRETIONS

Herd *et al.* (1975) injected mature mongrel dogs four times subcutaneously against *E. granulosus* using 5.0 mg secretory antigens from *E. granulosus* worms cultured *in vitro*. The antigen was incorporated in Freund's complete adjuvant for the first injection, and in Freund's incomplete adjuvant for the subsequent injections, which were given at intervals of 12, 3 and 2 weeks. A significant reduction in worm numbers (mean of 2037 in six immunised dogs versus mean of 5662 in five control dogs, $P<0.05$) was induced, and the percentage of egg-bearing worms was markedly suppressed (7.4 per cent versus 77.6 per cent).

In an attempt to improve the response to the secretory antigen, Herd (1977) immunised 10-week-old pups with a single subcutaneous injection of 10 mg antigen emulsified with 2×10^{10} killed *Bordetella pertussis* organisms and Freund's complete adjuvant. Eight weeks later a second injection of 5 mg antigen without the *B. pertussis* was given. No significant protection resulted from this preparation.

It is possible that the low reactivity found by Turner *et al.* (1936) and Gemmell (1962) in young pups was the cause of the lack of response here. There is little information on the effects, or mode of action of Freund's adjuvant or *B. pertussis* in dogs. Hence, further experiments with worm secretions and various adjuvants are required.

ONCOSPHERES

Coman and Rickard (1975) observed that eggs of *T. ovis*, *T. hydatigena* and *T. pisiformis*, released from proglottides detached from worms located in the anterior half of the dog small intestine, may hatch and the oncospheres become activated. If these oncospheres penetrate the epithelium of the intestine, they may release immunising antigens. The same principle may apply to *E. granulosus* worms, but has not been tested. Rickard *et al.* (1977a) then examined the effect of various treatments on the resistance of beagle pups to *T. pisiformis*. Studies were made of repeated infections terminated by anthelmintic, long standing infection, daily dosing with 100 000 *T. pisiformis* eggs, and the effect of age. However, apart from increasing age being associated with smaller worms, no immunity was induced. The effects of long standing infection, and of daily dosing with eggs, have not been tested with *E. granulosus* in dogs.

Immunity induced by a heterologous species was examined by Smyth *et al.* (1970), who concluded that no immunity against *E. granulosus* was induced by immunising dogs with a graded series of *T. hydatigena* oncospheres (20 000, 30 000, 50 000 at 2 d intervals intramuscularly). When Rickard *et al.* (1975) implanted *T. hydatigena* oncospheres intraperitoneally in diffusion chambers in dogs, again no immunity was induced to *E. granulosus* challenge infection.

In a more exhaustive study by Gemmell *et al.* (1985), 170 dogs aged 3–12 months were used to determine their susceptibility to *E. granulosus* infections following the ingestion of *T. hydatigena* eggs, or the sequential injection of 20 000, 30 000, and 50 000 *T. hydatigena* oncospheres intramuscularly or intravenously, at 3 d intervals. A challenge infection 3 months later was removed after 4 weeks, and was followed by a further challenge given 7 weeks later. No effect of ingestion of eggs, and no effect due to injected oncospheres was observed on the first challenge. However, there was a significant increase in the number of dogs with <400 worms in the injected groups after the second challenge.

Gemmell *et al.* (1985) then compared the effect of injecting homologous or heterologous oncospheres on worm numbers, growth and oogenesis of *E. granulosus* in dogs. Each group of dogs received the same series of injections to that described above, and a number of consecutive challenges, each terminated by purgation with arecoline hydrobromide. No immunity was induced by *T. serialis*, *T. pisiformis* or *T. multiceps* oncospheres, but a significant short-lived degree of immunity resulted from *E. granulosus*, *T. hydatigena* and *T. ovis*. As measured by the proportion of the dogs in each group with worm counts of <400, immunity was no greater for the homologous oncospheres than the heterologous. Immunity was also manifested by decreased growth and oogenesis of the established worms, but the duration of this effect was not tested.

ECHINOCOCCUS METACESTODES

Immunobiology

VARIATION BETWEEN ANIMALS

Within species Gemmell *et al.* (1985 and see Ch. 7) infected sheep with 25, 250 or 2500 eggs of *E. granulosus* and examined the sheep at post mortem 2–8 years later. The number of larvae found did not change with increasing age, and the mean number of dead, calcified larvae remained relatively constant, indicating that these lesions are very slow to resolve. Protoscoleces were seen in some cysts at 2 years, and the proportion of viable larvae containing protoscoleces increased subsequently with time. It was estimated that 50 per cent of viable larvae contained protoscoleces by the age of 6 years. There was no evidence that higher dose rates of eggs resulted in proportionally fewer cysts establishing or developing. The distribution of cysts between animals conformed to the negative binomial distribution, indicating overdispersion, and a considerable heterogeneity in the susceptibility of sheep to *E. granulosus*.

A similar study does not appear to have been undertaken with *E. multilocularis* using infections with oncospheres. However, the development of secondary *E. multilocularis* from protoscoleces or from an 'acephalic' (sterile) cyst injected intraperitoneally has been examined (Rau & Tanner 1972, Baron *et al.* 1974). In cotton rats there was a sigmoid growth curve with an upper limit of parasite mass being attained. Baron *et al.* (1974) attributed this to immunological control by the host of proliferation and metastasis. The variation between animals has not usually been documented, but in one example given by Rau and Tanner (1972) it was quite small. Mean differences of 10 g of larval cyst mass between groups of seven to 10 rats were statistically significant.

Between species The rate of growth of *E. granulosus* cysts in different genera of animals has been reviewed by Heath (1973). Most mammals can be infected experimentally with eggs of *E. granulosus*, and the rate of cyst development does not show consistent differences between genera. However, there are strain differences that develop within particular host–parasite ecosystems and these are discussed in Chapters 1 and 2 of this book. Whether these differences have an immunological basis has not been determined. Neither has there been an explanation for the situation (reviewed by Heath 1970) whereby the susceptibility to secondary infection in experimental animals appears to depend on the source of the injected protoscoleces. Homologous serial passage is usually successful, but the diffusion of host proteins into cysts (e.g. Coltorti & Varela-Diaz 1975) may mean that protoscoleces can acquire host determinants. This could then render them liable to lysis by complement activation at the site of recognition of heterologous host antigen. Ermolin and Til'tin (1975) showed that different antigens of parasite origin occurred in *E. granulosus* cysts from sheep and pigs, and this will also have to be considered.

The multivesicular (alveolar) hydatid cysts of *E. multilocularis* develop as a solid tumour-like vascularised mass in the organs of man and a number of rodent species. Growth is progressive or restrictive, and is determined by the species or strains of hosts concerned (Rausch & Schiller 1956, Yamashita *et al.* 1958, Lubinsky 1964, Ohbayashi *et al.* 1971, Ali-Khan 1974a, Kamiya *et al.* 1980a). Whereas the refractory or partially susceptible hosts evidently restrict or abort the larval cyst mass, hypersusceptible hosts are ultimately debilitated or killed (Rausch 1954, Ohbayashi *et al.* 1971). The immunological parameters that may regulate cyst proliferation have not been delineated sufficiently to explain the course of infection in progressive and restrictive types (Ali-Khan & Siboo 1980a). However, there is strong evidence that regulation is, to some extent, manifested by an antibody-dependent, cell-mediated cytotoxicity.

THE HOST RESPONSE

Two parasite antigens used for diagnostic purposes, antigen 5 and antigen B (reviewed by Williams and Sandeman 1982 and see Ch. 8) leak from, or are eliminated by, hydatid cysts, and a specific host IgG or IgE response to these antigens can be measured in humans. Eight other antigens of parasite origin have been demonstrated in hydatid cyst fluid by Chordi and Kagan (1965). A glycoprotein antigen with blood group P_1 activity can also be isolated from hydatid cyst membrane (Russi *et al.* 1974). In infected animals a variable number of antibodies can be detected, sometimes related to the degree of viability and integrity of the cyst (Todorov and Jeleva 1979, Todorov *et al.* 1979). Hyperglobulinemia has been observed in *E. granulosus* infected sheep, especially following the appearance of brood capsules and scoleces (Aminzhanov 1977, Katsova 1979). Circulating antigens can sometimes be detected (Zvolinskiene 1978, Richard-Lenoble *et al.* 1978).

The host cellular response to echinococcosis has been reviewed by Smyth and Heath (1970), and summarised by Ali-Khan and Siboo (1980a), Slais and Vanek (1980), Richards *et al.* (1983a), and Ali-Khan *et al.* (1983). The pathology varies somewhat, depending upon whether an invading oncosphere or experimental secondary echinococcosis is being studied. With oncospheres, necrosis of surrounding cells is followed by infiltration of neutrophils and macrophages. Eosinophils may become involved. If the oncosphere is able to resist the cellular attack by maintaining a zone of necrosis during development of the laminated layer, a range of cell types accumulate close to the periphery of the laminated layer. Mast cells, eosinophils and histiocytes tend to be found outside the inner zone of fibroblasts. In larger cysts, the inflammatory reaction is outside the connective tissue sheath and the laminated layer remains in contact with a thick layer of hyaline degenerated fibrous connective tissue. With secondary *E. granulosus*, small, free cysts show a primary macrophage invasion, overlaid by fibroblasts and a layer of mesothelial cells. With secondary *E. multilocularis*, the larval cyst mass grows progressively and metastasises in rodents despite a marked lymphoproliferative activity in the B-cell areas of lymphoid tissues and intense infiltration of the paracortex and medulla by plasmacytoid cells. The progressive growth of the mass in the host results in or from depression of the cytotoxic cellular response involving macrophages, eosinophils and neutrophils, but the humoral mechanism remains functional. Around the cysts a preponderance of neutrophils is slowly replaced by histiocytes bound to the laminated layer of the cyst, peripheral plasmacytes and giant cells.

Immunological responses

ANTIBODY

There is no evidence that antibody has a restricting role on the growth of the cysts but Heath and Lawrence (1976) pointed out that *E. granulosus* cysts developed *in vitro* in the absence of antibody at a rate commensurate with the most rapid recorded in mammalian intermediate hosts.

The sequential development of antibody to *E. granulosus* oncospheres in sheep has been studied by Yong *et al.* (1984). Oncospheres developed into small infertile cysts during the 12 months of the study. The earliest detection of antibody depended on the antigen used. For instance, sheep hydatid cyst fluid, when used as an antigen, detected antibody within 2 weeks of infection, whereas boiled sheep hydatid cyst fluid did not detect antibodies until 8–10 weeks after infection. The humoral responses detected using eight different antigens showed various distinct peaks of antibody responses, suggesting the production of antibodies of different specificity in response to the qualitative and quantitative changes in excretory, secretory and somatic antigens during the various phases of parasite development. When *E. granulosus* protoscoleces were injected into mice, Araj *et al.* (1977a), found that with hydatid cyst fluid antigen, the first detectable antibody occurred 10 weeks after injection. Similarly, Torres-Rodriguez and Wisnivesky (1978) could not demonstrate a serological response in mice infected with *E. granulosus* oncospheres until 11 weeks after infection. Precipitating antibodies to antigen 5 were the first to appear, and other antibodies detectable by agglutination reactions were not present until 18–20 weeks after infection. They suggested that the presence of circulating antibodies was connected with the presence of fluid in cysts.

In humans infected with *E. granulosus*, elevated levels of IgE antibody could be detected in all patients, but no change was found in levels of IgG, IgM or IgA (Dessaint *et al.* 1975). Much of the IgE antibody was specific for fraction 5 in 23 out of 39 patients tested. Perez Esandi (1970) detected predominantly IgG to sheep hydatid cyst fluid in infected humans, but IgA and IgM were also present.

In experimental secondary *E. multilocularis* infections, antibody level is related to the initial and resultant parasite biomass (Hinz 1973, Ali-Khan 1974b). Antibody stimulation apparently reaches a plateau with a 20 cyst inoculum, and a 100 cyst inoculum did not stimulate a higher level of antibody. The larval cyst mass grows progressively and metastasises (Ali-Khan 1978a, Ali-Khan & Siboo 1980b). The humoral mechanism remains functional, as shown by the fact that infected mice can respond to an injection of sheep erythrocytes by producing raised levels of haemagglutinins and plaque-forming cells when challenged with sheep erythrocytes (Ali-Khan 1974a, 1979). Specific antibodies of high (IgG_{2a} and IgG_{2b}) and low (IgM and IgG_1) affinities, as well as C3 have been detected on the surface of the cysts (Ali-Khan & Siboo 1981). IgM and IgG_1 increase markedly during the course of rapid cyst biomass increase (6–14 weeks). More IgM is produced than IgG_1, but much of it is of low specificity or not specific, as measured by absorption experiments with *E. multilocularis* antigen (Ali-Khan & Siboo 1982). In contrast, the specific IgG_1 increases to form 86–93 per cent of total circulating IgG_1. The significance of this high level of specific IgG_1, and its antiparasite role, has not been determined. Of the other antibody classes, only IgG_{2b} showed a slight increase in concentration and specificity with time.

COMPLEMENT

The protoscoleces of *E. multilocularis* and *E. granulosus* are lysed by fresh serum of many different species of mammals (Kassis & Tanner 1976, Herd 1976). Tegumental disruption occurred within 5 min (Kassis *et al.* 1976). The effect could be removed by heating serum to 56°C for 30 min. (Rau & Tanner 1976), by EDTA or by cobra venom factor. The activation of complement by the surface of protoscoleces may occur with or without specific immunoglobulins, thus involving either the classical or the alternative pathway (Kassis & Tanner 1976, Herd 1976, Rickard *et al.* 1977b, Kamiya *et al.* 1980b). Either mechanism results in the creation of transmembrane channels, which are probably the primary cause of cell lysis (Bhakdi 1982).

The presence of *Echinococcus* cysts appears to deplete host complement (Kassis & Tanner 1977b). They found that the rapid development stage of *E. multilocularis* infection was associated with depletion of serum complement. Conversely, the use of cobra venom factor to deplete complement resulted in a faster growth rate of *E. multilocularis* cyst masses. Depletion of complement may be due to lysis of some protoscoleces, releasing calcareous corpuscles which have been shown to have a direct anticomplementary effect. Also, *E. granulosus* cyst fluid interacts with complement, resulting in its depletion (Hammerberg *et al.* 1977) and the failure of complement to lyse protoscoleces in intact cysts has been attributed by Kassis and Tanner (1976) to the inactivation of C3 as it enters the cyst.

Kamiya *et al.* (1980b) examined the resistance to experimental secondary *E. multilocularis* infection of a number of different species of host, and also of different strains of inbred mouse. The host resistance was closely correlated with the extent of lysis of the protoscoleces in fresh serum *in vitro*. Because they were unable to demonstrate host immunoglobulins on the parasite tegument, but did demonstrate C3, they concluded that host resistance was correlated with serum complement levels.

LYMPHOID CELLS

When sheep were infected with eggs of *E. granulosus*, a neutrophilia was observed 3–5 d after infection (Petrova 1968). This was followed by a leucocytosis peaking between days 25–30. The predominant cells were eosinophils, lymphocytes and monocytes. Devouge and Ali-Khan (1983) found these latter three cell types accumulating in the peritoneal cavity of mice during the first 6 weeks of infection with *E. multilocularis*, when the host was able to restrict the growth rate of the parasite cyst mass.

Peritoneal cells from rats with massive *E. multilocularis* infections rapidly killed protoscoleces *in vitro* (Rau & Tanner 1976) but cells from uninfected or lightly infected animals had no effect. Simultaneous injection of protoscoleces and sensitised spleen cells into mice decreased the number and size of cysts that resulted (Araj *et al.* 1977b). Baron and Tanner (1977) considered that the activated macrophage was the key cell, because they could be seen to adhere to the parasite, and this adhesion was enhanced by 'immune' serum. The macrophages could be activated by previous infection, injection of BCG, or infection with *Taenia crassiceps* larvae. The stimulatory effect of BCG or its derivatives on resistance to infection, growth and metastasis has been shown for both *E. multilocularis* (Rau & Tanner 1975, Reuben *et al.* 1978, Reuben *et al.* 1979, Reuben & Tanner 1979) and *E. granulosus* (Thompson 1976). Phytohaemagglutinin (PHA) injected into the peritoneal cavity of cotton rats can also elevate cellular responses and protect against infection with *E. multilocularis* (Reuben & Tanner 1983). The protection can be abrogated by carrageenan, an anti-macrophage agent.

T cells may also be important in the immunological control of *E. multilocularis*. Baron and Tanner (1976) found that depletion of T cells enhanced metastasis of *E. multilocularis*. In congenitally athymic nude mice, *E. multilocularis* developed very rapidly, and the host tissue reaction was slight compared to that of heterozygous mice (Kamiya *et al.* 1980a).

Possible mechanisms of immune evasion

IMMUNOPROTECTION

Chordi and Kagan (1965) recognised host-derived gamma-globulin and albumin in sheep hydatid fluid, and specific identification of host IgG was described by Coltorti and Varela-Diaz (1972). They showed that the contaminants were of host origin and had probably diffused through the parasite membranes. A similar conclusion was drawn by Ermolin and Til'tin (1975), Kassis and Tanner (1977b), Khorsandi and Tabibi (1978) and Edwards (1982). Host IgG will bind to the laminated layer of hydatid cysts from mice and sheep (Varela-Diaz & Coltorti 1973, Coltorti & Varela-Diaz 1974) and it has been postulated that this constitutes a barrier to host immune cells, thus protecting the germinal layer (Coltorti & Varela-Diaz 1974). Ali-Khan and Siboo (1981) found non-specific antibodies in the germinal layer and within the cyst, but specific antibodies were only detected on or in the laminated layer. *In vitro*, low affinity antibodies (IgG_1 and IgM) were eluted from the laminated layer, but not the high affinity antibodies (IgG_{2a} and IgG_{2b}). The transplantation experiments of Coltorti and Varela-Diaz (1975), of *E. granulosus* cysts from one host species to another, also showed that the new host immunoglobulins did not appear in most cysts, even after 2 years, and those that did contain heterologous immunoglobulins may have been mechanically damaged.

It is tempting to suggest that during early development of the hydatid cyst it is possible for non-specific host serum components to diffuse into it. However, with the mounting of a specific host reaction to antigenic determinants in the laminated layer, specific immunoglobulins bind to this layer and may perhaps limit the further diffusion of host macromolecules into the cyst.

The deposition of immunoglobulins in the outer layers of developing *E. granulosus* cysts *in vitro* has been observed at the light microscope level by Heath and Lawrence (1976, 1981). In the presence of specific anti-hydatid immunoglobulins, cysts were protected once the first layer of the laminated layer had formed. The deposition of specific immunoglobulins was very obvious when compared to the light delineation of laminations in serum from uninfected sheep, and the lack of any delineation when grown in immunoglobulin-free foetal calf serum.

IMMUNOSUPPRESSION

Suppression of a cell-mediated response Heath (1970, 1973) reported that healthy *E. granulosus* cysts in sheep at one month after infection with eggs, were surrounded by a zone of necrotic cells between the laminated layer and the host chronic inflammatory reaction. It appeared that a toxic product from the juvenile cyst was able to destroy host lymphoid cells in close contact, and in cases where cells were closely applied to the laminated layer the cysts appeared degenerate, Annen *et al.* (1981) have now shown that *E. granulosus* cyst fluid contains a cytotoxic ingredient that is heat stable and of low molecular weight. They assumed that this substance could easily penetrate through the hydatid cyst wall and interfere locally with immunocompetent cells, facilitating the long term survival of the parasite. Such a substance has not been looked for in *E. multilocularis*.

Devouge and Ali-Khan (1983) have shown that when mice were inoculated intraperitoneally with *E. multilocularis* cysts, the growth rate of the larval cyst mass was restricted for the first 6 weeks, and that this was followed, between 7 and 14 weeks, by a progressive increase in cyst mass. During the restrictive phase there was an increase in the peritoneal cavity of lymphocytes, monocytes and eosinophils. Ali-Khan *et al.* (1983) used ultrastructural techniques to study this phase and found the following sequence of events:

> '(a) binding of leucocytes (eosinophils, neutrophils, macrophages) to the laminated layer or plasma membrane of the germinal layer; (b) disintegration and phagocytosis of the laminated layer by macrophages and/or eosinophils; (c) engulfment of microtriches by leucocytes; (d) areas of focal lesions in the form of gaps in the plasma membrane adjacent to the leucocytes, and (e) finally infiltration of the germinal layer and cyst lumen by leucocytes'.

They referred to the literature confirming the fact that eosinophils, neutrophils and macrophages possess Fc and C3 receptors which facilitate their binding to opsonised targets, and to the fact that Ali-Khan and Siboo (1980a) found that epitopes on the laminated layer of cysts bind antibodies and that the split products of C3 are found between the laminated and germinal layers. They suggested that there was a strong likelihood that cystolysis was brought about by an antibody-dependent cell cytotoxicity mechanism.

During the proliferative phase of *E. multilocularis* in mice, Devouge and Ali-Khan (1983) found that the peritoneal lymphocytes, monocytes and eosinophils declined and were replaced by neutrophils. There was also splenomegaly and involution of the thymus. Ali-Khan (1979) reported that during this phase there was depression of the cell-mediated immune response to homologous antigen but not to heterologous antigens. The lymph nodes draining the cyst mass were depleted of T cells, the paracortex area was disorganised and there was an intense plasmacytosis. Ali-Khan and Siboo (1980a,b) concluded that early in the infection T cell-mediated immunity may control the growth of the larval cyst mass, but as the antigenic load increases the paracortex becomes rapidly disorganised in the draining nodes and a humoral response predominates. A similar pathology was recorded for secondary *E. granulosus* infections in mice (Ali-Khan 1978b).

Allan *et al.* (1981) found also that there was a significant reduction in thymus-derived cells in mice infected with *E. granulosus*. By adoptive transfer of lymph node cells to syngeneic mice they showed substantial interference with ability of the recipient mouse to respond to an injection of sheep erythrocytes (which stimulate both T and B cells). They suggested that chronic infection with *E. granulosus* over a period of 13 months had altered the composition of the T cell population in favour of non-specific T cell suppressor activity.

In vitro studies of murine lymph node–cell interactions with living protoscoleces of *E. granulosus* (Dixon *et al.* 1982) have shown that contact with cells from normal uninfected mice results in blastic transformation of the cells, especially of T cells. The stimulus was not released from the parasite surface, and intimate contact was necessary. They suggested that the blastic transformation may be the *in vitro* representation of an immunosuppressive mechanism favouring the survival of the parasite.

Anticomplementary effects Cyst fluid from *E. granulosus* is known to be anticomplementary in the presence of freshly collected sera and activates the alternative pathway via C3 (Hammerberg *et al.* 1977, Perricone *et al.* 1980). A glycolipid, considered to be a polyhexosamine ceramide, can be extracted from hydatid cyst fluid and germinal layer. Only that from cyst fluid is anticomplementary (Ehrlich & Hrzenjak 1978, Hrzenjak *et al.* 1979).

Complement-rich sera have no harmful effect *in vitro* on protoscoleces contained within cysts, indicating the presence of a barrier which prevents the complement proteins from making effective contact with the protoscoleces (Kassis & Tanner 1976). They speculate that the barrier may be the cyst wall or the effect may lie in the anticomplementary action of calcareous corpuscles found free in hydatid fluid. With respect to the cyst wall, ultrastructural studies of Richards *et al.* (1983b) have shown the accumulation of electron-dense bodies in the laminated layer of *E. granulosus* cysts. These can be induced further by *in vitro* culture, and the authors suggest that these bodies may play an active role in the resistance of the cyst to complement attack.

Immunoprophylaxis

EVIDENCE FOR ACQUIRED IMMUNITY

Some resistance to the establishment of an *E. granulosus* infection in sheep following a single oral exposure to homologous eggs or oncospheres has been reported. Sweatman *et al.* (1963) found that approximately 70 per cent of a challenge infection was prevented from establishing following oral infections of from 10 to 10 000 eggs given 9 months earlier. A similar level of protection has also been recorded by Yarulin (1968) and Aminzhanov (1976). With secondary *E. granulosus* in mice, De Rycke and Pennoit-De Cooman (1973) found that a successful primary infection usually resulted in the rejection of a challenge infection. Similarly, with *E. multilocularis* in cotton rats, Rau and Tanner (1973) showed that subcutaneous cysts that weighed more than 5 g effectively suppressed the establishment, growth and transperitoneal dissemination of challenging infections.

PASSIVE IMMUNISATION

Passive immunisation of lambs with the serum from sheep with *E. granulosus* cysts did not protect lambs against experimental infection (Ramazanov 1979). Lambs were not protected, when challenged at 2 weeks of age, against *E. granulosus* infection even though their dams were heavily infected with cysts (D. D. Heath & W. K. Yong unpublished). A range of passively acquired antibodies against *E. granulosus* were demonstrated by immunoelectrophoresis, but none were associated with protection. Similar results were obtained for *E. multilocularis* in mice, in that no resistance was passed from infected mothers to their offspring (Hinz and Domm 1980). However, in none of the cases quoted was it shown that the donors of the serum or colostrum were themselves immune to reinfection.

IMMUNISATION WITH SOMATIC ANTIGENS (INCLUDING CYST FLUID)

Against primary infection with eggs Turner *et al.* (1937) immunised sheep against *E. granulosus* using various injection regimes of dried powdered protoscoleces and germinal layer. At necropsy 12 months later it was found that immunisation did not prevent infection, but sometimes reduced the number of cysts establishing. However, there was a marked host reaction to the developing cysts, resulting in a thick pericystic membrane and calcification of the laminated layer. In many cases this led to death of the cysts. Similar pathology has been described by Sweatman *et al.* (1963) and Gemmell (1966). Penfold (1938) carried out a similar experiment, except that he gave more injections, and the antigen was 'carbolised' rather than dried. No reduction in number of cysts or viability was observed at necropsy 9 months later.

After immunisation of five sheep with hydatid cyst fluid for 8 weeks, Dada and Belino (1981) recorded a significant decrease in numbers of cysts per sheep. Immunisation with extract of *E. granulosus* worms was less effective. All immunised sheep were infected with some cysts. Moya and Blood (1964) also immunised sheep with hydatid cyst fluid. At necropsy, similar numbers of sheep were infected in the immunised and control groups. They did not report on whether cyst numbers or viability were affected.

Against secondary infection with protoscoleces Dévé (1934) immunised mice and rabbits with *E. granulosus* cystic membrane, but did not find any resistance to secondary echinococcosis. A more detailed study by Pauluzzi and De Rosa (1969), immunising mice with extract of *E. granulosus* membrane or cyst fluid, showed that less cysts established, but those that did establish had greater weight than the controls. Little resistance using cyst fluid has been seen in other experiments (De Rycke & Pennoit-De Cooman 1973, De Rosa *et al.* 1974, 1977). However, protoscolex antigens have generated some resistance. De Rycke and Pennoit-De Cooman (1973) found significant immunity after immunising mice with protoscolex extract, and complete protection if living material was used. The successful establishment of living *E. granulosus* cysts in a subcutaneous site resulted in unsuccessful establishment of an intraperitoneal challenge infection. A similar result was obtained with *E. multilocularis* (Rau & Tanner 1973, Hinz 1979).

Using extracts of *E. granulosus* protoscoleces, Tassi and Dottorini (1980) fractionated the material on an ion-exchange column. They found that the crude extract, and a 0.8 M fraction, resulted in fewer cysts in mice, while 1.6 M and 5.0 M fractions resulted in similar numbers of cysts to controls, but the cysts were heavier.

Clearly, immunisation with protoscolex antigens has some effect on challenge with protoscoleces. In some cases the mechanism of resistance may be non-specific, because Reuben *et al.* (1978) protected cotton rats against *E. multilocularis* infections by activating macrophages with BCG, or with phytohaemagglutinin (Reuben and Tanner 1983).

IMMUNISATION WITH ONCOSPHERE ANTIGENS

***E. granulosus* oncospheres** Gemmell (1966) immunised lambs against *E. granulosus* by an intramuscular injection of oncospheres. Immunising doses of 1000–50 000 oncospheres did not significantly alter the approximately 90 per cent rejection of a challenge infection. All sheep were infected, but in most cases the cysts were dead at necropsy after 30 months. Heath *et al.* (1981) found that if two or more injections of oncospheres were given at 14 d intervals, the degree of resistance was significantly higher than that resulting from a single injection, and also most immunised sheep were fully protected against the establishment of cysts.

Oncosphere products have also been used to immunise against infection with oncospheres. Xylinas *et al.* (1976) protected mice against intraperitoneal *E. granulosus* infection by injection of an antigen prepared from *E. granulosus* eggs, and Osborn and Heath (1982) protected lambs against oral infection with *E. granulosus* eggs by injecting the used culture medium in which *E. granulosus* oncospheres had been incubated for 14 d. Figure 6.1 demonstrates the difference between developing larvae of *E. granulosus* cultured *in vitro* for 3 d in the presence of 'non-immune' and 'immune' serum without complement. Antibody precipitating on the plasma membrane cannot exert lethal effects in the absence of complement, and is pushed away from the surface of the developing larva by the first layer of the laminated layer.

Oncospheres of other taeniid species Immunisation of sheep with *T. ovis* oncospheres gave variable results after *E. granulosus* challenge infection. Gemmell (1966) obtained a non-significant reduction in cyst

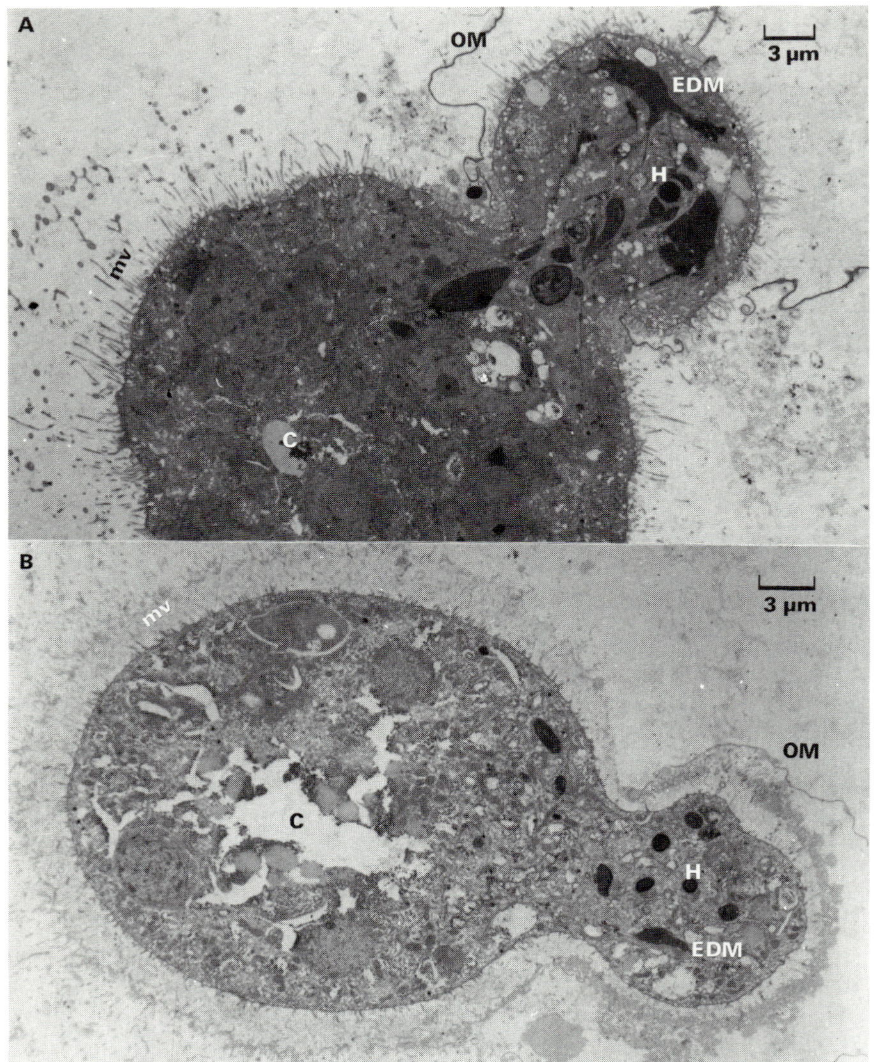

Figure 6.1 *Echinococcus granulosus* oncospheres cultured *in vitro* for 3 d, following the method described by Heath and Lawrence (1976, 1981). (A) Culture medium contains inactivated normal sheep serum. (B) Culture medium contains inactivated serum from a sheep immunised with the secretions of developing *E. granulosus* oncospheres, as described by Osborn and Heath (1982). The serum was obtained at necropsy following a challenge infection with *E. granulosus* eggs. No cysts were found in the sheep, but control sheep were heavily infected. Ultrastructural work was carried out by A. Harris, using the technique of Harris and Heath (1983). *Abbreviations*: OM, oncospheral membrane; EDM, electron-dense material; H, hook; C, incipient central cavity; MV, microvilli.

numbers, whereas in the experiment described by Heath *et al.* (1979), the reduction was significant. Immunisation with *T. hydatigena* oncospheres in both cases gave non-significant reductions in cyst numbers. Immunisation of sheep with very large doses of *T. pisiformis* eggs gave partial protection against *E. granulosus* (Ramazanov 1979) but 5000 *T. pisiformis* eggs were not enough to be effective.

Immunotherapy

Evranova (1970, 1972) described experiments on immunotherapy of *E. granulosus* cysts in sheep. She used an antigen prepared from *E. granulosus* cysts and injected it with thymol palmitate or vitamin B_{12} as adjuvants. Cysts in treated sheep showed abnormally thickened adventitia, heavy calcification of the cyst wall, and degeneration of the germinal layer.

Many similar trials in humans infected with *E. granulosus* have been carried out (e.g. Petroff 1923, Calcagno 1940) and these have been reviewed by Marchevsky (1973) and Varela-Diaz (1973). They conclude that there is no unequivocal evidence for the effectiveness of injected hydatid antigens against cysts of *E. granulosus*, and that such treatments are likely to result in hypersensitivity.

CONCLUSIONS

The general pattern which has emerged in this chapter is one of limited but increasing understanding of immunobiological processes, little success with immunotherapy, but encouraging progress with immunoprophylaxis.

Protoscoleces of *E. granulosus* appear to be the most effective immunogen for immunisation of dogs against *E. granulosus* worms. Variations in number and size of *E. granulosus* worms resulting from infection of non-immunised dogs have been described, and it is now possible to devise an experiment to test antigen preparations, with the expectation of an unequivocal result.

Immunity of sheep to *E. granulosus* cysts can be acquired or artificially induced. A single injection of *E. granulosus* oncospheres results in significant resistance to a challenge infection, and after two injections a significantly greater resistance is engendered. A very high degree of resistance is also induced by the injection of the secretory products of oncospheres cultured into 14 d old cysts *in vitro*. However, the limited availability of *E. granulosus* eggs may preclude any development of large-scale immunisation procedures. If immunisation is to be used in a campaign to control *E. granulosus* it may be necessary to identify the functional antigen using monoclonal antibody technology, and to synthesise the antigen by recombinant DNA techniques.

REFERENCES

Ali-Khan, Z. 1974a. Host–parasite relationship in echinococcosis. I. Parasite biomass and antibody response in three strains of inbred mice against graded doses of *Echinococcus multilocularis* cysts. *J. Parasitol.* **60**, 231–5.

Ali-Khan, Z. 1974b. Host–parasite relationship in echinococcosis. II. Cyst weight, hematologic alterations, and gross changes in the spleen and lymph nodes of C57L mice against graded doses of *Echinococcus multilocularis* cysts. *J. Parasitol.* **60**, 236–42.

Ali-Khan, Z. 1978a. *Echinococcus multilocularis*: cell mediated immune response in early and chronic alveolar murine hydatidosis. *Exp. Parasitol.* **46**, 157–65.

Ali-Khan, Z. 1978b. Pathological changes in the lymphoreticular tissue of Swiss mice infected with *Echinococcus granulosus* cysts. *Z. ParasitKde* **58**, 47–54.

Ali-Khan, Z. 1979. Humoral response to sheep red blood cells in C57L/J mice during early and chronic stages of infection with *Echinococcus multilocularis* cysts. *Z. ParasitKde* **59**, 259–65.

Ali-Khan, Z. and R. Siboo 1980a. Pathogenesis and host response in subcutaneous alveolar hydatidosis. I. Histogenesis of alveolar cyst and a qualitative analysis of the inflammatory infiltrates. *Z. ParasitKde* **62**, 241–54.

Ali-Khan, Z. and R. Siboo 1980b. Pathogenesis and host response in subcutaneous alveolar hydatidosis. II. Intense plasmacellular infiltration in the paracortex of draining lymph nodes. *Z. ParasitKde* **62**, 255–65.

Ali-Khan, Z. and R. Siboo 1981. *Echinococcus multilocularis*: Distribution and persistence of specific host immunoglobulins on cyst membranes. *Exp. Parasitol.* **51**, 159–68.

Ali-Khan, Z. and R. Siboo 1982. *Echinococcus multilocularis*: immunoglobulin and antibody response in C57BL/6J mice. *Exp. Parasitol.* **53**, 97–104.

Ali-Khan, Z., R. Siboo, M. Gomersall and M. Faucher 1983. Cystolytic events and the possible role of germinal cells in metastasis in chronic alveolar hydatidosis. *Ann. Trop. Med. Parasitol.* **77**, 497–512.

Al-Khalidi, N. W. 1982. Investigations of the immunity of dogs to *Echinococcus granulosus* (Batsch 1786) during the prepatent infection. *Dissert. Abstr. Int. B* **43**, 62.

Allan, D., P. Jenkins, R. J. Connor and J. B. Dixon 1981. A study of immunoregulation of BALB/c mice by *Echinococcus granulosus equinus* during prolonged infection. *Parasite Immunol.* **3**, 137–42.

Aminzhanov, M. 1975. [The life-span of *Echinococcus granulosus* in the dog.] *Veterinariya, Moscow* **12**, 70–2 (in Russian).

Aminzhanov, M. 1976. [The biology of hydatids in sheep.] *Veterinariya, Moscow* **7**, 68–70 (in Russian).

Aminzhanov, M. 1977. [Haematological changes in sheep infected with *Echinococcus*.] *Veterinariya, Moscow* **12**, 86–8 (in Russian).

Aminzhanov, M. 1980. [Immunoprophylaxis of hydatidosis in animals.] *Trudy Uzbek. Nauchno-issled, Vet. Inst.* **30**, 15–8 (in Russian).

Annen, J. M., P. Kohler and J. Eckert 1981. Cytotoxicity of *Echinococcus granulosus* cyst fluid *in vitro*. *Z. ParasitKde* **65**, 79–88.

Araj, G. F., R. M. Matossian and G. J. Frayha 1977a. The host response in secondary hydatidosis of mice. I. Circulating antibodies. *Z. ParasitKde* **52**, 23–30.

Araj, G. F., R. M. Matossian and A. H. Malakian 1977b. The host response in secondary hydatidosis of mice. II. Cell mediated activity. *Z. ParasitKde* **52**, 31–8.

Baron, R. W. and C. E. Tanner 1976. The effect of immunosuppression on secondary *Echinococcus multilocularis* infections in mice. *Int. J. Parasitol.* **6**, 37–42.

Baron, R. W. and C. E. Tanner 1977. *Echinococcus multilocularis* in the mouse: the *in vitro* protoscolicidal activity of peritoneal macrophages. *Int. J. Parasitol.* **7**, 489–95.

Baron, R. W., M. E. Rau and C. E. Tanner 1974. Growth of secondary *Echinococcus multilocularis* in experimentally infected hosts. *Can. J. Zool.* **52**, 587–9.

Bhakdi, S. 1982. Effect of complement on cell membranes. In *Immune reactions to parasites*, W. Frank (ed.), 185–94. Jena: Verlag Gustav Fischer.

Calcagno, B. N. 1940. Terapeutica biologica de la hidatidosis. *Bol. Trab. Acad. Arg. Cirug.* **24**, 679–84, 754–6, 836–7.

Chappel, R. J., R. P. Herd and D. Biddell 1974. Characterization of the metabolic secretions of *Echinococcus granulosus. Proc. Aust. Biochem. Soc.* **7**, 31.

Chordi, A. and I. G. Kagan 1965. Identification and characterisation of antigenic components of sheep hydatid fluid by immunoelectrophoresis. *J. Parasitol.* **51**, 63–71.

Coltorti, E. A. and V. M. Varela-Diaz 1972. IgG levels and host specificity in hydatid cyst fluid. *J. Parasitol.* **58**, 753–6.

Coltorti, E. A. and V. M. Varela-Diaz 1974. *Echinococcus granulosus*: penetration of macromolecules and their localization on the parasite membranes of cysts. *Exp. Parasitol.* **35**, 225–31.

Coltorti, E. A. and V. M. Varela-Diaz 1975. Penetration of host IgG molecules into hydatid cysts. *Z. ParasitKde* **48**, 47–51.

Coman, B. J. and M. D. Rickard 1975. The location of *Taenia pisiformis, Taenia ovis* and *Taenia hydatigena* in the gut of the dog and its effect on net environmental contamination with ova. *Z. ParasitKde* **47**, 237–48.

Dada, B. J. O. and E. D. Belino 1981. Immunization of sheep against cystic hydatidosis with homologous and heterologous metacestode antigens. *Int. J. Zoonoses* **8**, 20–5.

De Rosa, F., S. Dottorini, G. R. Stagni and S. Pauluzzi 1974. Immunogenic fractions of *Echinococcus granulosus* – a preliminary report. In *Third International Congress of Parasitology, Munich, Proceedings*, Vol. 1, 561–2. FACTA Publication.

De Rosa, F., S. Dottorini and S. Pauluzzi 1977. Tentativi di vaccinazione contro l'idatidosi sperimentale secondaria del topo BALB/C con liquidi cystici e loro frazioni. *Annali Sclavo* **19**, 470–7.

De Rycke, P. H. and E. Pennoit-De Cooman 1973. Experimental secondary echinococcosis of *Echinococcus granulosus.* IV. Vaccination of host mice. *Z. ParasitKde* **42**, 49–59.

Dessaint, J. P., D. Bout, P. Wattre and A. Capron 1975. Quantitative determination of specific IgE antibodies to *Echinococcus granulosus* and IgE levels in sera from patients with hydatid disease. *Immunology* **29**, 813–23.

Dévé, F. 1934. Essai d'immunisation anti-échinococcique par injections sous-cutanées de membranes hydatiques broyées a L'état frais. *C. R. Seanc. Soc. Biol.* **115**, 1025–6.

Devouge, M. and Z. Ali-Khan 1983. Intraperitoneal murine alveolar hydatidosis: relationship between the size of the larval cyst mass, immigrant inflammatory cells, splenomegaly and thymus involution. *Tropmed. Parasitol.* **34**, 15–20.

Dixon, J. B., P. Jenkins and D. Allan 1982. Immune recognition of *Echinococcus granulosus* 1. Parasite-activated, primary transformation by normal murine lymph node cells. *Parasite Immunol.* **4**, 33–45.

Edwards, G. T. 1982. Host IgG in equine hydatid cyst fluid. *Ann. Trop. Med. Parasitol.* **76**, 485–7.

Ehrlich, I. and T. Hrzenjak 1978. Immunokemijska osnova antigenosti helmintoparazita: antigenost hidatidne tekućine cestoda Echinoccocus granulosus larv. *Vet. Arhiv.* **48** (Suppl.), S21–S23.

Elowni, E. E. 1982. *Hymenolepis diminuta*: source of protective antigens as determined by irradiation and chemical elimination of immunizing worms. *Exp. Parasitol.* **54**, 1–6.

Ermolin, G. A. and B. P. Til'tin 1975. [Parasitic antigens and molecular mimicry of hydatid cysts.] In *Antropozoogel'mintozy i perspektivy ikh likvidatsii, Moskow.* 24–6 (in Russian).

Evranova, B. G. 1970. [Prophylactic and therapeutic immunization of animals against tissue helminths.] *Uchen. Zap. Kazan. Vet. Inst. Baum.* **107**, 193–6 (in Russian).

Evranova, V. G. 1972. [Immunisation of animals against tissue helminths.] *Mater. Nauch. Issled. Chlenov Vsesoy. Obshch. Gel'mint. 1970–71* **24**, 226–31 (in Russian).

Gemmell, M. A. 1962. Natural and acquired immunity factors interfering with development during the rapid growth phase of *Echinococcus granulosus* in dogs. *Immunology* **5**, 496–503.

Gemmell, M. A. 1966. Immunological responses of the mammalian host against tapeworm infections. IV. Species specificity of hexacanth embryos in protecting sheep against *Echinococcus granulosus. Immunology* **11**, 325–35.

Gemmell, M. A., R. J. Lawson and M. G. Roberts 1985. Population dynamics in echinococcosis and cysticercosis. I. Biological parameters of *Echinococcus granulosus* in dogs and sheep. (Submitted for publication.)

Gill, H. S. 1969. Vaccination trials against *Echinococcus granulosus* infection in dogs. *J. Commun. Dis.* **1**, 258–62.

Hammerberg, B., A. J. Musoke and J. F. Williams 1977. Activation of complement by hydatid cyst fluid of *Echinococcus granulosus. J. Parasitol.* **63**, 327–31.

Harris, A. and D. D. Heath 1983. Rapid processing of *in vitro* cultured microscopical metacestodes for ultrastructure studies. *J. Parasitol.* **69**, 998.

Heath, D. D. 1970. *The developmental biology of larval cyclophyllidean cestodes in mammals.* PhD thesis, The Australian National University, Canberra, Australia.

Heath, D. D. 1973. The life cycle of *Echinococcus granulosus* – a review. In *Recent Advances in Hydatid Disease – Proceedings of a Symposium presented by the Hamilton Medical Veterinary Association, Australia,* R. W. Brown, J. R. Salisbury, W. E. White (eds), 7–18, Hamilton, Victoria, Australia: Hamilton Medical Veterinary Association.

Heath, D. D. and S. B. Lawrence 1976. *Echinococcus granulosus*: development *in vitro* from oncosphere to immature hydatid cyst. *Parasitology* **73**, 417–23.

Heath, D. D. and S. B. Lawrence 1981. *Echinococcus granulosus* cysts: early development *in vitro* in the presence of serum from infected sheep. *Int. J. Parasitol.* **11**, 261–6.

Heath, D. D., S. B. Lawrence and W. K. Yong 1979. Cross-protection between the cysts of *Echinococcus granulosus, Taenia hydatigena* and *T. ovis* in lambs. *Res. Vet. Sci.* **27**, 210–12.

Heath, D. D., S. N. Parmeter, P. J. Osborn and S. B. Lawrence 1981. Resistance to *Echinococcus granulosus* infection in lambs. *J. Parasitol.* **67**, 797–9.

Herd, R. P. 1976. The cestocidal effect of complement in normal and immune sera *in vitro. Parasitology* **72**, 325–34.

Herd, R. P. 1977. Resistance of dogs to *Echinococcus granulosus. Int. J. Parasitol.* **7**, 135–8.

Herd, R. P., R. J. Chappel and D. Biddell 1975. Immunization of dogs against *Echinococcus granulosus* using worm secretory antigens. *Int. J. Parasitol.* **5**, 395–9.

Hinz, E. 1973. Befall mit *Echinococcus multilocularis* und Antikörpertiter bei intraperitoneal und subkutan infizierten NMRI-Mäusen. *Z. Tropenmed. Parasitol.* **24**, 198–206.

Hinz, E. 1979. *Echinococcus multilocularis*: Superinfektionen bei der experimentell infizierten Maus. *Tropmed. Parasitol.* **30**, 387–90.

Hinz, E. and S. Domm 1980. Die experimentelle *Echinococcus multilocularis* – Infektion von Muttermäusen und ihre Bedeutung für die Nachkommen. *Tropmed. Parasitol.* **31**, 135–42.

Hopkins, C. A. and I. F. Barr 1982. The source of antigen in an adult tapeworm. *Int. J. Parasitol.* **12**, 327–33.

Hrzenjak, T., V. Muie and I. Ehrlich 1979. [A comparative study of the polyhexosamine ceramide complex isolated from *Echinococcus granulosus* larvae and *Fasciola hepatica*.] *Vet. Arhiv* **49**, 21–32 (in Croation).

Isaak, D. D. 1983. *In vitro* tapeworm extract-induced proliferative responses of gut-associated lymphoid cells from *Hymenolepis diminuta* infected mice. *J. Helminthol.* **57**, 43–50.

Kamiya, H., M. Kamiya, M. Ohbayashi and T. Nomura 1980a. [Studies on the host resistance to infection with *Echinococcus multilocularis*. 1. Difference of susceptibility of various rodents, especially of congenitally athymic nude mice.] *Jap. J. Parasitol.* **29**, 87–100 (in Japanese).

Kamiya, H., M. Kamiya and M. Ohbayashi 1980b. [Studies on host resistance to infection with *Echinococcus multilocularis*. 2. Lytic effect of complement and its mechanism.] *Jap. J. Parasitol.* **29**, 169–79 (in Japanese).

Kassis, A. I. 1977. Humoral aspects of the immunity to hydatid disease: the role of complement and antibodies in the control of echinococcosis. *Dissert. Abstr. Int. B* **37**, 5602.

Kassis, A. I. and C. E. Tanner 1976. The role of complement in hydatid disease: *in vitro* studies. *Int. J. Parasitol.* **6**, 25–35.

Kassis, A. I. and C. E. Tanner 1977a. Host serum proteins in *Echinococcus multilocularis*: complement activation via the classical pathway. *Immunology* **33**, 1–9.

Kassis, A. I. and C. E. Tanner 1977b. *Echinococcus multilocularis*: complement's role *in vivo* in hydatid disease. *Exp. Parasitol.* **43**, 390–5.

Kassis, A. I., S. L. Goh and C. E. Tanner 1976. Lesions induced by complement *in vitro* on the protoscoleces of *Echinococcus multilocularis*: a study by electron microscopy. *Int. J. Parasitol.* **6**, 199–211.

Katsova, L. B. 1979. [Biochemical background to the pathogenesis of hydatidosis.] *Mater. Respub. Sem. Parazit. Bolez. Sel'skokoz. K. I. Skryabin* 79–85 (in Russian).

Khorsandi, H. O. and V. Tabibi 1978. Similarities of human hydatid cyst fluid components and the host serum. *Bull. Soc. Path. Exot.* **71**, 95–100.

Lubinsky, G. 1964. Growth of the vegetatively propagated strain of larval *Echinococcus multilocularis* in some strains of Jackson mice and their hybrids. *Can. J. Zool.* **42**, 1099–103.

Lübke, R. 1973. Invasionsversuche durch Scolices von *Echinococcus granulosus* bei Hunden. *Tier. Umschau* **28**, 646–9.

Machnicka, B. and L. Choromanski 1983. Immune response and immunodepression in *Hymenolepis diminuta* infection in rats. *Z. ParasitKde* **69**, 239–45.

Marchevsky, N. 1973. Revision de la literatura sobre tratamiento biologico de la hidatidosis. *Bol. Centro Panam. Zoon.* **15**, 186–205.

Movsesijan, M. and Z. Mladenović 1970. [Active immunisation of dogs against *Echinococcus granulosus*.] *Vet. Glas.* **24**, 189–93 (in Croatian).

Movsesijan, M. and Z. Mladenović 1971. [The possibility of using different developmental stages of *E. granulosus* for detection of specific antibodies against this parasite.] *Vet. Glas.* **25**, 159–63 (in Croatian).

Movsesijan, M., A. Sokolić and Z. Mladenović 1968. Studies on the immunological potentiality of irradiated *Echinococcus granulosus* forms: immunization experiments in dogs. *Br. Vet. J.* **124**, 425–32.

Moya, V. and B. D. Blood 1964. Actividad inmunogenica de un producto biologico ensayado como vacuna contra la hidatidosis ovina. *Bol. Chil. Parasit.* **19**, 7–10 (English summary p. 7).

Ohbayashi, M., R. L. Rausch and F. H. Fay 1971. On the ecology and distribution of *Echinococcus* spp. (Cestoda: Taeniidae) and characteristics of their development in the intermediate host. II. Comparative studies of the development of larval *E. multilocularis*, Leuckart, 1863, in the intermediate host. *Jap. J. Vet. Res.* **19** (Suppl.) 1–53.

Osborn, P. J. and D. D. Heath 1982. Immunisation of lambs against *Echinococcus granulosus* using antigens obtained by incubation of oncospheres *in vitro*. *Res. Vet. Sci.* **33**, 132–3.

Pauluzzi, S. and F. De Rosa 1969. L'idatidosi sperimentale. V. Vaccinoprofilassi contro l'idatidosi sperimentale secondaria da *Echinococcus granulosus* del topo BALB/C. *Annali Sclavo* **11**, 518–30.

Penfold, H. B. 1938. An attempt to immunise lambs against hydatid disease. *Med. J. Aust.* **1**, 375–7.

Perez Esandi, M. V. 1970. Isolation and characterization of antibodies from sera of humans infected with *Echinococcus granulosus*. *J. Parasitol.* **56**, 336–9.

Perricone, R., L. Fontana, C. De Carolis and P. Ottaviani 1980. Activation of alternative complement pathway by fluid from hydatid cysts. *New Engl. J. Med.* **302**, 808–9.

Petroff, N. N. 1923. Ein vaccinetherapieversuch bei der *Echinococcus* – krankheit der lungen. *Zbl. Chir.* **50**, 1322–5.

Petrova, R. F. 1968. [Blood picture in experimental hydatidosis in sheep.] *Materiali Seminara-Soveshch. Borbe Gel'mint. Zhivot. Chimk. Alma-Ata* 115–6 (in Russian).

Ramazanov, V. T. 1979. [Experimental chemoprophylaxis, active and passive immunization in experimental hydatidosis in sheep.] *Mater. Respub. Sem. Parazit. Bolez. Sel'skokoz. K. I. Skryabin* 117–21 (in Russian).

Rau, M. E. and C. E. Tanner 1972. *Echinococcus multilocularis* in the cotton rat. Asexual proliferation following the intraperitoneal inoculation of graded doses of protoscolices. *Can. J. Zool.* **50**, 941–6.

Rau, M. E. and C. E. Tanner 1973. *Echinococcus multilocularis* in the cotton rat. The effect of preexisting subcutaneous cysts on the development of a subsequent intraperitoneal inoculum of protoscolices. *Can. J. Zool.* **51**, 55–9.

Rau, M. E. and C. E. Tanner 1975. BCG suppresses growth and metastasis of hydatid infections. *Nature, Lond.* **256**, 318–9.

Rau, M. E. and C. E. Tanner 1976. *Echinococcus multilocularis* in the cotton rat: the *in vitro* protoscolicidal activity of peritoneal cells. *Int. J. Parasitol.* **6**, 195–8.

Rausch, R. 1954. Studies on the helminth fauna of Alaska. XX. The histogenesis of the alveolar larva of *Echinococcus* species. *J. Infect. Dis.* **94**, 178–86.

Rausch, R. and E. L. Schiller 1956. Studies on the helminth fauna of Alaska. XXV. The ecology and public health significance of *Echinococcus sibiricensis*, Rausch and Schiller, 1954, on St Lawrence Island. *Parasitology* **46**, 395–419.

Reuben, J. M. and C. E. Tanner 1979. Immunoprophylaxis with BCG of experimental *Echinococcus multilocularis* infections. *Aust. Vet. J.* **55**, 105–8.

Reuben, J. M. and C. E. Tanner 1983. Protection against experimental echinococcosis by non-specifically stimulated peritoneal cells. *Parasite Imm.* **5**, 61–6.

Reuben, J. M., C. E. Tanner and V. Portelance 1979. Protection of cotton rats against experimental *Echinococcus multilocularis* infections with BCG cell walls. *Infect. Immun.* **23**, 582–6.

Reuben, J. M., C. E. Tanner and M. E. Rau 1978. Immunoprophylaxis with BCG of experimental *Echinococcus multilocularis* infections. *Infect. Immun.* **21**, 135–9.

Richard-Lenoble, D., M. D. Smith, M. Loisy and P. J. Verroust 1978. Human hydatidosis: evaluation of three serodiagnostic methods, the principal subclass of specific immunoglobulin and the detection of circulating immune complexes. *Ann. Trop. Med. Parasitol.* **72**, 553–60.

Richards, S. K., C. Arme and F. J. Bridges 1983a. *Echinococcus granulosus equinus*: an ultrastructural study of murine tissue response to hydatid cysts. *Parasitology* **86**, 407–17.

Richards, S. K., C. Arme and F. J. Bridges 1983b. *Echinococcus granulosus equinus*: an ultrastructural study of the laminated layer, including changes on incubating cysts in various media. *Parasitology* **86**, 399–405.

Rickard, M. D., B. J. Coman and R. M. Cannon 1977a. Age resistance and acquired immunity to *Taenia pisiformis* infection in dogs. *Vet. Parasitol.* **3**, 1–9.

Rickard, M. D., S. N. Parmeter and M. A. Gemmell 1975. The effect of development of *Taenia hydatigena* larvae in the peritoneal cavity of dogs on resistance to a challenge infection with *Echinococcus granulosus*. *Int. J. Parasitol.* **5**, 281–3.

Rickard, M. D., L. M. Mackinlay, G. J. Kane, R. M. Matossian and J. D. Smyth 1977b. Studies on the mechanism of lysis of *Echinococcus granulosus* protoscoleces incubated in normal serum. *J. Helminthol.* **51**, 221–8.

Russi, S., A. Siracusano and G. Vicari 1974. Isolation and characterisation of a blood P_1 active carbohydrate antigen of *Echinococcus granulosus* cyst membrane. *J. Immunol.* **112**, 1061–9.

Slais, J. and M. Vanek 1980. Tissue reaction to spherical and lobular hydatid cysts of *Echinococcus granulosus* (Batsch, 1786). *Folia Parasitol.* **27**, 135–43.

Smyth, J. D. 1964. Observations on the scolex of *Echinococcus granulosus*, with special reference to the occurrence and cytochemistry of secretory cells in the rostellum. *Parasitology* **54**, 515–26.

Smyth, J. D. and D. D. Heath 1970. Pathogenesis of larval cestodes in mammals. *Helminthol. Abstr. A* **39**, 1–23.

Smyth, J. D., M. A. Gemmell and M. M. Smyth 1970. Establishment of *Echinococcus granulosus* in the intestine of normal and vaccinated dogs. *H. D. Srivastava commemorative volume* 167–78.

Sokolov, V. A., G. P. Averkin and V. I. Osipov 1975. [Some features of the agent of echinococcosis in the Altai.] *Mater. Nauch. Konf. Vsesoy. Obshch. Gel'mint.* **27**, 140–6 (in Russian).

Sweatman, G. K. and R. J. Williams 1963. Comparative studies on the biology and morphology of *Echinococcus granulosus* from domestic livestock, moose and reindeer. *Parasitology* **53**, 339–90.

Sweatman, G. K., R. J. Williams, K. M. Moriarty and T. C. Henshall 1963. On acquired immunity to *Echinococcus granulosus* in sheep. *Res. Vet. Sci.* **4**, 187–98.

Tassi, C. and S. Dottorini 1980. Vaccinoprofilassi dell'idatidosi sperimentale e movimento anticorpale contro diverse frazioni antigeniche degli scolici. *Giorn. Mall. Inf. Parassitol.* **32**, 809–10.

Thompson, R. C. A. 1976. Inhibitory effect of BCG on development of secondary hydatid cysts of *Echinococcus granulosus*. *Vet. Rec.* **99**, 273.

Thompson, R. C. A. and J. Eckert 1983. Observations on *Echinococcus multilocularis* in the definitive host. *Z. ParasitKde* **69**, 335–45.

Thompson, R. C. A., J. D. Dunsmore and A. R. Hayton 1979. *Echinococcus granulosus*: secretory activity of the rostellum of the adult cestode *in situ* in the dog. *Exp. Parasitol.* **48**, 144–63.

Todorov, T. and R. Jeleva 1979. Nachweis prazipitierender Antikorper bei der Eckinokokkose mit der Gegenstrom-Immunelektrophorese. *Tropenmed. Parasitol.* **30**, 182–8.

Todorov, T., I. Dakov, M. Kosturkova, S. Tenev and A. Dimitrov 1979. Immunoreactivity of pulmonary echinococcosis. 1. A comparative study of immunodiagnostic tests. *Bull. Wld Hlth Org.* **57**, 735–40.

Torres Rodriguez, J. M. and C. Wisnivesky 1978. Cinética de la repuesta serólógica del ratón trás la infección primaria experimental con embrióforos de *Echinococcus granulosus*. *Annls Parasitol. Hum. Comp.* **53**, 479–86.

Turner, E. L., D. A. Berberian and E. W. Dennis 1933. Successful artificial immunization of dogs against *Taenia echinococcus*. *Proc. Soc. Exp. Biol. Med.* **30**, 618–9.

Turner, E. L., D. A. Berberian and E. W. Dennis 1936. The production of artificial immunity in dogs against *Echinococcus granulosus J. Parasitol.* **22**, 14–28.

Turner, E. L., E. W. Dennis and D. A. Berberian 1937. The production of artificial immunity against hydatid disease in sheep. *J. Parasitol.* **23**, 43–61.

Varela-Diaz, V. M. 1973. Aspectos immunologicos del tratamiento biologico de la hidatidosis. *Bol. Cent. Panam. Zoon.* **15**, 20–39.

Varela-Diaz, V. M. and E. A. Coltorti 1973. The presence of host immunoglobulins in hydatid cyst membranes. *J. Parasitol.* **59**, 484–8.

Williams, J. F. and R. M. Sandeman 1982. Antigens of taeniid cestodes. In *Cysticercosis: present state of knowledge and perspectives*, A. Flisser, K. Willms, J. P. Laclette, C. Larralde, C. Ridaura, F. Beltrán (eds) 525–37. New York: Academic Press.

Wolfe, J. H. and R. E. W. Halliwell 1980. Total hemolytic complement values in normal and diseased dog populations. *Vet. Immunol. Immunopath.* **1**, 287–98.

Xylinas, M. E., J. T. Papavassiliou and U. Marcelou-Kinti 1976. [Active immunisation of mice against *Echinococcus granulosus*.] *Acta Microbiol. Hell.* **21**, 86–90 (in Greek).

Yamashita, J., M. Ohbayashi, Y. Kitamura, K. Suzuki and M. Okugi 1958. Studies on *Echinococcosis*. VIII. Experimental *Echinococcosis multilocularis* in various rodents; especially on the difference of susceptibility among uniform strains of the mouse. *Jap. J. Vet. Res.* **6**, 135–55.

Yarulin, G. R. 1968. [Study of the development of hydatid cysts during experimental infection of lambs.] *Moscow: Izdat. Akad. Nauk. SSSR*, 378–82 (in Russian).

Yong, W. K., D. D. Heath and F. Van Knapen 1984. Comparison of cestode antigens in an enzyme-linked immunosorbent assay for the diagnosis of *Echinococcus granulosus*, *Taenia hydatigena* and *T. ovis* infections in sheep. *Res. Vet. Sci.* **36**, 24–31.

Zvolinskiene, V. 1978. The demonstration of the circulating antigens of hydatid cyst (*Echinococcus granulosus*) in the blood serum of patients ill with echinococcosis and their diagnostic importance. In *4th International Congress of Parasitology, Warsaw*, Section E, 106.

7 Epidemiology and control of hydatid disease

M. A. GEMMELL AND J. R. LAWSON

INTRODUCTION

Kuchenmeister, in 1852, determined the general characteristics of the life history of cestodes by demonstrating that when fed to dogs, larval *Taenia pisiformis* were transformed into tapeworms. Von Siebold, in 1853, however, must be recognised as the person who first defined the life history of *Echinococcus granulosus.* He fed the protoscoleces of '*Echinococcus veterinorum*' (*E. granulosus*), from cattle, to dogs. Subsequent studies during the remainder of the 19th century by such distinguished biologists as Kuchenmeister, Naunyn, Nettleship, Krabbe, Leuckart, Thomas and many others, confirmed the life-cycle and established that the hydatid cysts observed in man were the same as those in animals. The life-cycle became well known throughout the world before the turn of the century and many medical and veterinary authorities made formal recommendations for the prevention of the feeding of raw offal and the need to treat dogs with areca nut.

The first control programme was initiated in Iceland and followed the classic 16-page booklet written by Krabbe in 1864. This described the life histories of three important cestodes of dogs and sheep in great detail as well as the measures available to counteract infection. This booklet, together with the Bible and the Icelandic sagas, were among the very few pieces of literature written in the Icelandic language. The long winter nights and a literate community ensured that it was read and its messages were understood. This can be regarded as one of the first experiences of health education for the control of hydatid disease.

Survey work undertaken during the first 60 years of the 20th century revealed a high prevalence of *E. granulosus* in many countries including those colonised during the preceding century, such as Australia and New Zealand (Gemmell 1960, 1961a, Rausch 1967, Schantz & Schwabe 1969, Williams *et al.* 1971, Matossian *et al.* 1977, see Chs 2 & 3).

Along with measurements of progress in control programmes, there has been a considerable upsurge in epidemiological research over the past 25 years. This has enhanced knowledge of the dynamics of transmission and of the methods required for control. A definition of the factors that contribute to determining the basic reproductive rate (Macdonald 1965, Anderson 1982a,b, May 1982) is of central importance to an understanding of both parasite population biology and control strategies. This research is described in this review.

With respect to studies on the dynamics of transmission in echinococcosis/hydatidosis, all parasitologists are aware of the health hazards involved in working with these organisms. Sometimes information vital to an understanding of the survival processes cannot readily be obtained by direct experimentation with this parasite. Parasitologists have often used *Taenia hydatigena, T. ovis* and *T. pisiformis* as models for investigating those factors which may enhance or reduce transmission. This we have done where data for *Echinococcus* are not available.

GENERAL EPIDEMIOLOGICAL CONSIDERATIONS

The natural focus

There are situations where *E. granulosus* occurs naturally without involving domestic animals or man other than as accidental hosts (see Ch. 2). One of the best known examples is the dingo–wallaby life-cycle (Durie & Riek 1952, Gemmell 1959). This is a natural predator–prey relationship. It has been suggested that the pulmonary location of the larvae reduces the ability of wallabies (*Wallabia* spp.) to escape capture by the dingo and thereby enhances the chances of successful transmission (Durie & Riek 1952).

In endemic areas sufficient eggs are available in the environment to ensure that some of the population of intermediate hosts ingest eggs. These wallabies survive long enough for the larvae to reach maturity and become available to a proportion of the dingo population. Although this has been known for some time, very little is understood of the spatial and temporal relationships between the host populations and the factors which influence the survival of the parasite.

An important aspect of this life-cycle is the unfavourable environment for the survival of eggs (see below). However, it has been observed that the proportion of heavily infected dingoes is higher than that of naturally infected dogs in areas with generally cooler weather patterns where a dog–sheep cycle predominates. This has also been found to be the case among Turkana dogs in northern Kenya. In that region, as pointed out by Nelson and Rausch (1963), 'most of the infections were readily detected, but only in the Turkana dogs were the infections so heavy that the intestines were "furred" with thousands of worms'. It is, therefore, likely that in hot climates successful transmission only occurs if there is a strong infection pressure and a highly susceptible definitive host population.

The domestic focus

The life-cycle may involve sheep, cattle, pigs, goats, camels, buffaloes or horses as intermediate hosts (see Chs 2 & 3). Strains differ and these differences may be of epidemiological significance (see Ch. 1). The biological parameters described in this chapter refer only to the dog–sheep strain in mainland Australia and New Zealand.

The dynamics of transmission of *Echinococcus* spp. is made much more complex by human activities (see Ch. 3). These influences are summarised in Fig. 7.1.

Wildlife and synanthropic foci

In some cases domestic and wildlife foci are interconnected. An example of this is *E. multilocularis* in the arctic fox (*Alopex lagopus*) and vole (*Microtus oeconomus*) cycle in the tundra zone of Alaska, and on St Lawrence Island (Rausch 1967, Fay 1973). The domestic part of the cycle involves dogs and voles (see Ch. 2). In this situation, the abundance of parasites is associated with a 3–4 year cycle of host populations. Under the conditions prevailing on St Lawrence Island, hyperendemic synanthropic foci may be produced when voles exist as commensals in settlements where sled dogs are numerous (Rausch & Schiller 1956, Rausch 1972, Fay 1973). While the host population fluctuations may restrict transmission from time to time, many of the infected foxes may still have burdens of between 10 000 and 25 000 worms (Rausch & Richards 1971). Another factor that assists transmission is the rapid development of the larvae in intermediate hosts whose life expectancy does not exceed one year (Rausch 1967).

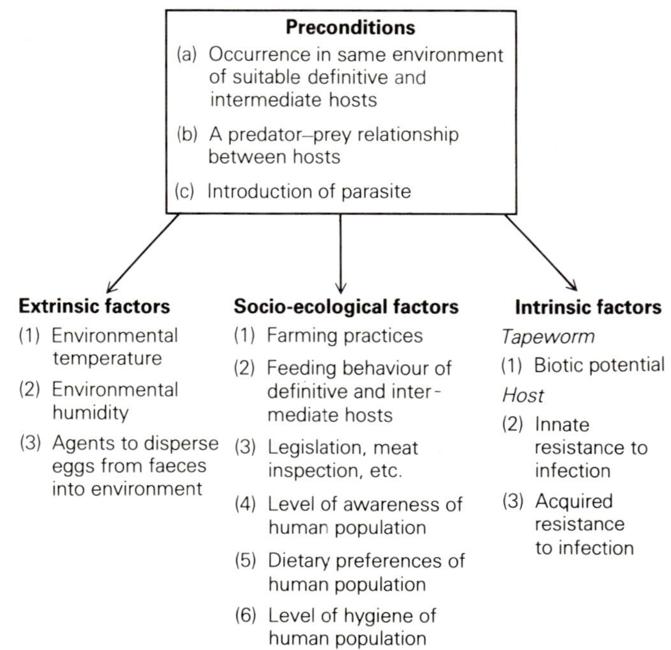

Figure 7.1 Factors influencing the domestic life-cycles of Taeniidae.

BASIC REPRODUCTIVE RATE

If the numbers of a parasite population are stable, the total numbers emigrating from the population, by death or other losses into the environment, are equal to the numbers entering the population through asexual and sexual reproduction. Expressed another way it means that each individual in the population replaces itself by giving rise to an average of precisely one other individual during its life-span. If the numbers in the population are increasing this figure will be greater than one, and if the numbers are decreasing, less than one. This concept has been termed the basic or intrinsic reproductive rate (R_0) (Macdonald 1965, Anderson 1982a,b, May 1982) and is a function of the net reproduction, expected life-span and the infection pressure of the parasite in each phase of its life-cycle. In many natural situations the theoretical basic reproductive rate of *Echinococcus* spp. would seem to be above unity. Thus in the absence of density-dependent constraints, the population should increase. This does not seem to happen. The constraints that prevent this are described below.

DENSITY-DEPENDENT REGULATION

Bradley (1972, 1974) outlined three methods by which parasite populations may be constrained. These are:

(a) Type I, which is a form of transmission with no negative feedback operating. This is mainly density-independent and involves extrinsic factors, e.g. weather.
(b) Type II, which involves regulation at the level of the host population either (i) through a density-dependent immune response that eliminates the parasites in individual hosts, thereby preventing reinfection, or (ii) through over-dispersion of the parasite population within the host population with subsequent death of the heavily infected individuals.
(c) Type III, to which we shall show that *Echinococcus* spp. potentially belong, is a density-dependent regulation by the host through an immune system. In this system only the surplus parasites are eliminated and death of the host through hyper-parasitism is unusual.

Types I and II are basically unstable.

STABILITY

The stability of a biological system describes its ability to withstand perturbation; and afterwards to return to the previous equilibrium or reach a new one (Fig. 7.2).

Investigation of the dynamics of transmission of the *Echinococcus* spp. system and of its stability, must in the first instance be based on a literary

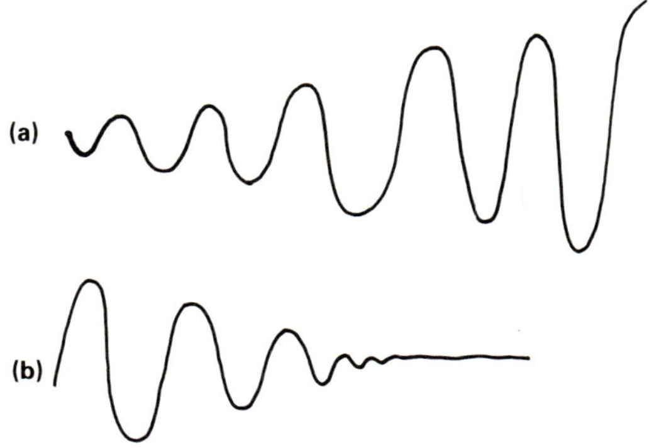

Figure 7.2 Diagrammatic representation of fluctuations in numbers after perturbation in (a) an unstable parasite population and (b) a stable parasite population.

description of the population parameters of the three stages – the adult, the egg and the larva. It is only when the parameters for each stage are known that it is possible to determine the stability of the whole system. In recent years, mathematical models for *Echinococcus* have been constructed (Harris *et al.* 1980, Keymer 1982). These may indicate stability characteristics and help to identify particular aspects of the life history which are poorly understood and require further research.

BIOLOGICAL PARAMETERS

The adult sub-population in dogs

NUMBER AND LONGEVITY OF WORMS

When dogs were experimentally infected with equal amounts (0.25 ml) of fresh protoscoleces of *E. granulosus*, worm counts varied from 0 to 100 000. Of 213 dogs experimentally infected, 5.6 per cent failed to become infected. Of the infected dogs, 17 per cent had less than 100, 11 per cent had between 100 and 1000, and 72 per cent had more than 1000 worms (Gemmell *et al.* 1985).

In contrast, in the field situation, surveys involving rural dogs have shown that both the proportion infected and the proportion having high worm counts is much less than this. For example, in New South Wales and Victoria where 20 per cent of 590 and 3 per cent of 792 dogs harboured *E. granulosus*, only 2.5 per cent and 0.3 per cent of the infected animals had more than 1000 and 100 worms respectively (Gemmell 1957, Jackson & Arundel 1971).

The life-span of adult *E. granulosus* has been variously cited as 6–20 months (Sweatman & Williams 1963a, Aminzhanov 1975, Harris *et al.* 1980), but we have, however, been unable to find any definitive study describing the longevity of any *Echinococcus* spp. This parameter still, therefore, needs to be defined.

DISTRIBUTION AND GROWTH CHARACTERISTICS

The numerical distribution of worms in dogs fed 17 500, 87 500 and 175 000 protoscoleces of sheep origin are illustrated in Figure 7.3a. It was found that at all dose rates the variance was greater than the mean (i.e. was over-dispersed). The index of dispersion increased linearly with the number of protoscoleces fed. Neither age nor sex of host modified this distribution. At all dose levels, the proportion of protoscoleces which developed into adult tapeworms remained constant and was on average less than one in 20 (Gemmell *et al.* 1985).

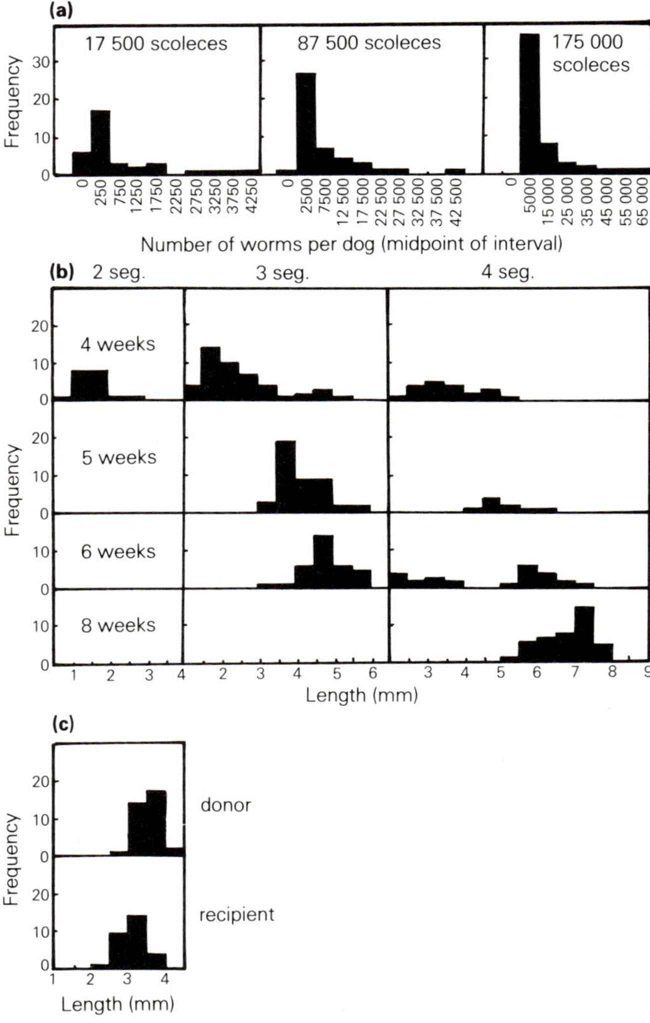

Figure 7.3 Distribution of *Echinococcus granulosus* in dogs following the feeding of (a) 17 500, 87 500 and 175 000 protoscoleces; (b) lengths of two-, three-, and four-segmented worms at specified ages; and (c) worms with arrested growth transferred at 11 weeks from donor to recipient.

The growth patterns of *E. granulosus* derived from protoscoleces in sheep are illustrated in Figure 7.3b. Two growth characteristics were observed: 'normal' and 'retarded'. With normal growth the three- and four-segmented worms increased in length up to 70 and 56 d, respectively. The first eggs were observed in four-segmented organisms at 35 d, and in the faeces at 42 d with the first major discharge occurring between days 56 and 63.

When retarded growth occurred the worm size of 77 d old worms remained similar to that of two-segmented worms of about 28 d. When these were transferred to naive recipients they failed to grow over a period of 14 d (Fig. 7.3c). This suggests that a permanent suppression of growth may take place in some dogs before 28 d (Gemmell *et al.* 1985). Arrested growth has also been reported by Herd (1977).

ACQUIRED RESISTANCE

Evidence for immunity to *E. granulosus* by dogs has been reviewed by Gemmell (1976a), Rickard (1983) and Heath (Ch. 6). This evidence is conflicting. Several studies described in these reviews suggest that dogs injected with homologous somatic antigens or with secretory products or dosed with irradiated protoscoleces, showed, when challenged, some degree of altered susceptibility to either the number of parasites establishing, their growth and/or their fecundity.

The difficulty in interpretation may be due to the wide variation in susceptibility of dogs to *E. granulosus*. Most dogs, however, do acquire a degree of resistance associated with the frequency of ingestion of protoscoleces (Fig. 7.4) (Gemmell *et al.* 1985). This is manifested by a reduction from the expected in the worm burdens at consecutive challenge

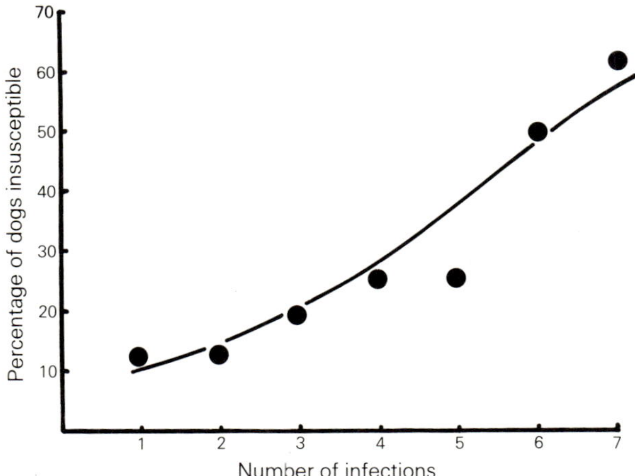

Figure 7.4 Percentage of dogs becoming insusceptible to *Echinococcus granulosus* at a specified number of infections (line represents best fit to the probit transformation).

exposures and a reduction in the size of the worms. However, oogenesis of these worms is not necessarily affected. It has been estimated from the probit transformed data that 50 per cent of dogs may develop a degree of resistance by the sixth infection and an extrapolation suggests that 99 per cent may do so by the 12th infection (Gemmell *et al.* 1985).

Dogs, by their lingual-anal grooming habits have access to tapeworm eggs. However, unlike sheep, they do not appear to acquire resistance to *E. granulosus* by ingesting eggs (Gemmell *et al.* 1985).

The egg sub-population in the environment

EGG OUTPUT

As previously described, the distribution of *E. granulosus* is over-dispersed in experimental and natural infections in dogs and only a small proportion of them harbour very heavy infections. The number of eggs in each proglottid has been estimated to vary from 200 to 800 (Rausch & Schiller 1956, Arundel 1972 and see Ch. 1). A daily peak of only 71 000 eggs has been observed from a dog harbouring 12 767 worms (Sweatman & Williams 1963a). It is the number of heavily infected animals (super-spreaders) in an area, and their movements, which influence the distribution of the larvae in the intermediate host.

EGG DISPERSAL

Rhythmic contractions of the proglottid may assist in egg expulsion (Fay 1973) and lead to the migration of proglottids for several centimetres from the faecal mass (Mattoff & Kolev 1964). It is now evident, however, that eggs may disperse over a much wider area than can be explained by proglottid movement (Gemmell & Johnstone 1977, Gemmell & Lawson 1982a, Lawson & Gemmell 1983).

Using *T. hydatigena* and *T. ovis* as models, it has been found that eggs spread up to 80 m from the site of deposition within 10 d (Gemmell & Johnstone 1976). It was also found that eggs spread equally in all directions in the summer and that this was independent of the height of the grass, the prevailing wind, and the slope of the ground (Gemmell *et al.* 1978). In contrast to the symmetry of summer dispersion, dispersion in the winter has been observed to be asymmetrical (Lawson & Gemmell 1985). The explanation for the variation is discussed below. In all these experiments, cyst counts observed in sheep showed marked over-dispersion, and this may indicate that eggs were dispersed in clusters.

It is difficult to determine the extent of the spread of eggs in endemic regions because 'wild' eggs may interfere with the interpretation of the data, but there is good circumstantial evidence that some eggs may travel long distances. This evidence comes from an investigation of an epidemic outbreak of *T. ovis* at the field station of the Hydatid Research Unit, in New Zealand, where dispersal up to 175 m was confirmed (Lawson & Gemmell 1983). An investigation of an epidemic of *T. hydatigena* in the

Styx field trial (Gemmell 1978c) and of *T. ovis* in the Otago/Southland regional surveillance programme in New Zealand (described later) showed that heavy concentrations of eggs may occur within an area of 10 ha following their deposition by the dog, and a few eggs may disperse up to 10 km, thereby involving an area of 30 000 ha. An illustration of the effects of this dispersion combined with the longevity of the eggs in the field is given for *T. ovis* in Figure 7.5.

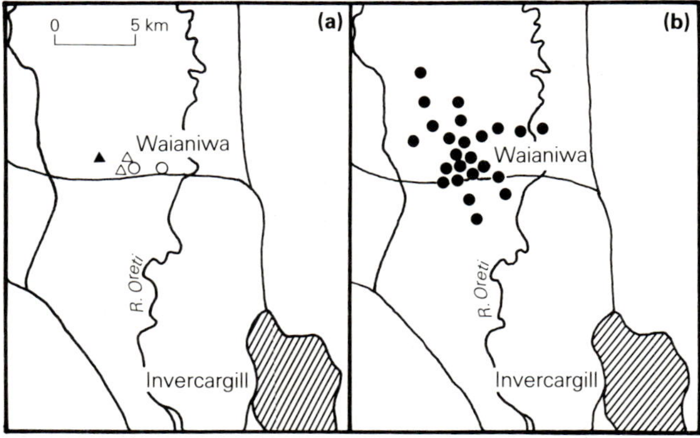

Figure 7.5 An example of egg dispersal and survival. The prevalence of *Taenia ovis* in lambs from farms in Waianiwa, Southland, New Zealand between 1979 (a) and 1980 (b). ▲, ®15 per cent; △, 10–14.9 per cent; ○, 5–9.9 per cent; ●, 1–4.9 per cent. The farms with more than 5 per cent may have kept one or more infected dogs at one time in 1979.

MECHANISMS OF EGG DISPERSAL

That tapeworm eggs spread from the site of deposition is now well documented, but the mechanisms by which they spread are not well understood. Many agents have been implicated, including wind, rainfall, birds, arthropods, earthworms and molluscs, as well as on the feet of animals (for reviews on dispersal of other cestode eggs see Gemmell & Johnstone 1977, Gemmell & Lawson 1982a, Lawson & Gemmell 1983).

With regard to wind and air currents, Sweatman and Williams (1963b) sprayed eggs of *E. granulosus* and *T. hydatigena* on to pasture and measured the effects downwind by grazing sentinel sheep. They confirmed that eggs were picked up by the sheep. Unfortunately, similar measurements were not made upwind. Thus, the evidence for wind or air currents being a factor in egg dispersal still remains controversial.

With regard to insects, Schiller (1954) provided unequivocal evidence that *Phormia regina* (blowfly) can transmit the eggs of *E. multilocularis* from the faeces of the arctic fox (*A. lagopus*) to red-backed voles (*Chlethrionomys rutilis dawsoni*), and Heinz and Brauns (1955) recovered the eggs of *E. granulosus* from the bodies of *Sarcophaga tibialis* (fleshfly). Fontana and

Severino-Brea (1961) observed the eggs of *E. granulosus* undamaged in the gut of blowfly maggots of *Lucilia* and *Calliphora* spp. that had fed on egg-contaminated faeces.

Lawson and Gemmell (1985) have shown that between 5 and 34 per cent of four species of blowfly found in the South Island of New Zealand (*Calliphora quadrimaculata*, *C. hortona*, *C. stygia* and *Hybopygia varia*) ingest eggs of *T. hydatigena* when naturally attracted to feed on dog faeces containing this parasite. The maximum number of eggs ingested was 860 (mean 113 per fly). After feeding naturally on contaminated faeces, all four species of fly transmitted infection to lambs when administered to them. Laboratory experiments showed that the majority of eggs (82.4 per cent) were excreted within 24 h of ingestion by flies.

Many studies have been undertaken on fly dispersal. Maximum distances travelled by *Musca domestica, Chrysomya macellaria, P. regina, Lucilia serricata* and *Sarcophaga* spp. have been determined at 21, 24, 18, 1.6, and 5 km respectively (Bishopp & Laake 1921), and *Phaenicia serricata* 6 km, *P. regina* 13 km and *M. domestica* 19 km by Lindquist *et al.* (1951). However, most flies when caught within 24 h were within 1.6 km of the release point. Flies display a random dispersal pattern, with frequent reversals (Schoof & Siverly 1954, Schoof 1959) and aggregations at specific sites attractive to them.

The symmetrical distribution of the eggs of *T. hydatigena* in the summer (Gemmell *et al.* 1978) and asymmetrical distribution in the winter (Lawson & Gemmell 1985) can be explained by high fly activity in summer and a trend for the less active flies to disperse downwind from dog faeces in winter.

WEATHER FACTORS AND LONGEVITY OF EGGS

Both *in vitro* and *in vivo* studies have been used to evaluate the likely effects of weather on the longevity of the eggs of *Echinococcus* spp. (for a description of information on other Taeniidae see Gemmell 1978a).

LONGEVITY IN TEMPERATE ZONES

When eggs of *E. granulosus* were stored in the presence of moisture at 21°C, the embryos (oncospheres) could be activated after 28 d but not after 56 d. In contrast, when stored at 70°C under the same conditions, some eggs survived for 294 d (Fig. 7.6) (Gemmell 1977). This is consistent with the observations made for other taeniid tapeworms that longevity is greater at lower temperatures. Field trials support the concept that eggs may survive for about one year; heavy rains may, however, wash them deep into the soil profile rendering them unavailable to grazing animals (Sweatman & Williams 1963b).

LONGEVITY UNDER EXTREME CLIMATIC CONDITIONS

High temperature effects Eggs of *E. granulosus* stored at 60°C, 70°C and 100°C failed to activate after 10, 6 and 1 min exposure, respectively (Meymerian & Schwabe 1962). No data are available for *E. granulosus* at

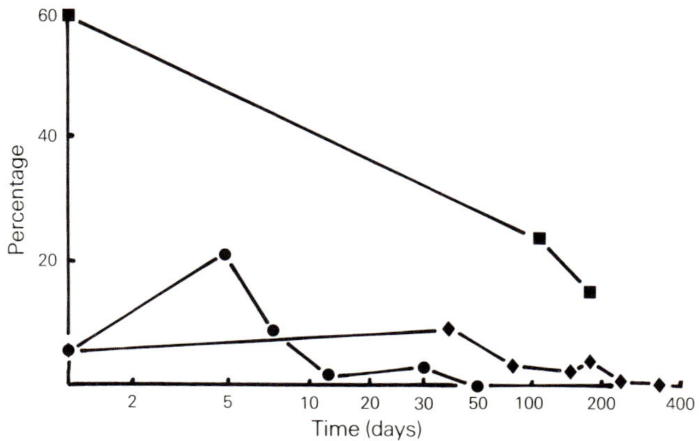

Figure 7.6 Percentage of embryos of *Echinococcus granulosus* which are activated *in vitro* after storage of eggs at 21 °C (●—●) and 7 °C (◆—◆) and decrease in infectivity of eggs of *Taenia hydatigena* to sheep in the natural environment (■—■).

lower temperatures, but the eggs of *T. hydatigena* and *T. ovis* failed to activate after storage for a few hours at 45°C or 4 d at 38°C (Gemmell 1977).

Low temperature effects After storage at −10°C for 4 months eggs of *E. granulosus* were still infective to a pig (Dévé 1910). Red-backed voles (*C. rutilis*) were infected with eggs of *E. multilocularis* which had been stored at −26°C for about 2 months and at −51°C for 24 h (Schiller 1955). Eggs of *E. granulosus* stored for 24 h at −35°C or occasionally at −50°C, were infective to rodents, but eggs were killed at −70°C (Colli & Williams 1972). It seems that the eggs of *Echinococcus* spp. can withstand the low temperatures that occur in the natural environment.

Desiccation effects At relative humidities of 60 and 80 per cent the eggs of *E. granulosus* failed to activate *in vitro* after 1 and 2 d exposure, respectively (Laws 1968). This author concluded that desiccation was 'likely to dominate all other natural restrictions on the survival of taeniid eggs in nature'. It seems that the eggs of *Echinococcus* spp. cannot withstand desiccation at any temperature.

EFFECT OF MATURATION AND AGEING ON LONGEVITY

In vitro, it has been observed that the activity of the embryos of *E. granulosus* increased after eggs had been stored in water at 21°C for 1 week (Fig. 7.6). A similar phenomenon has been reported for *T. hydatigena* (Gemmell 1977).

It has been shown that the eggs of *E. granulosus* stored at 10°C and 21°C for up to 32 d were infective to mice but that thereafter, although invasive, they did not survive (Batham 1957). Evidence for an ageing process has been provided under natural conditions with *T. hydatigena*. Here the proportion of embryos that developed into cysticerci declined from 60 to 25 to 15 per cent at 0, 3 and 6 months after the eggs had been deposited on the pasture (Fig. 7.6b; Gemmell & Macnamara 1976). Ageing affects not only the number of larvae that will establish, but also the number of these that survive within the intermediate host.

Based on these observations, it seems that proglottids at the time of expulsion contain eggs ranging in maturity (Gemmell 1977). During the free-living phase, temperatures between 7°C and below 38°C may permit some juveniles to mature. Sub-zero temperatures may limit the number of juveniles reaching maturity, but may not necessarily increase the life-span of the organism. The higher the temperature the greater the acceleration of the maturation and ageing processes (Gemmell 1977). This may account for 'sterile' immunity in animals that have been exposed to senescent eggs (Gemmell 1977).

The larval sub-population in sheep

NUMBER AND LONGEVITY

When sheep were fed with 25, 250 or 2500 eggs it was found that the proportion which developed into cysts was constant. About one in every 70 embryos established, but fewer than one in every 250 embryos survived and developed into a cyst (Gemmell *et al.* 1985).

In New Zealand prior to the introduction of control about 75 per cent of adult sheep were infected. The mean number and range of *E. granulosus* cysts in 5-year-old female sheep were seven and 0–38, respectively (Gemmell 1961b). This may imply that these sheep ingested on average at least 500 eggs during the period that they were susceptible to infection.

Deaths of larvae rarely occur in sheep once they have been established for 2 years and the life-span of the successful organisms can be regarded as the same as that of the host (Gemmell *et al.* 1985).

DISTRIBUTION AND GROWTH CHARACTERISTICS

When 2500 eggs of *E. granulosus* were administered to sheep the numerical distribution of larvae was found to be over-dispersed (Fig. 7.7a). The index of dispersion increased as the size of the egg dose increased (Gemmell *et al.* 1985). The percentages of sheep that remained uninfected after being given 25, 250 or 2500 eggs were 38, 13 and 7 per cent, respectively. The percentages with no viable cysts 2 years after infection were 88, 75 and 35 per cent, respectively (Gemmell *et al.* 1985). This indicates that the size of the egg dose is important in establishing an infection, but that not all sheep are equally susceptible.

In New Zealand, prior to control, the distribution was also over-dispersed and 25 per cent of 5-year-old ewes were uninfected (Gemmell 1961b). This distribution will arise not only from heterogeneity within the

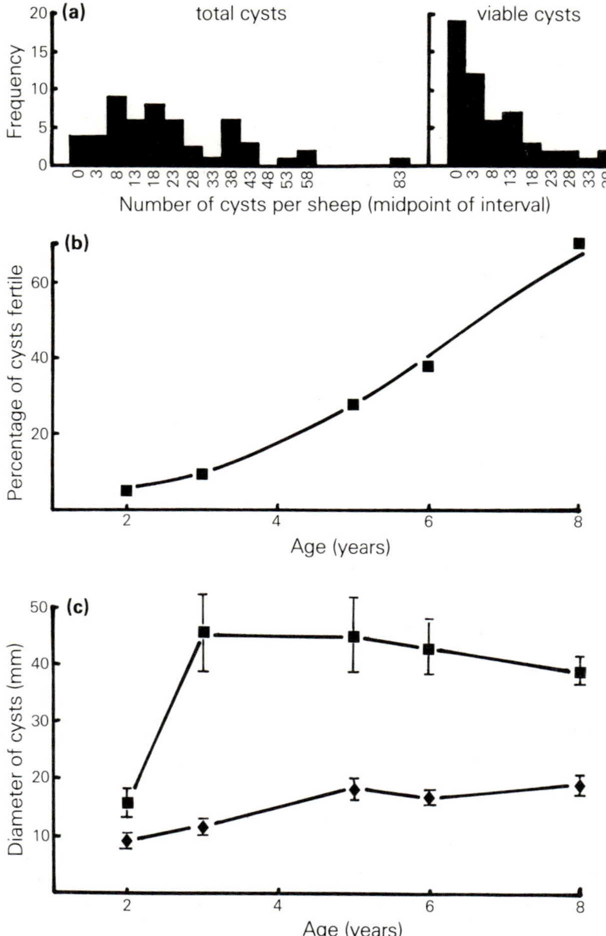

Figure 7.7 Distribution and development of *Echinococcus granulosus* in sheep (n = 54): (a) distribution of total and viable cysts from 2500 eggs; (b) percentage of larvae with protoscoleces at specified ages (line represents best fit to the probit transformation); (c) diameter of fertile (■—■) and non-fertile (◆—◆) larvae at specified ages.

egg and sheep populations, but also from spatial heterogeneity in egg distribution.

Protoscoleces were observed in cysts 2 years after infection and the proportion of viable larvae containing protoscoleces increased with the age of the larvae (Gemmell *et al.* 1985). The proportion of larvae that developed protoscoleces over time was normally distributed and half of the viable cysts contained protoscoleces at 6 years (Fig. 7.7b). An extrapolation suggests that 99 per cent of larvae would contain protoscoleces at 17 years.

The larvae with protoscoleces were significantly larger than those without protoscoleces at the same age (Fig. 7.7c). This suggests that the development of fertility is associated with a rapid growth phase.

ACQUIRED RESISTANCE

There is clear evidence for all species of taeniid tapeworm so far studied that strong immunity is acquired by the intermediate host following ingestion or injection of eggs of the homologous species (Gemmell & Soulsby 1968, Gemmell & Macnamara 1972, Gemmell 1976a, Gemmell & Johnstone 1977, Flisser *et al.* 1979, Williams 1979, Rickard 1983, Rickard & Williams 1982, Gemmell & Lawson 1982b, Lawson & Gemmell 1983).

There is good evidence that strong immunity to *E. granulosus* can be induced by the injection of homologous eggs (Gemmell 1966, Heath *et al.* 1979a). The mechanisms involved are reviewed in Chapter 6. The evidence for the acquisition of immunity through the ingestion of eggs is, however, less well documented. This is because it is difficult to distinguish between the primary and challenge infections. Sweatman *et al.* (1963) attempted to solve this problem by using an interval of 9 months between the egg doses. They were able to demonstrate a strong immunity to *E. granulosus* in sheep when 50 000–100 000 eggs were given, but only a partial immunity at lower egg doses. There is some evidence, for *T. hydatigena*, that the immunity is stronger when the challenge infection is given 3 rather than 9 months after the primary infection, suggesting a loss of immunity over time (Gemmell & Johnstone 1981). This can account for the limited immunity at the low egg-dose levels of *E. granulosus* administered by Sweatman *et al.* (1963).

Immunity can also be induced to *E. multilocularis* in *C. rutilis* by an injection of homologous eggs (R. L. Rausch & M. A. Gemmell unpublished data). A slight degree of reciprocal immunity can be induced between *E. granulosus* and either *T. hydatigena* or *T. ovis* in sheep (Gemmell 1966). There appear to be no reciprocal effects between *E. granulosus* and *E. multilocularis* in *C. rutilis* (R. L. Rausch & M. A. Gemmell unpublished data).

Transmission between hosts

As previously pointed out, the infection pressure, which describes the rate of transmission between hosts, is a fundamental parameter determining the basic reproductive rate. Exposed to a constant rate of infection, the proportion of animals that become infected as a function of time can be described by the equation $Y = 1 - e^{-kt}$, where k is a constant called the infection pressure, t is the duration of exposure and e is the base of natural logarithms (Gemmell & Johnstone 1977).

LARVAE TO ADULTS

Unfortunately, the important measurement of the infection pressure (k)

which describes the rate of flow has not been made for any species of *Echinococcus*.

In order to measure *k* for *E. granulosus* in any endemic situation, it would be necessary to survey the dog population with arecoline hydrobromide at specified intervals while leaving their feeding and scavenging patterns undisturbed.

EMBRYOS TO LARVAE

Here the method for estimating *k* involves infecting definitive hosts with adult worms and placing them on an egg-free pasture. The number of naive intermediate hosts that become infected at each grazing interval can then be measured. Several studies have been undertaken using *T. hydatigena* infections (Gemmell 1976b,c, Gemmell & Macnamara 1976). Lambs gradually acquire grazing competence over the first 5 weeks after birth and it was found that when reared close to dogs infected with *T. hydatigena*, they usually ingested small numbers of eggs and became lightly infected. In contrast, when immunologically naive weaned lambs were introduced to egg-contaminated pasture, they became heavily infected and displayed a highly aggregated distribution of larvae. It was estimated that 60 per cent of the lambs ingested eggs every day (k = 1.4/day). When the dogs were removed and the equilibrium between immigration and emigration of eggs was disturbed, the number of lambs ingesting eggs every day declined slowly to 6.5 per cent (k = 0.067) and 3 per cent (k = 0.03) after 3 months and 6 months, respectively. Within 10 d of reintroducing infected dogs, the original infection pressure was restored.

The only information on the infection pressure for *E. granulosus* in endemic areas is from surveys defining the age-specific prevalence. In one base-line survey carried out in New Zealand, where up to 37 per cent of the dogs were infected with *E. granulosus*, it was found that there was a significant increase ($P<0.001$) in the prevalence of *E. granulosus* and *T. hydatigena* in sheep associated with age (Gemmell 1961b). With *E. granulosus*, the upper asymptote of infection was not reached until 5 years in female sheep; however, with *T. hydatigena* all susceptible animals were infected by 6 months of age (Fig. 7.8). Furthermore, the age-specific prevalence of *E. granulosus* at all ages studied was higher in female than male sheep. This can be attributed to different infection pressures associated with different proximities to the dog kennels. This evidence suggests, therefore, that in the natural environment *E. granulosus*, while producing sufficient eggs to infect almost all susceptible sheep during their lifetime, has a much lower excess of transmission than that of the large tapeworms.

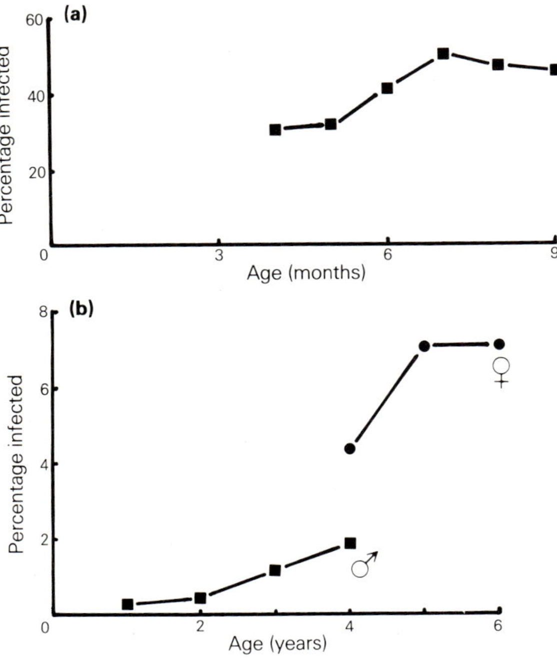

Figure 7.8 Acquisition of larvae of (a) *Taenia hydatigena* and (b) *Echinococcus granulosus* by sheep in endemic areas of New Zealand prior to the introduction of control.

Density-dependent constraints

IN THE DEFINITIVE HOST

Resistance acquired by dogs acts as a negative feedback mechanism that serves to regulate the number of adults that develop and hence the rate of flow of parasites through the system. The extent to which acquired resistance occurs in dogs is dependent on the density of the larval sub-population in the intermediate host and frequency of contact. Thus, in highly endemic regions, the mean level of parasites within the dog population may be lower than expected. This is supported by the previously described surveys of *E. granulosus* in New South Wales and Victoria where most of the dogs were uninfected or carried very few worms even though fed on a diet composed almost exclusively of raw sheep offal.

IN THE INTERMEDIATE HOST

In the hyperendemic situation, the basic reproductive rate is greater than unity and intermediate hosts may ingest many more eggs than will develop into larvae. If these infections were successful and cumulative, many animals would become overloaded with larvae and might die.

However, due to the acquired immunity, death from *E. granulosus* in animals in hyperendemic regions is very rare.

With *T. hydatigena* and *T. ovis* the role of acquired immunity in regulating parasite numbers is well documented (Gemmell & Macnamara 1972, Gemmel 1976a). Unfortunately, for *Echinococcus* spp. little is known of the effects of acquired immunity on the regulation of larval populations in any predator–prey system. The missing information includes (a) age at which the intermediate host acquires immunological competence to the various larval antigens; (b) role of colostrum; (c) time interval required for the induction of immunity following the ingestion of eggs; (d) size of the egg dose required to induce immunity; and (e) duration of immunity in the absence of eggs being ingested.

To gain some insight into these processes for *Echinococcus* spp., comparable information is provided here for *T. hydatigena* or *T. ovis*. With these models it has been found that: (a) lambs gradually acquire grazing ability (Fig. 7.9a) and competence to the full range of larval antigens within about 5 and 8 weeks, respectively, after birth (Gemmell *et al.* 1968a, Gemmell 1976c); (b) some immunity may be transferred by colostrum to the offspring and its effects may last about 6 to 8 weeks (Gemmell *et al.* 1969, Rickard & Arundel 1974, Sutton 1979, Heath *et al.* 1979b); (c) in immunologically competent animals strong immunity is acquired within 2 weeks of the ingestion of the first eggs (Fig. 7.9b) (Gemmell *et al.* 1968b); (d) this immunity may be acquired following the ingestion of as few as 10–50 eggs (Sweatman 1957, Gemmell 1969); and (e) it is lost with consequent superinfection if eggs are not ingested within about 12 months, irrespective of the presence of larvae from a previous infection (Fig. 7.9c) (Gemmell & Johnstone 1981).

The epidemiological events described above indicate that in areas where the infection pressure from eggs is high there may be a period of only 14 d within the lifetime of the intermediate host when it is susceptible to infection with larval tapeworms. It is the epidemiological situation during that period, together with the variability in natural susceptibility within the flock, which will determine the infective pattern (Gemmell 1976a, Gemmell & Johnstone 1977, Gemmell & Lawson 1982b). This mechanism operates as a strong negative feedback and the higher the infection pressure the stronger it will be.

CONTROL

If control measures reduce the basic reproductive rate below unity, numbers will decrease and control can be regarded as being effective. The force needed to reduce R_0 below 1 will depend on the stability of the parasite population. Measures applied at any point in the life-cycle may contribute to reducing R_0. The lower the value of R_0 the easier it will be to control the parasite population. The question with respect to *E. granulosus* is; ‘Can control by attacking only one stage be effective, or is

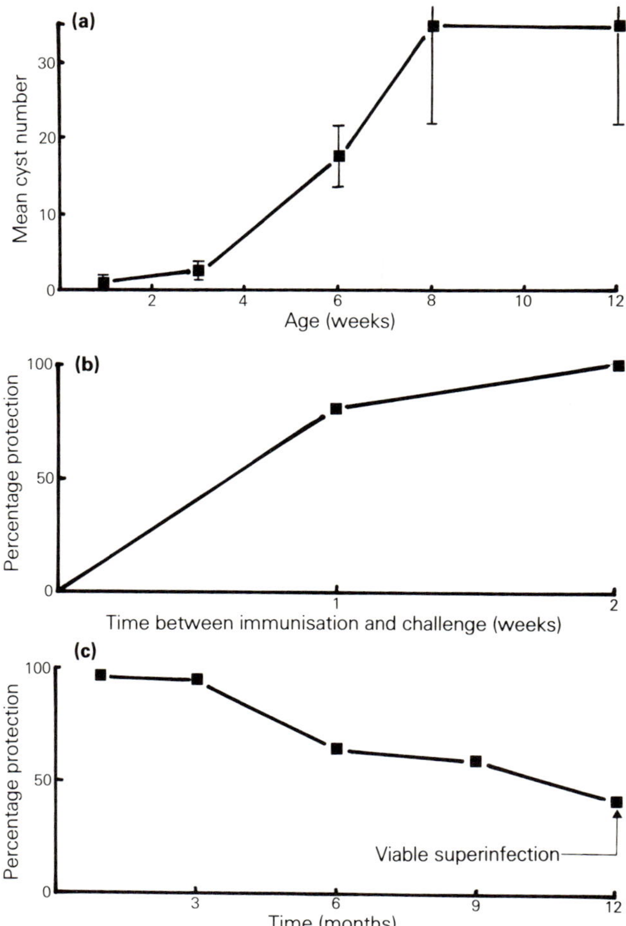

Figure 7.9 The ingestion of eggs, and the acquisition and loss of immunity to *Taenia hydatigena* by sheep: (a) ability of lambs to pick up eggs at specified ages; (b) time interval for acquisition of immunity; (c) time interval for loss of immunity.

the stability so great that more than one stage must be attacked simultaneously?' Control programmes and field trials provide the only practical means of testing this stability.

The points in the life-cycle of *E. granulosus* at which control could be applied are illustrated in Figure 7.10. However, the only method available at the present time is the prevention of larval development into patent tapeworms in the dog. This can be achieved either by denying dogs raw infected offal or by treating them with anthelmintics (Gemmell 1978b, 1979). Field trials as well as national control programmes have been implemented using these methods. Changes in the prevalence of *E. granulosus* in sheep can be used to evaluate the stability of the system. We propose in the subsequent section to compare the stability of *E. granulosus*

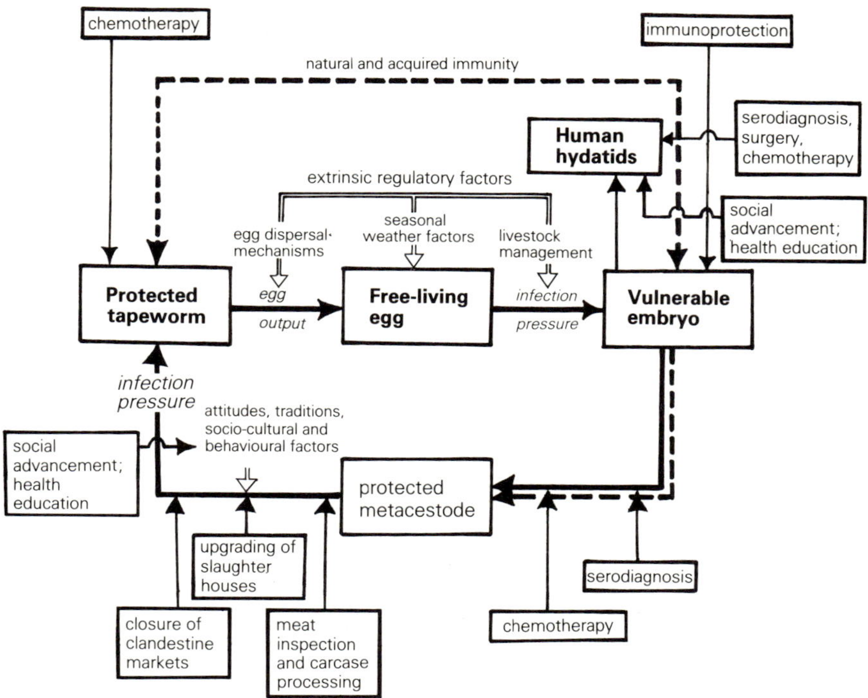

Figure 7.10 Flow chart of the life-cycle of *Echinococcus granulosus* showing points at which control may be applied.

with that of *T. hydatigena* and *T. ovis* by examining the changes in prevalence of the larvae in sheep which take place following the implementation of control.

Testing stability by field trials

The Styx field trial was initiated in 1943 in an isolated valley of the Maniototo Plain of the South Island of New Zealand (Gemmell 1968, 1978c). There were 48 farms in the original trial (1943–51), but from 1958 this was reduced to 11 in order to study the dynamics of transmission of *E. granulosus, T. hydatigena* and *T. ovis* in more detail. In 1978, this trial was expanded to include monitoring of the control programme on all 10 000 farms of the provinces of Otago and Southland with a computerised surveillance system. This involved examination for *E. granulosus* and *T. ovis* infections of all sheep that were submitted for slaughter through killing establishments.

THE STYX FIELD TRIAL

For the first 9 years of the Styx field trial all dog owners were requested not to feed raw offal to their dogs, which were treated every 3 months with arecoline hydrobromide. During this period (1943–51), there was a decline in taeniid cysts in the livers of sheep from about 80 to 40 per cent, but this included both *E. granulosus* and *T. hydatigena*. However, there was no decline in the prevalence of the latter in lambs and almost all susceptible animals were parasitised by 6 months of age. This suggested that *E. granulosus* was less stable than *T. hydatigena*.

From 1958, a strong educational campaign, backed up with an arecoline-based surveillance scheme, was introduced. The object was to test the effects on transmission of educating owners in preventing their dogs gaining access to raw sheep offal. When the age cohorts born prior to the trial were removed by slaughter at about 6 years of age, the prevalence of *E. granulosus* declined virtually to zero in the sheep population (Fig. 7.11a). In contrast, no effects were observed on the prevalence of *T.*

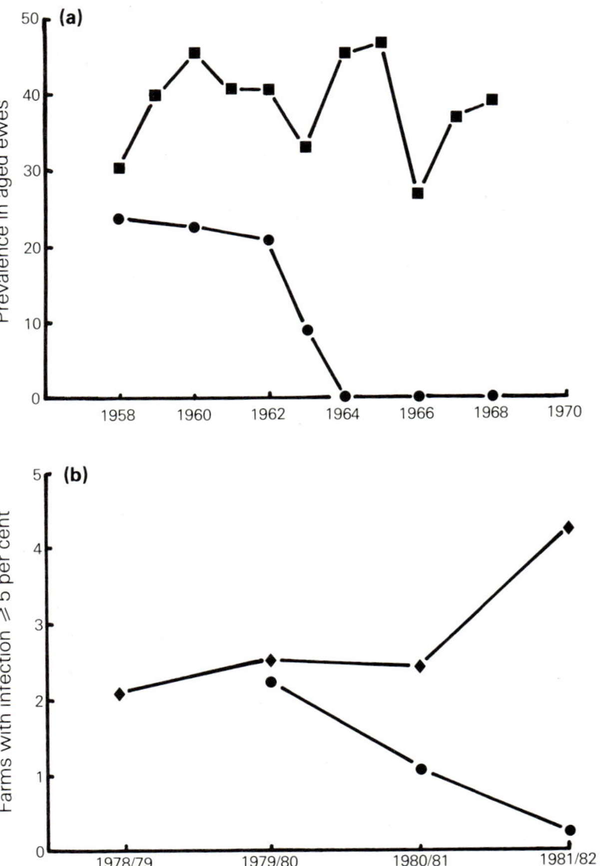

Figure 7.11 Differences in response by *Echinococcus granulosus, Taenia hydatigena* and *T. ovis* to control by (a) arecoline surveillance in the Styx field trial; (b) 6-weekly dog-dosing with praziquantel in Otago and Southland, New Zealand. ●—●, *E. granulosus*; ■—■, *T. hydatigena*; ◆—◆, *T. ovis*.

hydatigena in the same sheep and superinfection was observed. This provided further evidence that the rate of transmission of *E. granulosus* was much less than that of *T. hydatigena*.

OTAGO/SOUTHLAND SURVEILLANCE PROGRAMME

The Otago and Southland provinces have 10 000 farms with 40 000 dogs and 12 million sheep. For 6 years before surveillance was undertaken, the dogs had been treated every 6 weeks with niclosamide, which, having no effect on *E. granulosus*, can be regarded as a placebo. There had, however, been a continuing educational control programme since 1959 and there was evidence of a continuing decline in prevalence. Praziquantel was introduced in 1978. The decline continued and the proportion of farms harbouring adult sheep with more than 5 per cent *E. granulosus* fell from 2.6 to 1.2 to 0.2 per cent between the years 1979, 1980 and 1981, respectively (Fig. 7.11b). In contrast, the proportion of farms harbouring lambs infected with *T. ovis* remained relatively constant at about 40 per cent, with the number of epidemic outbreaks stabilised at between 2 and 4 per cent (Fig. 7.11b).

The results from the Styx field trial and the Otago/Southland surveillance programme demonstrate that control in the definitive host can destabilise the whole *E. granulosus* system. In contrast, with *T. hydatigena* and *T. ovis* the epidemiological pattern transformed from hyperendemic to focal epidemic, and R_0 was not reduced below 1. Therefore, *E. granulosus* populations can be regarded as less stable than those of the large taeniids.

Control programmes

There are at present six national or provincial programmes for which longitudinal prevalence data on echinococcosis in sheep are available (Fig. 7.12). All show a marked reduction in prevalence over time, thereby indicating that R_0 has been reduced below 1.

New Zealand, Tasmania, Cyprus and Argentina (Neuquén) have all relied on an arecoline surveillance and educational programme. New Zealand relied on a laboratory test for its educational campaign. All others have used a field test with the direct demonstration of infected dogs. Tasmania quarantined infected dogs, and more recently infected sheep flocks (Meldrum & McConnell 1968, McConnell & Green 1979). Cyprus reduced its dog population drastically, thereby reducing the habitat for the adult tapeworms (Polydorou 1976, 1980). Argentina, on the other hand, treated with praziquantel only those dogs shown to be infected by arecoline surveillance.

The rate of decline in prevalence of echinococcosis in aged sheep is similar for New Zealand and Tasmania, although that of the latter, which includes both lung and liver cysts, declined to less than 1 per cent more quickly than that for the former. The rate of decline for Cyprus was much greater than that of either New Zealand or Tasmania. That for Argentina has shown periods of sharp decline followed by periods of plateau. During

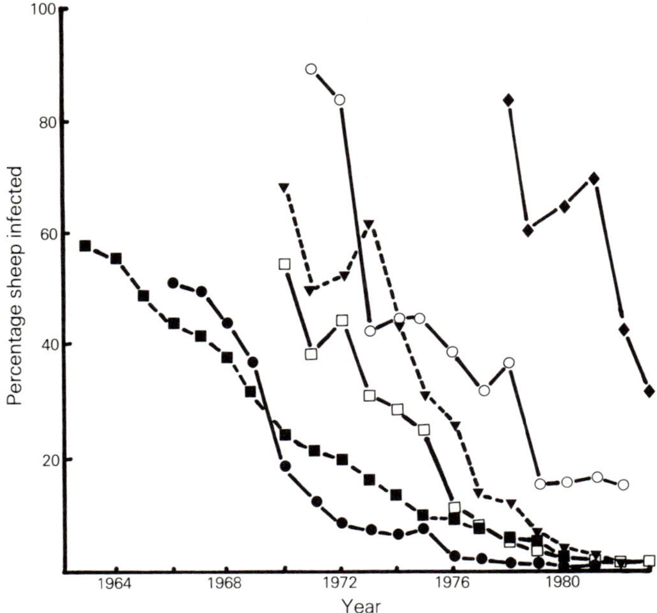

Figure 7.12 Changes in prevalence of *Echinococcus granulosus* in aged sheep during control programmes in New Zealand (■—■), Tasmania (●—●), Cyprus (▼- - - ▼), the Falkland Islands (□—□), Argentina (Neuquén) (○—○) and Chile (Region XII) (◆—◆). *Sources*: New Zealand: New Zealand National Hydatids Council 1982, *22nd annual report* for the year ended 31 March 1982. Tasmania: Tasmanian Hydatids Eradication Council 1982, *Annual report and Statement of Accounts* for the year ending 30 June 1982. Cyprus: K. Polydorou, personal communication. Falkland Islands: *Falkland Islands Hydatid News* No. 16. Argentina: O. De Zavaleta and A. S. Thakur, personal communications. Chile: O. Campano Díaz and A. S. Thakur, personal communications.

these latter periods it seems that the parasite population stabilised at lower levels than previously.

Both Region XII in Chile and the Falkland Islands have used a 6-weekly drug treatment programme with praziquantel and in each case the initial decline in the prevalence has been consistently rapid. Indeed, this rate is similar to that for Cyprus but was achieved without a dog destruction policy.

CONCLUSIONS

The overall stability of a host–parasite system involves complex interactions between stabilising and destabilising forces (Anderson 1978). Several theoretical studies have implicated a variety of factors influencing stability (Crofton 1971a,b, Bradley 1972, Anderson 1978, 1982a,b,

Anderson & May 1978, May & Anderson 1978, May 1982, Anderson & Gordon 1982). These include over-dispersion of parasites within the host population, immunological response of the host, time delays in reproduction and transmission, and reproduction of the parasite within the host. All the above studies involved systems where the parasite induces mortality in the host population. This is not the case with *Echinococcus* spp., in which the adult parasite is well tolerated by the definitive host and the powerful immune response of the intermediate host prevents lethal numbers of larvae maturing.

We recognise that many of the relevant biological parameters are not yet known for *E. granulosus* and we have had to extrapolate from studies using *T. hydatigena* and *T. ovis*. From an evaluation of the measurements of the biological parameters of each sub-population, we consider that the factors which may confer overall stability in the *E. granulosus* system include (a) heterogeneity in all three parasite stages and both hosts leading to an over-dispersed distribution of parasites within the hosts and in the environment; (b) a relatively short maturation time within the definitive host measured in weeks; (c) tolerance of eggs to a relatively wide range of weather factors; (d) tolerance to pathology by both hosts; (e) a strong negative feedback in the intermediate host which wanes in the absence of egg ingestion.

Biological parameters that tend to destabilise this system may include (f) a small number of eggs per proglottid (but this may be compensated for by high worm burdens in some definitive hosts, i.e. 'superspreaders') and (g) a long time delay of several years for maturation of the larvae in the intermediate host population.

There is strong evidence that it is only necessary to attack one stage in order to destabilise the whole *E. granulosus* system. In contrast, it seems that the cysticercoses with their high egg production and shorter developmental period in the larval phase – and a potentially higher R_0 than *E. granulosus* – may require an attack at more than one stage to bring about effective control. *E. multilocularis* appears to have some of the attributes of the large taeniid systems. It may, with its generally large worm burdens and short maturation time for the larvae, prove to be more stable than *E. granulosus* given stable host population densities. This may also be the case with the Turkana dog and Australian dingo systems with their large worm burdens and thus high egg output.

REFERENCES

Aminzhanov, M. 1975. [The lifespan of *Echinococcus granulosus* in the dog.] *Veterinariya, Moscow* **12**, 70–2 (in Russian).

Anderson, R. M. 1978. The regulation of host population growth by parasitic species. *Parasitology* **76**, 119–57.

Anderson, R. M. 1982a. Host–parasite population biology. In *Parasites – their world and ours*, D. F. Mettrick and S. S. Desser (eds) 303–12. Amsterdam: Elsevier.

Anderson, R. M. 1982b. Transmission dynamics and control of infectious disease agents. In *Population biology of infectious diseases*, R. M. Anderson and R. M. May (eds) 149–76. Berlin: Springer-Verlag.

Anderson, R. M. and D. M. Gordon 1982. Processes influencing the distribution of parasite numbers within host populations with special emphasis on parasite-induced host mortalities. *Parasitology*, **85**, 373–98.

Anderson, R. M. and R. M. May 1978. Regulation and stability of host–parasite population interactions. 1. Regulatory processes. *J. Anim. Ecol.* **47**, 219–47.

Arundel, J. H. 1972. A review of cysticercoses of sheep and cattle in Australia. *Aust. Vet. J.* **48**, 140–55.

Batham, E. J. 1957. Notes on viability of hydatid cysts and eggs. *N.Z. Vet. J.* **5**, 74–6.

Bishopp, F. C. and E. W. Laake 1921. Dispersion of flies by flight. *J. Agric. Res.* **21**, 729–66.

Bradley, D. J. 1972. Regulation of parasite populations. A general theory of the epidemiology and control of parasitic infections. *Trans. R. Soc. Trop. Med. Hyg.* **66**, 697–708.

Bradley, D. J. 1974. Stability in host–parasite systems. In *Ecological stability*, M. B. Usher and M. H. Williamson (eds) 71–87. London: Chapman and Hall.

Colli, C. W. and J. F. Williams 1972. Influence of temperature on the infectivity of eggs of *Echinococcus granulosus* in laboratory rodents. *J. Parasitol.* **58**, 422–6.

Crofton, H. D. 1971a. A quantitative approach to parasitism. *Parasitology*, **62**, 179–94.

Crofton, H. D. 1971b. A model of host–parasite relationships. *Parasitology*, **63**, 343–64.

Dévé, F. 1910. Echinococcose primitive expérimentale. Résistance des oeufs du échinocoque à la congélation. *C. R. Séanc. Soc. Biol.* **69**, 568–70.

Durie, P. H. and R. F. Riek 1952. The role of the dingo and wallaby in the infestation of cattle with hydatids *Echinococcus granulosus* (Batsch, 1786) Rudolphi, 1805 in Queensland. *Aust. Vet. J.* **28**, 249–54.

Fay, F. H. 1973. The ecology of *Echinococcus multilocularis* Leuckart, 1863 (Cestoda: Taeniidae) on St Lawrence Island, Alaska. 1. Background and rationale. *Annls Parasitol. Hum. Comp.* **48**, 523–42.

Flisser, A., R. Pérez-Montfort and C. Larralde 1979. The immunology of human and animal cysticercosis: a review. *Bull. Wld Hlth Org.* **57**, 839–56.

Fontana, V. P. and R. Severino-Brea 1961. Centro estudio profilaxis hidatidosis. *Archs Int. Hidat.* **20**, 283–6.

Gemmell, M. A. 1957. Hydatid disease in Australia. II. Observations on the geographical distribution of *Echinococcus granulosus* (Batsch, 1786) Rudolphi, 1805 in the dog in New South Wales. *Aust. Vet. J.* **33**, 217–26.

Gemmell, M. A. 1959. Hydatid disease in Australia. VI. Observations on the carnivora of New South Wales as definitive hosts of *Echinococcus granulosus* (Batsch, 1786) Rudolphi, 1805 and their role in the spread of hydatidiasis in domestic animals. *Aust. Vet. J.* **35**, 450–5.

Gemmell, M. A. 1960. Advances in knowledge on the distribution and importance of hydatid disease as world health and economic problems during the decade 1950–1959. *Helminthol. Abs.* **29**, 355–69.

Gemmell, M. A. 1961a. Hydatid disease in Australasia. *Bull. Off. Int. Epiz. C* **614**, 1–21.

Gemmell, M. A. 1961b. An analysis of the incidence of hydatid cysts (*Echinococcus granulosus*) in domestic food animals in New Zealand, 1958–1959. *N.Z. Vet. J.* **9**, 29–37.

Gemmell, M. A. 1966. Immunological responses of the mammalian host against tapeworm infections. IV. Species specificity of hexacanth embryos in protecting sheep against *Echinococcus granulosus*. *Immunology* **11**, 325–35.

Gemmell, M. A. 1968. The Styx Field-Trial. A study on the application of control measures against hydatid disease caused by *Echinococcus granulosus*. *Bull. Wld Hlth Org.* **39**, 73–100.

Gemmell, M. A. 1969. Hydatidosis and cysticercosis. 1. Acquired resistance to the larval phase. *Aust. Vet. J.* **45**, 521–4.

Gemmell, M. A. 1976a. Immunology and regulation of the cestode zoonoses. In *Immunology of parasitic infections*, S. Cohen and E. Sadun (eds) 333–58. Oxford: Blackwell Scientific Publications.

Gemmell, M. A. 1976b. Factors regulating tapeworm populations: estimations of the build-up and dispersion patterns of eggs after the introduction of dogs infected with *Taenia hydatigena*. *Res. Vet. Sci.* **21**, 220–2.

Gemmell, M. A. 1976c. Factors regulating tapeworm populations: the changing opportunities of lambs for ingesting the eggs of *Taenia hydatigena*. *Res. Vet. Sci.* **21**, 223–6.

Gemmell, M. A. 1977. Taeniidae: modification to the life span of the egg and the regulation of tapeworm populations. *Exp. Parasitol.* **41**, 314–28.

Gemmell, M. A. 1978a. The effect of weather on tapeworm eggs and its epidemiological implications. In *Weather and parasitic animal disease*, Wld Met. Org. Tech. Note No. 159, 83–94.

Gemmell, M. A. 1978b. Perspective on options for hydatidosis and cysticercosis control. *Vet. Med. Rev.* **1**, 3–48.

Gemmell, M. A. 1978c. The Styx Field-Trial: Effect of treatment of the definitive host for tapeworms on larval forms in the intermediate host. *Bull. Wld Hlth Org.* **56**, 433–43.

Gemmell, M. A. 1979. Hydatidosis control – a global view. *Aust. Vet. J.* **55**, 118–25.

Gemmell, M. A. and P. D. Johnstone 1976. Factors regulating tapeworm populations: dispersion of eggs of *Taenia hydatigena* on pasture. *Ann. Trop. Med. Parasitol.* **70**, 431–4.

Gemmell, M. A. and P. D. Johnstone 1977. Experimental epidemiology of hydatidosis and cysticercosis. *Adv. Parasitol.* **15**, 311–69.

Gemmell, M. A. and P. D. Johnstone 1981. Factors regulating tapeworm populations: estimations of the duration of acquired immunity by sheep to *Taenia hydatigena*. *Res. Vet. Sci.* **30**, 53–6.

Gemmell, M. A. and J. R. Lawson 1982a. Ovine cysticercosis: an epidemiological model for the cysticercoses. I. The free-living egg phase. In *Cysticercosis: present stage of knowledge and perspectives*, A. Flisser, K. Willms, J. P. Laclette, C. Larralde, C. Ridaura and F. Beltrán (eds), 87–98. New York: Academic Press.

Gemmell, M. A. and J. R. Lawson 1982b. Ovine cysticercosis: an epidemiological model for the cysticercoses. II. Host immunity and regulation of the parasite population. In *Cysticercosis: present state of knowledge and perspectives*, A. Flisser, K. Willms, J. P. Laclette, C. Larralde, C. Ridaura and F. Beltrán (eds), 647–60. New York: Academic Press.

Gemmell, M. A. and F. N. Macnamara 1972. Immune responses to tissue parasites. II. Cestodes. In *Immunity to animal parasites*, E. J. L. Soulsby (ed.), 235–72. New York: Academic Press.

Gemmell, M. A. and F. N. Macnamara 1976. Factors regulating tapeworm populations: estimations of the infection pressure and index of clustering from

Taenia hydatigena before and after the removal of infected dogs. *Res. Vet. Sci.* **21**, 215–9.

Gemmell, M. A. and E. J. L. Soulsby 1968. The development of acquired immunity to tapeworms and progress towards active immunization with special reference to *Echinococcus* spp. *Bull. Wld Hlth Org.* **39**, 45–55.

Gemmell, M. A., S. K. Blundell and F. N. Macnamara 1968a. Immunological responses of the mammalian host against tapeworm infections. V. The development of artificially induced immunity to *Taenia hydatigena* in young lambs. *Proc. Univ. Otago Med. Sch.* **46**, 4–5.

Gemmell, M. A., S. K. Blundell and F. N. Macnamara 1968b. Immunological responses of the mammalian host against tapeworm infections. VII. The effect of the time interval between artificial immunization and the ingestion of eggs on the development of immunity by sheep to *Taenia hydatigena. Exp. Parasitol.* **23**, 83–7.

Gemmell, M. A., S. K. Blundell and F. N. Macnamara 1969. Immunological responses of the mammalian host against tapeworm infections. IX. The transfer *via* colostrum of immunity to *Taenia hydatigena. Exp. Parasitol.* **26**, 52–7.

Gemmell, M. A., P. D. Johnstone and C. C. Boswell 1978. Factors regulating tapeworm populations: dispersion patterns of *Taenia hydatigena* eggs on pasture. *Res. Vet. Sci.* **24**, 334–8.

Gemmell, M. A., J. R. Lawson and M. G. Roberts 1985. Population dynamics in echinococcosis and cysticercosis. I. Biological parameters of *Echinococcus granulosus* in dogs and sheep. (Submitted for publication.)

Harris, R. E., K. J. A. Revfeim and D. D. Heath 1980. Simulating strategies for control of *Echinococcus granulosus, Taenia hydatigena* and *T. ovis. J. Hyg., Camb.* **84**, 389–404.

Heath, D. D., S. B. Lawrence and W. K. Yong 1979a. Cross-protection between the cysts of *Echinococcus granulosus, Taenia hydatigena* and *T. ovis* in lambs. *Res. Vet. Sci.* **27**, 210–2.

Heath, D. D., W. K. Yong, P. J. Osborn, S. N. Parmeter, S. B. Lawrence, and H. Twaalfhoven 1979b. The duration of passive protection against *Taenia ovis* larvae in lambs. *Parasitology,* **79**, 177.

Heinz, H. J. and W. Brauns 1955. The ability of flies to transmit ova of *Echinococcus granulosus* to human foods. *S. Afr. J. Med. Sci.* **20**, 131–2.

Herd, R. P. 1977. Resistance of dogs to *Echinococcus granulosus. Int. J. Parasitol.* **7**, 135–8.

Jackson, P. J. and J. H. Arundel 1971. The incidence of tapeworms in rural dogs in Victoria. *Aust. Vet. J.* **47**, 46–53.

Keymer, A. 1982. Tapeworm infections. In *Population dynamics of infectious diseases. Theory and applications.* R. M. Anderson (ed.) 109–38. London: Chapman and Hall.

Laws, G. F. 1968. Physical factors influencing survival of taeniid eggs. *Exp. Parasitol.* **22**, 227–39.

Lawson, J. R. and M. A. Gemmell 1983. Hydatidosis and cysticercosis: the dynamics of transmission. *Adv. Parasitol.* **22**, 261–308.

Lawson, J. R. and M. A. Gemmell 1985. Dispersal of taeniid eggs with particular reference to the role of blowflies. *Parasitology* (in press.)

Lindquist, A. W., W. W. Yates and R. A. Hoffman 1951. Studies of the flight habits of three species of flies tagged with radioactive phosphorus. *J. Econ. Ent.* **44**, 397–400.

McConnell, J. D. and R. J. Green 1979. The control of hydatid disease in Tasmania. *Aust. Vet. J.* **55**, 140–5.

Macdonald, G. 1965. The dynamics of helminth infections, with special reference to schistosomes. *Trans. R. Soc. Trop. Med. Hyg.* **59**, 489–506.

Matoff, D. and G. Kolev 1964. The role of the hairs, muzzle and paws of echinococcic dogs in the epidemiology of echinococcosis. *Z. Tropenmed. Parasitol.* **15**, 452–60.

Matossian, R. M., M. D. Rickard and J. D. Smyth 1977. Hydatidosis: a global problem of increasing importance. *Bull. Wld Hlth Org.* **55**, 499–507.

May, R. M. 1982. The impact, transmission and evolution of infectious diseases. *Nature, Lond.* **297**, 539–40.

May, R. M. and R. M. Anderson 1978. Regulation and stability of host–parasite population interactions. II. Destabilizing processes. *J. Anim. Ecol.* **47**, 249–67.

Meldrum, G. K. and J. D. McConnell 1968. The control of hydatid disease in Tasmania. *Aust. Vet. J.* **44**, 212–7.

Meymerian, E. and C. W. Schwabe 1962. Host–parasite relationships in echinococcosis. VII. Resistance of the ova of *Echinococcus granulosus* to germicides. *Am. J. Trop. Med. Hyg.* **11**, 360–4.

Nelson, G. S. and R. L. Rausch 1963. *Echinococcus* infection in man and animals in Kenya. *Ann. Trop. Med. Parasitol.* **57**, 136–49.

Polydorou, K. 1976. The control of the dog population in Cyprus as the first objective of the anti-*Echinococcus* campaign. *Bull. Off. Int. Epiz.* **86**, 705–15.

Polydorou, K. 1980. The control of echinococcosis in Cyprus, *FAO Wld Animal Rev.* No. 33, 19–25.

Rausch, R. L. 1967. On the ecology and distribution of *Echinococcus* spp. (Cestoda: Taeniidae) and characteristics of their development in the intermediate host. *Annls Parasitol. Hum. Comp.* **42**, 19–63.

Rausch, R. L. 1972. Observations on some natural-focal zoonoses in Alaska. *Arch. Environ. Hlth*, **25**, 246–52.

Rausch, R. L. and S. H. Richards 1971. Observations on parasite–host relationships of *Echinococcus multilocularis* Leuckart, 1863, in North Dakota. *Can. J. Zool.* **49**, 1317–30.

Rausch, R. L. and E. L. Schiller 1956. Studies on the helminth fauna of Alaska. XXV. The ecology and public health significance of *Echinococcus sibiricensis* Rausch & Schiller, 1954, on St Lawrence Island. *Parasitology* **46**, 395–419.

Rickard, M. D. 1983. Immunity. In *Biology of the Eucestoda*, C. Arme and P. W. Pappas (eds), London: Academic Press.

Rickard, M. D. and J. H. Arundel 1974. Passive protection of lambs against infection with *Taenia ovis* via colostrum. *Aust. Vet. J.* **50**, 22–4.

Rickard, M. D. and J. F. Williams 1982. Hydatidosis/cysticercosis: immune mechanisms and immunization against infection. *Adv. Parasitol.* **21**, 229–96.

Schantz, P. M. and C. W. Schwabe 1969. Worldwide status of hydatid disease control. *J. Am. Vet. Med. Ass.* **155**, 2104–21.

Schiller, E. L. 1954. Studies on the helminth fauna of Alaska. XIX. An experimental study on blowfly (*Phormia regina*) transmission of hydatid disease. *Exp. Parasitol.* **3**, 161–6.

Schiller, E. L. 1955. Studies on the helminth fauna of Alaska. XXVI. Some observations on the cold-resistance of eggs of *Echinococcus sibiricensis* Rausch and Schiller, 1954. *J. Parasitol.* **41**, 578–82.

Schoof, H. F. 1959. How far do flies fly, and what effect does flight pattern have on their control? *Pest Cont.* **27**, 16–18, 20, 22, 66.

Schoof, H. F. and R. E. Siverly 1954. Urban fly dispersion studies with special reference to movement pattern of *Musca domestica*. *Am. J. Trop. Med. Hyg.* **3**, 539–47.

Sutton, R. J. 1979. The passive transfer of immunity to *Taenia ovis* in lambs via colostrum. *Res. Vet. Sci.* **27**, 197–9.

Sweatman, G. K. 1957. Acquired immunity in lambs infected with *Taenia hydatigena*, Pallas 1766. *Can. J. Comp. Med.* **21**, 65–71.

Sweatman, G. K. and R. J. Williams 1963a. Comparative studies on the biology and morphology of *Echinococcus granulosus* from domestic livestock, moose and reindeer. *Parasitology* **53**, 339–90.

Sweatman, G. K. and R. J. Williams 1963b. Survival of *Echinococcus granulosus* and *Taenia hydatigena* eggs in two extreme climatic regions of New Zealand. *Res. Vet. Sci.* **4**, 199–216.

Sweatman, G. K., R. J. Williams, K. M. Moriarty and T. C. Henshall 1963. On acquired immunity to *Echinococcus granulosus* in sheep. *Res. Vet. Sci.* **4**, 187–98.

Williams, J. F. 1979. Recent advances in the immunology of cestode infections. *J. Parasitol.* **65**, 337–49.

Williams, J. F., H. L. Adaros and A. Trejos 1971. Current prevalence and distribution of hydatidosis with special reference to the Americas. *Am. J. Trop. Med. Hyg.* **20**, 224–36.

8 Immunodiagnosis of hydatid disease

M. D. RICKARD AND M. W. LIGHTOWLERS

INTRODUCTION

Hydatid disease in humans usually comes to the attention of the clinician for four major reasons: when a large cyst has some mechanical effect on body function; when allergic phenomena or other miscellaneous symptoms such as eosinophilia occur; the accidental traumatic rupture of a cyst with consequent acute allergic reactions; and the incidental finding of cysts during roentgenography, body scanning or surgery for other clinical reasons. Most physical diagnostic aids available to the clinician such as roentgenography, radioisotopic and ultrasonic scanning and computerised axial tomography (CAT scanning) can determine the location, size and physical appearance (i.e. fluid-filled, calcified) of a mass lesion, but often cannot make a precise diagnosis as to its nature. Closed aspiration of cysts should be avoided because of the danger of leakage of protoscoleces and the development of secondary cysts or anaphylaxis. Sometimes cyst membranes, protoscoleces or hooklets can be demonstrated in sputum when cysts have ruptured in the lung. The frequent difficulty in obtaining a definitive diagnosis by other means is the reason why immunological methods have played such an important role in the diagnosis of hydatid disease. Rickard and Williams (1982) point out that

> despite significant increases in the amount of research in helminth immunoparasitology in recent years, on the whole few practical tools have been put into the hands of clinicians, pathologists, epidemiologists and others who directly confront parasitic diseases in man and animals. In cestodiasis, the present-day success of serodiagnostic methods in human hydatidosis respresents a remarkable, and very welcome, exception to this rule.

By comparison with investigations in humans, relatively little research has been directed toward the development of immunodiagnostic techniques for hydatid infection in domesticated animals, despite their potential usefulness in control programmes. Accurate serological diagnosis of infection by *Echinococcus* spp. is difficult due to serological cross-reactions with the several species of taeniid cestodes having both definitive and intermediate hosts in common with *E. granulosus*. The occurrence of naturally acquired infection with hydatids is highly likely to be associated with transmission of these other taeniid species. Lightowlers *et al.* (1984)

stressed that polyparasitism with taeniid cestodes made the use of correct control animals of vital importance for research on hydatid serodiagnosis in sheep, and that many analyses of immunodiagnostic procedures for hydatid infection are difficult to interpret owing to the lack of appropriate age-matched controls in which the extent of infection with all larval cestodes was known. A further problem in immunodiagnosis of hydatid infection in animals is the apparently poor antibody response to infection in many natural intermediate hosts. This poor response contrasts with the typically high levels of specific antibody seen in human infections.

The history of advances in the immunodiagnosis of hydatid disease largely reflects increased characterisation of parasite antigens. Definition of specific antigens and fractionation techniques remain crucial to maximising the usefulness of immunodiagnosis in man and animals. The literature on hydatid antigens has not been reviewed in detail since Kagan and Agosin (1968) and, because of the importance of antigen characterisation in immunodiagnostic techniques, information on *Echinococcus* antigens is reviewed here with particular emphasis on the more recent findings.

ANTIGENS OF *ECHINOCOCCUS* SPP.

Human or animal intermediate hosts of *Echinococcus* spp. are exposed to a variety of antigenic determinants on parasite-derived or parasite-modified molecules to which a host immune response may be evoked. Each of these various sources of antigenic stimulation may be relevant to immunodiagnosis. Initially the host is exposed to the invading oncosphere. A period of post-oncospheral development follows, leading to the formation of an immature cyst and finally to the fertile metacestode stage. Both somatic tissues of the parasite as well as excretory or secretory molecules are potential antigens. Many factors may influence the repertoire of antigens to which the host is exposed including species or strain of parasite, host species or strain, host immunocompetence, organ parasitised, cyst fertility, cyst viability, integrity of the cyst wall, etc.

Investigations of *Echinococcus* antigens have predominantly involved analysis based on the production of specific antibody. These studies have analysed antibody responses of hosts with *Echinococcus* infection as well as antibody responses in animals hyperimmunised with parasite cyst fluid or tissue extracts. Some of the antigens recognised by an artificially immunised animal may not necessarily be immunogenic in an infected host. Similarly, some molecules antigenic in an infected host, particularly excretory or secretory antigens, may not be recognised by artificially immunised animals. However, the dominant parasite antigens which elicit antibody production in infected hosts are recognised by antibodies in the sera of immunised animals. For this reason sera from immunised animals have played an important role in the characterisation of *Echinococcus* antigens and continue to be used in the standardisation of serodiagnostic tests (Varela-Díaz & Coltorti 1976).

In the definitive host a variety of potential sources of antigenic stimulation are also possible. These include excretory or secretory molecules or parasite break-down products absorbed directly from the gut lumen, antigens deposited directly into the gut mucosa at the site of scolex attachment and antigens released during abortive invasion of oncospheres hatching prematurely in the definitive host.

The majority of investigations into *Echinococcus* spp. antigens have been with *E. granulosus* and, unless otherwise specifically stated, the following discussion of hydatid antigens refers to this species. Early research on the composition of hydatid cyst fluid, protoscoleces and cyst membranes concentrated on analysis of biochemical composition and was reviewed by Kagan and Agosin (1968).

Source of antigens for diagnostic tests

Hydatid cyst fluid, protoscoleces and cyst membranes from a variety of hosts have been used as sources of antigen in diagnostic tests. Comparison of both quantitative and qualitative aspects of the antigenic components of cyst fluid have been reported including data on fluid from various hosts, different parasitised organs and from fertile and infertile cysts. Fluid from fertile cysts, irrespective of host species, contains higher concentrations of antigens than sterile cysts (Bensted & Atkinson 1953, Hariri *et al.* 1965). However, viable but non-fertile cysts with healthy germinal layers contain antigens suitable for diagnostic tests so that antigenicity is not exclusively associated with cyst fertility (Hariri *et al.* 1965). Musiani *et al.* (1978) examined the concentration of two major antigens in cyst fluid and found that sheep and human cyst fluids contained higher concentrations of these antigens than cyst fluids from either cattle or pigs and that the amount of antigen was greater in hepatic than in pulmonary cysts. Similarly, Hariri *et al.* (1965) found the highest concentration of hydatid antigens in sheep liver cysts, although both liver and lung cysts from other hosts were also adequate antigen sources. Hydatid protoscoleces and cyst membranes, either intact or as extracts, have also been evaluated as sources of antigen for diagnostic tests (Kagan & Norman 1961, Hariri *et al.* 1965, Fischman 1968, Garabedian 1971, Dottorini & Tassi 1978, Craig & Rickard 1981b). Generally hydatid cyst fluid has been found to be a superior source of parasite antigen for diagnostic tests (Kagan & Norman 1961, Hariri *et al.* 1965, Tassi *et al.* 1981, Craig & Rickard 1981b).

Oncospheral antigen has not been evaluated for the serological diagnosis of hydatid infection in the intermediate host. Anti-oncospheral antibodies can be detected in the sera of animals infected with other larval taeniid parasites (Craig & Rickard 1981a) and for this reason oncospheres may be a useful antigen source particularly for serological diagnosis of recent infection. Oncospheres are known to be the target of protective immune responses in infection with various taeniid cestodes (reviewed by Rickard & Williams 1982).

Cysts of *E. multilocularis* have been reported to be poor sources of antigens for serological diagnosis of infection with either *E. multilocularis* or *E. granulosus* (Kagan *et al.* 1960a, Kagan & Norman 1961), although they have been used successfully in the diagnosis of both *E. multilocularis* and *E. granulosus* infections in man (Leykina *et al.* 1981, Gottstein *et al.* 1983) and *E. multilocularis* infection in mice (Ali-Khan 1974, Ali-Khan & Siboo 1982). The large amount of parasite material which can be obtained from laboratory infection of rodents makes *E. multilocularis* an attractive potential antigen supply.

Cross-reactivity between crude antigen extracts of various taeniid species has enabled antigen preparations from heterologous taeniid parasite species to be used in serological tests (Hariri *et al.* 1965, Kagan & Agosin 1968, Yong *et al.* 1978, 1984).

Characterisation of antigens

Characterisation of specific antigen components of hydatid metacestodes has been achieved largely through the application of gel diffusion and immunoelectrophoresis techniques using sera from infected hosts or immunised animals. Hydatid cyst fluid and extracts of cyst membranes and protoscoleces are composed of complex mixtures of antigens. Kagan and Norman (1961) identified 23 different antigenic components in *E. granulosus* and 27 components in *E. multilocularis* preparations using sera from immunised rabbits. Comparison of precipitation patterns of parasite preparations with sera from rabbits immunised with host serum or tissue components demonstrated several antigens common to the host and parasite (Kagan & Norman 1961, Norman *et al.* 1964, Chordi & Kagan 1965, Capron *et al.* 1968, Varela-Díaz *et al.* 1974, Gomez-Garcia *et al.* 1980). It was speculated that these common antigens may have been due to antigen sharing or mimicry as a mechanism by which the parasite avoided the host immune responses (Capron *et al.* 1968). However, Coltorti and Varela-Díaz (1972) demonstrated that albumin, immunoglobulin and various other host serum components were present in hydatid cyst fluid obtained from four different hosts, and found that the albumin to immunoglobulin ratio was the same as that in serum although at a much reduced concentration. Further evidence for the host origin of the shared antigens was provided by experiments demonstrating the penetration of serum components into hydatid cysts either following their transplantation into a different host species (Varela-Díaz & Coltorti 1972, 1973, Coltorti & Varela-Díaz 1975b) or *in vitro* (Coltorti & Varela-Díaz 1974). Not all hydatid cysts take up host molecules (Coltorti & Varela-Díaz 1972, Hustead & Williams 1977) and temporary leaks in cyst membranes (Coltorti & Varela-Díaz 1975b) and cyclic uptake activity (Hustead & Williams 1977) have been suggested as possible mechanisms to account for this variable uptake. Cysts incubated in ^{125}I-labelled macromolecules rapidly take up the label but it is present as dialyzable fragments in the cyst which suggests that enzymatic degradation of proteins occurs (Hustead & Williams 1977). If this were the case, an additional interpretation of the variable uptake of macromolecules by cysts may be that it is an artefact created by the rapid degradation of absorbed molecules so that they are not recognised by anti-sera probes.

MAJOR ANTIGENS

Several parasite-specific antigens have been described in hydatid fluid and tissue extracts (Kagan & Norman 1961, Norman *et al.* 1964, Chordi & Kagan 1965, Varela-Díaz *et al.* 1974). Kagan and Norman (1961) identified four parasite components in antigen preparations from cyst fluid and tissues of *E. granulosus* and *E. multilocularis*. Three bands which were found most frequently with the sera of infected patients were identified in Ouchterlony by Kagan and Norman (1963) and their molecular weights estimated from diffusion coefficients. The most frequently found band, designated P_1, occurred in nine out of 10 diagnostic sera, and the most immunoreactive components were partially purified using diethylaminoethyl (DEAE) cellulose. Kent (1963) also purified a fraction from cyst fluid which reacted in Ouchterlony with the sera from patients with hydatid infection. Subsequently, more sensitive immunoelectrophoretic techniques were applied to the analysis of *Echinococcus* antigens (Biguet *et al.* 1962, Norman *et al.* 1964, Chordi & Kagan 1965). Using the sera from 16 patients with hydatid infection and sheep hydatid cyst fluid as antigen, Chordi and Kagan (1965) were the first to analyse antibody responses in human hydatid infection by immunoelectrophoresis (IEP). Two particular precipitation bands were found to be produced by diagnostic sera. These were designated band 4 and band 5. Band 4 was produced by all sera which showed any bands in IEP and this band was suggested to recognise the same antigen component as the P_1 band in Ouchterlony. The next most frequently occurring precipitate was band 5. Band 4 and band 5 antigens were shown clearly to be parasite components by analyses using sera from rabbits immunised with either cyst fluid antigen or host serum. Capron *et al.* (1967, 1970) used a different numbering system for identifying arcs formed in IEP with hydatid antigens and sera from hydatid patients. They identified a precipitation line designated fraction 5 or arc 5 which was not seen using antigen preparations from other parasites and which occurred frequently with sera from patients with hydatid infection. Arc 5 did not occur with sera from patients without hydatid infection and was not found in six sera from patients with *E. multilocularis* infection.

There are problems associated with the use of crude hydatid antigens in serological tests and Oriol *et al.* (1971) developed a simple technique for the partial purification of parasite antigens from hydatid cyst fluid. Like Chordi and Kagan (1965) they found two dominant parasite antigens in cyst fluid although no attempt was made to relate the purified antigens to Chordi and Kagan's (1965) band 4 and band 5 or Capron *et al.*'s (1967) fraction 5. They designated the two antigens antigen A and antigen B. The purified preparation containing these antigens was composed of approximately equal portions of lipid and protein with a minor carbohydrate component, and less than 2 per cent of the purified fraction was contaminant host protein. By using very high antigen concentration in IEP, they found an additional minor antigen in the purified preparation. Antigenic activity of antigens A and B was retained after delipidisation. Separation profiles on Sephadex G-200 showed that both antigens were present in the first major peak, but that only antigen B was present in the peak eluting at the same position as immunoglobulin. The approximate molecular weight for antigen B was estimated to be 160 000 daltons. Purified antigen B was shown to aggregate, suggesting that the antigen existed in several distinct forms in reversible equilibrium. Antigen B was thermostable and resisted boiling for 15 min without loss in antigenicity whereas antigen A was heat labile. Subsequently Oriol and Oriol (1975) estimated the molecular weight of antigen B to be 120 000 daltons by sedimentation equilibrium and found the antigen to be composed of approximately 50 per cent α-helix with optical properties corresponding to those of a secreted biological metabolite.

The use of the purified lipoprotein antigens A and B for the immunodiagnosis of human hydatid infection was evaluated by Williams *et al.* (1971). Antibodies to antigen A were detected most frequently, and antibodies to antigen A and/or antigen B were found in 45 out of 52 serum samples which had been shown previously to react with crude hydatid cyst fluid antigens. Sera from 80 donors without hydatid infection, but which included patients infected with a variety of other parasites, were all serologically negative to both antigens.

Chromatographic separation of cyst fluid antigens by Pozzuoli *et al.* (1972) again demonstrated two major antigens which they identified as being the antigens 4 and 5 of Chordi and Kagan (1965). The chromatographic behaviour of these two antigens was identical to that previously described for antigens A and B (Oriol *et al.* 1971). Further studies evaluated the immunoreactivity of these antigens with sera from patients with hydatid infection, and developed techniques for the preparation of purified antigens (Pozzuoli *et al.* 1974, 1975, Piantelli *et al.* 1977, Musiani *et al.* 1978, Lauriola *et al.* 1978). The larger MW component, antigen 4, had the greatest immunoreactivity with sera from patients with hydatid disease, and all sera from patients with *E. granulosus* infection which had antibodies to cyst fluid antigens demonstrable in IEP had antibodies to this antigen. Most sera also had antibodies to antigen 5. False positive reactions to antigen 4 occurred with the sera of some individuals apparently free from hydatid infection. Antigen 4 was found to be heat labile and antigen 5 heat stable. Estimates of the molecular weights of the antigens on the basis of chromatographic behaviour were more than 400 000 daltons for antigen 4 and 150 000 daltons for antigen 5. Analysis of purified antigens in sodium dodecylsulphate polyacrylamide gel electrophoresis (SDS-PAGE) showed that antigen 4 had a molecular weight of 67 000 daltons and antigen 5 included three components of between 20 000 and 10 500 daltons. Under reducing conditions, antigen 4 was shown to be composed of two components of 47 000 and 20 000 daltons. Antigen subunits recovered from gels stimulated antibody production against antigens 4 and 5 when used to immunise rabbits.

Bout *et al.* (1974) prepared specific antisera to fraction 5 (Capron *et al.* 1967) and purified the antigen by antibody affinity chromatography and determined the elution profile of fraction 5 in Sephadex G-200. Fraction 5 appeared in the high molecular weight material excluded from the gel as well as in a peak corresponding to the elution of albumin. On this latter basis, the molecular weight of fraction 5 was estimated to be 60 000 daltons and the higher molecular weight material was suggested to be either polymers or antigen–antibody complexes [Piantelli *et al.* (1977) described the occasional presence of antigen 4 in the albumin peak and indicated that this occurred most frequently in material which had been preserved for a long time]. Fraction 5 was found to be heat labile. Hydatid antigens prepared by Bout *et al.* (1974) according to the technique of Oriol *et al.* (1971) were shown to contain fraction 5 in addition to another component described as '*lipoproteine ubiquitaire*'. Using chromatographic techniques, Dottorini and Tassi (1977) isolated the fraction 5 which was found to have a molecular weight ranging from 100 000 to 300 000 daltons. This antigen co-eluted with at least three other antigens. A fraction of cyst fluid enriched for fraction 5 was obtained from sucrose gradient ultracentrifugation. The complexity of this fraction with respect to contaminant host proteins or the presence of other parasite antigens was not assessed. Analysis of fraction 5 in SDS-PAGE under reducing conditions revealed a single band of 69 000 daltons.

Tassi *et al.* (1980, 1981) described other fractions of hydatid cyst fluid prepared by salt precipitation and density sedimentation which were useful for serological diagnosis of hydatid infection in sheep and man, and one particular fraction designated 'band 7' showed high sensitivity and specificity in diagnosis. The relationship between this preparation and other characterised hydatid antigens is unclear. The refractive index at which band 7 sedimented (n = 1.3858) was outside the range (n = 1.3725 – 1.3750) in which fraction 5 was detected by Dottorini and Tassi (1977).

P_1 BLOOD GROUP ANTIGEN

There is a component of hydatid cyst fluid and tissue extracts that has antigenic activity similar to the human red blood cell P_1 antigen (Cameron & Staveley 1957). This antigen is responsible for the presence of high levels of anti-P_1 antibodies seen in P_2 blood group patients with hydatid infection (Merritt & Hardy 1955, Cameron & Staveley 1957). Anti-P_1 antibodies have also been reported in sera of patients infected with *Fasciola hepatica* (Ben-Ismail *et al.* 1980). The antigen is present in hydatid membranes as a glycoprotein with the antigenic determinant associated with the carbohydrate moiety (Russi *et al.* 1974). Antibodies to this antigen were detected in 11 out of 21 sera from hydatid patients by Russi *et al.* (1974) and in nine out of 58 cases by Bombardieri *et al.* (1974). Any relationship between this antigen and the other major antigens is unclear. Yarzabal *et al.* (1977b) showed that the localisation of antigen B in hydatid protoscoleces corresponded exactly to that of the PAS-positive substance described by Kilejian *et al.* (1961). Immunofluorescence studies identified the PAS-positive substance as the P_1 human blood group antigen and showed that when protoscoleces were cultured *in vitro* the culture fluid becomes strongly positive for anti-P_1 inhibiting substances (Smyth, Morgan, Morgan & Watkins unpublished data, cited by Smyth 1968). There is no correlation evident between the presence of anti-P_1 antibodies and antibodies to fraction 5 or antigen B in the sera of patients with hydatid infection (Bombardieri *et al.* 1974).

OTHER ANTIGEN FRACTIONS AND ANTIGENIC ACTIVITY

Various other techniques have been used to obtain fractions of crude hydatid antigens for immunodiagnostic tests. Early works have been reviewed by Kagan and Agosin (1968) and more recent antigen fraction techniques include those of Muntyan (1971), Pauluzzi and Dottorini (1972), Pauluzzi *et al.* (1972a,b), Ballad *et al.* (1977), Hrženjak *et al.* (1977, 1979) and Leykina *et al.* (1981). Hamel and Ris (1982) described an antigen termed 'cathodic antigen' which was apparently useful for diagnosis of hydatid infection in sheep. The precipitation line formed in IEP with antibody and this antigen has similarities to that formed with the P_1 active polysaccharide antigen of Bombardieri *et al.* (1974). Affinity chromatography purification or depletion of hydatid antigens using polyclonal or monoclonal antisera have recently been applied to processing of cestode antigens (Craig *et al.* 1980, 1981, Craig & Rickard 1981b, Gottstein *et al.* 1983, Lightowlers *et al.* 1984, Rickard *et al.* 1984). While these techniques have been useful for the preparation of antigens for particular diagnostic tests the antigens involved have not been characterised.

Components of crude hydatid antigens initiate host lymphocyte blast transformation *in vitro* (Miggiano *et al.* 1966, Yusuf *et al.* 1975), and crude hydatid antigen can also be used to demonstrate immediate type hypersensitivity *in vivo*. Studies on purified antigens have shown that both fraction 5 (Capron *et al.* 1967) and antigen B (Oriol *et al.* 1971) elicit positive skin reactions in hydatid patients and that specific IgE antibody is produced against these antigens in man and animals with hydatid infection (Oriol *et al.* 1971, Williams *et al.* 1971, Williams 1972, Dessaint *et al.* 1975, Yarzábal *et al.* 1975, Bout *et al.* 1977).

Nomenclature of hydatid antigens

Three separate terminologies have been and continue to be used for the major antigens of *E. granulosus* metacestodes. The probable synonyms for the two major antigens and the characteristics of these antigens are summarised in Table 8.1. On the basis of their abundance in cyst fluid and tissue extracts, characteristic precipitations in IEP, chromatographic behaviour and temperature sensitivities, antigen 4 of Chordi and Kagan (1965), 'fraction 5' (antigen 5) of Capron *et al.* (1967) and antigen A of Oriol *et al.* (1971) are the same parasite antigen. For the same reasons,

Table 8.1 Characteristics of the two major antigens of hydatid cyst fluid

	Synonyms	Principal composition	Molecular weight	Sub-unit molecular weight	Antigenic stability at 100°C	Relative concentration in sheep hydatid cyst fluid
antigen 5	antigen A[1,5] antigen 4[4,6–10] arc 5, F_5, fraction 5, antigen 5[2,3,11,12]	lipoprotein[1]	≥400 000[6] 100 000–300 000[12]	67 000 (47 000 + 20 000)[8] 60 000[3] 69 000[12]	labile[1,3,10,12]	1[9]
antigen B	antigen B[1,5] antigen 5[4,6–10]	lipoprotein[1]	160 000[1] 120 000[5] 150 000[6]	three components 10 500–20 000[8]	stable[1,10]	10[9]

[1] Oriol *et al.* 1971; [2] Capron *et al.* 1967; [3] Bout *et al.* 1974; [4] Chordi & Kagan 1965; [5] Oriol & Oriol 1975; [6] Pozzuoli *et al.* 1972; [7] Pozzuoli *et al.* 1975; [8] Piantelli *et al.* 1977; [9] Musiani *et al.* 1978; [10] Lauriola *et al.* 1978; [11] Varela-Díaz *et al.* 1974; [12] Dottorini & Tassi 1977.

antigen 5 of Chordi and Kagan (1965) and antigen B of Oriol *et al.* (1971) are identical. Although this situation is well recognised (Piantelli *et al.* 1977, Schantz & Gottstein 1985), many of the studies of antigen characterisation have used one terminology (antigens 4 and 5) and the majority of the diagnostic serology studies have used another (antigen 5 and antigen B). A case can be made for using each of the three terminologies: that of Chordi and Kagan (1965) on the basis of priority, of Capron *et al.* (1967) on the basis of current international acceptance in serology, and of Oriol *et al.* (1971) on the basis of their characterisation of the antigens associated with precipitation arcs with antibody in IEP. The nomenclature antigen 5 ('fraction 5', Capron *et al.* 1967) and antigen B (Oriol *et al.* 1971) will be used throughout the remainder of this chapter. International standardisation of nomenclature of the defined antigens is necessary. We believe that the preferable terminology would be antigens A and B and that the diagnostic arc identified in immunoelectrophoresis with antigen A continue to be termed 'arc 5'. However, there is as yet no unequivocal demonstration that the molecules referred to by their various 'synonyms' are absolutely identical.

Tissue localisation of antigen 5 and antigen B

Localisation of antigen 5 and antigen B on cyst membranes and protoscoleces has been investigated using indirect immunofluorescence (Yarzabal *et al.* 1976, 1977b) and immunocytochemistry in light (Rickard *et al.* 1977) and electron microscopy (Davies *et al.* 1978). Antigen 5 occurs in the inner portion of the germinal layer, the brood capsule wall and the parenchyma of the protoscoleces. The parenchymal cells in the subtegumental region of the protoscoleces are probably involved in the synthesis of the antigen. The antigen is also found on the osmoregulatory collecting ducts which may be involved in antigen excretion. The major source of antigen B is tegumental cells of protoscoleces anterior to the suckers. Antigen B also occurs diffusely throughout the laminated layer and on the germinal layer with denser areas on the tegument and in the sub-tegumental region of protoscoleces, on calcareous corpuscles and in the interstitial substance of brood capsules.

Antigens of adult *Echinococcus* tapeworms

Little is known concerning the antigens of adult *Echinococcus* worms. Using indirect fluorescent antibody techniques, Movsesijan and Mladenović (1971) were able to identify antibodies to the adult tapeworms in the sera of dogs experimentally infected with *E. granulosus*. Other studies on immunodiagnosis in the definitive host have used antigens from the metacestode. Jenkins and Rickard (1985) have found that antibodies to hydatid antigens are readily detected in the serum of infected dogs. In addition, sera from dogs infected with *T. hydatigena* were found to recognise oncosphere-specific determinants from the beginning of patency. Antigenicity of defined hydatid antigens in dogs has not been assessed.

IMMUNOLOGICAL DIAGNOSIS OF HYDATID DISEASE IN HUMANS

The following account of immunological diagnosis of hydatid disease in man is not intended to be a comprehensive review but rather a summary of current approaches. For further discussion of the literature the reader is referred to other comprehensive reviews (Kagan 1968, Matossian 1977, Kagan 1978, Rickard 1979, Schantz & Kagan 1980, Schantz & Gottstein 1985).

The parasites

Three species of *Echinococcus* are known to occur in humans, namely *E. granulosus, E. multilocularis* and *E. vogeli*. The geographic distribution and biological characteristics of these parasites are described in Chapters 1 and 2. *E. granulosus* is by far the most common and widespread of these species in man and most of the studies on serodiagnosis have been carried out on patients with hydatid disease due to this organism. Where these various species co-exist sympatrically, confusion can occur in serological diagnosis. There is increasing evidence that different 'strains' of *E. granulosus* occur (see Ch. 1), and this may influence the efficacy of various tests. There is no direct evidence of such an effect at the present time, although the apparent lack of serological response to *E. granulosus* infection in the Turkana people of Kenya (Anon. 1981) may well reflect a novel immunological relationship between this particular 'strain' of parasite and its human host.

Antibody response to infection

Specific antibodies in all major classes of immunoglobulin, i.e. IgM, IgG, IgA and IgE, have been demonstrated in sera from humans with hydatid disease (Castagnari *et al.* 1968, Dessaint *et al.* 1975, Matossian *et al.* 1976, Richard-Lenoble *et al.* 1978). Because it is usually many years after initial infection that clinical symptoms become evident, studies on the dynamics of antibody production throughout infection are not available. Consequently it is not known how soon after infection antibodies can be detected in the serum. IgG is the predominant immunoglobulin produced in response to hydatid infection and increased levels of specific IgG can persist for several years after cysts have been removed. Elevated IgM levels tend to return to normal fairly rapidly after cure (Matossian *et al.* 1972), and where specific IgE levels are elevated, these also are reported to return to normal quite rapidly after successful treatment (Dessaint *et al.* 1975).

Immunological tests for hydatid disease

Almost all available serological tests have been used for the diagnosis of human hydatid disease. There are considerable differences between the various tests both in their ability to detect specific antibody in the sera of infected persons (sensitivity) and in their capacity to discriminate between persons with hydatid disease, infection with other parasites or with other clinical disorders (specificity). As the sensitivity of a test increases, so generally does the demand for improved antigens in order that sufficient specificity can be achieved to take advantage of the greater sensitivity. For example, the indirect haemagglutination (IHA) test is highly sensitive in detecting antibody against the hydatid parasite. However, when used with 'crude' cyst fluid antigens, significant cross-reactions occur with sera from patients with other parasitic diseases so that the lowest titre which can be taken as diagnostic for hydatid disease without compromising specificity becomes 1:64 to 1:1024 (Varela-Díaz *et al.* 1975b, Picardo & Guisantes 1981). Thus, much of the advantage gained by the higher sensitivity of this test is lost due to non-specific 'false positive' reactions at low titres.

CASONI INTRADERMAL TEST

The appearance of an immediate hypersensitivity reaction following the intradermal injection of hydatid cyst fluid antigen has been widely used in the immunodiagnosis of human hydatid disease since its demonstration by Casoni in 1912. Despite its widespread use, there is still confusion concerning which antigens to use, their dosage and the interpretation of the tests. The test is generally quite sensitive in patients with hydatid infection, but its value as a diagnostic aid is doubtful because of the poor specificity of the test (Kagan 1968, Schantz *et al.* 1975, Yarzábal *et al.* 1975). Attempts have been made to improve the performance of this test by varying the amount of antigen injected (Kagan *et al.* 1966, Williams 1972). Hydatid cyst fluid is known to contain substances which can non-specifically trigger components of the host inflammatory system (Hammerberg *et al.* 1977) and this may account for some of the non-specific reactions following intradermal injection of cyst fluid antigen.

COMPLEMENT FIXATION TEST

Since its introduction by Ghedini in 1906, the complement fixation test (CFT) has been used often in the serological diagnosis of human hydatid disease. There are serious doubts about the sensitivity and specificity of the CFT (Kagan 1968, Kertesz *et al.* 1979), even when the strictest attention is paid to standardisation procedures (Bradstreet 1969). In an analysis of the value of CFT, Dighero and Bradstreet (1979) showed that out of a total of 6328 sera submitted for diagnosis of hydatid disease, 1.2 per cent gave 'false positive' CFTs at titres of 1:8 or greater. Hydatid disease was confirmed in 191 patients out of the 6328 sera submitted, i.e. 3 per cent, and alongside this figure the 1.2 per cent CFT 'false positives' is quite significant.

INDIRECT AGGLUTINATION TESTS

In these tests antigen is coupled to inert particles so that when divalent antibody binds specifically with the antigen at certain antibody : antigen ratios it causes agglutination or clumping of the particles. Two such tests are in common use, namely, the indirect haemagglutination (IHA) test and the latex agglutination (LA) test.

The IHA test uses red blood cells as a passive carrier for antigen and was first adapted for the diagnosis of hydatid disease by Garabedian *et al.* (1957). Several variations of the IHA test have been employed, using erythrocytes from different species and various chemicals to facilitate antigen binding and/or preservation of the antigen sensitised cells. Many methods have been found to give satisfactory results, although Varela-Díaz *et al.* (1975b) concluded that the standard tannic acid technique was as useful as any others. The relative ease of performance and popularity of the IHA test is reflected in the ready availability of commercial kits.

The IHA test is one of the most sensitive in common use for hydatid disease diagnosis and will detect very low levels of antibody. The literature concerning this test is extensive and is documented by Kagan (1968) and Schantz & Gottstein (1985). Most workers have used crude cyst fluid antigens which results in significant reaction with sera from patients with other parasitic diseases or with other miscellaneous clinical disorders. Specific diagnostic titres of 1:64 to 1:1024 have been suggested (Varela-Díaz *et al.* 1975b,c, Picardo & Guisantes 1981), and using these criteria the test compares in sensitivity to other commonly used methods. Infection with the larval stages of *Taenia solium* can give rise to high IHA titres, indistinguishable from those of hydatid disease patients (Schantz *et al.* 1980).

The LA test (Fischman 1960, Szyfres & Kagan 1963, Williams & Prezioso 1970) uses latex particles as the inert antigen carrier. Dilutions of test serum are mixed with latex particles sensitised with crude cyst fluid antigens, and visible clumping can be seen in positive samples within 10 min (Varela-Díaz & Coltorti 1976). The test is easy to perform and excellent results regarding sensitivity and specificity have been achieved (Varela-Díaz *et al.* 1975c, Dighero & Bradstreet 1979, Picardo & Guisantes 1981). Some workers have reported lesser specificity for LA (Hoghooghi *et al.* 1976, Rickard 1984) but it is likely that variations in the procedures used, especially with respect to the type of latex particles, may account for this problem (Schantz & Gottstein 1985).

INDIRECT LABELLED-ANTIBODY TESTS

There are several variations of indirect labelled-antibody tests. In all cases, test serum is incubated with antigen bound to a solid phase. Specific antibody which binds to the antigen is visualised by using anti-immunoglobulin antisera which are conjugated with a marker allowing either quantitative or qualitative assessment of specific antibody present in the original test serum. The most commonly used markers are fluorescent chemicals which allow visual assessment by microscopy, enzymes which produce a colour change when reacted with their substrate and radioactively labelled antibody which can be quantitated using appropriate measuring equipment. These tests are typically capable of detecting minute quantities of specific antibody because of the amplification provided by the second antibody reaction. They have the additional advantage of allowing measurement of the immunoglobulin classes of the specific antibodies present in the test serum.

The indirect fluorescent antibody (IFA) test usually uses whole protoscoleces or protoscolex fragments as antigen (Fraga de Azevado & Rombert 1965, Fischman 1968, Matossian & Araj 1975) but soluble cyst fluid antigens have also been used by absorbing them on to a solid matrix such as cellulose (Gore *et al.* 1970) or sepharose beads (Matossian *et al.* 1979). The IFA test can detect low levels of anti-*Echinococcus* antibody, but non-specificity can be a significant problem (Mahajan *et al.* 1976, Eckert & Wissler 1978, Matossian *et al.* 1979) especially with cyst fluid antigen (Gore *et al.* 1970).

The enzyme-linked immunosorbent assay (ELISA) uses an anti-immunoglobulin reagent labelled with an enzyme which produces a colour change when incubated with its substrate. The colour change can be examined visually or more accurately quantitated using a spectrophotometer. Several different enzyme conjugates have been employed successfully in the diagnosis of echinococcosis, including peroxidase (Farag *et al.* 1975), alkaline phosphatase (Sorice *et al.* 1977) and urease (Rickard *et al.* 1984). The ELISA has been carried out in polystyrene tubes (Farag *et al.* 1975) and in polystyrene microtitre plates (Sorice *et al.* 1977, Ambroise-Thomas *et al.* 1978). Excellent results have been achieved using the tube method which appears to be more sensitive than the micro-ELISA (Iacona *et al.* 1980). However, with the automated equipment now available the micro-ELISA is more convenient to use, especially for any large-scale application. Felgner (1978) used the stick-ELISA with good results and this method may be adaptable for producing ELISA kits for screening in the field.

Using crude hydatid cyst-fluid antigens the ELISA test has given results which compare very favourably with IHA. Cross-reactions occur with sera from patients with unrelated parasite infections, notably schistosomiasis and filariasis, as well as with sera from patients infected with the more closely related parasite *T. solium* or with the various *Echinococcus* spp. (Sorice *et al.* 1977, Ambroise-Thomas *et al.* 1978, Matossian *et al.* 1979, Speiser 1980, Iacona *et al.* 1980, Guisantes *et al.* 1981, Tassi *et al.* 1982, Rickard *et al.* 1984) and this has to be taken into account when establishing specific diagnostic titres.

Iacona *et al.* (1980) and Rickard *et al.* (1984) reported experiments using hydatid cyst fluid antigens fractionated by salt precipitation (Oriol *et al.* 1971) in ELISA, and although increased sensitivity was achieved, more non-specific reactions occurred than with crude cyst fluid antigen. An antigen further purified by affinity chromatography gave increased specificity, although sensitivity was reduced (Rickard *et al.* 1984). Farag *et al.* (1975) reported excellent results using purified antigen 5 in ELISA, but their estimate of sensitivity may have been higher than normally expected because all of their serum samples were selected on the basis of the presence of the arc 5 in immunoelectrophoresis.

Radioimmunoassay tests use antibodies labelled with a radioactive marker, usually ^{125}I, and radiation measuring equipment is necessary to give a quantitative result. In the solid phase radioimmunoassay (RIA), antigens are bound to plastic tubes. This test is comparable in sensitivity and specificity to other serological methods, but does not appear to offer any particular advantage over them (Musiani *et al.* 1974, Richard-Lenoble *et al.* 1978, Matossian 1981). A modified radioimmunoassay, the radioallergosorbent test (RAST) has been used to determine levels of *Echinococcus*-specific IgE antibodies in sera from echinococcosis patients (Huldt *et al.* 1973, Dessaint *et al.* 1975, Ito *et al.* 1977, Sorice *et al.* 1979). Estimates of the numbers of patients with elevated levels of specific IgE varied from 30 to 90 per cent, and the levels bore no relationship to levels of other Ig classes. Multiple cyst infections or 'fissurated' cysts gave higher specific IgE levels. A significant number of persons infected with other parasites can give false positive results with RAST. The use of this test for postoperative surveillance of hydatid disease patients will be discussed later in this chapter.

PRECIPITATION TESTS

There are many tests which rely on visual assessment of precipitate formed by the reaction between antigen and antibody. The majority of the tests in common use are carried out by immunodiffusion or by electrophoresis in a gel matrix, but other methods have also been used with success. These tests are qualitative rather than quantitative, but have provided some of the most specific means for diagnosing echinococcosis.

Application of the immunoelectrophoresis (IEP) test to the analysis of antigens recognised by antibodies in sera from patients with hydatid disease was originally described by Chordi and Kagan (1965). Subsequently Capron *et al.* (1967) described the presence of a precipitation arc in IEP, designated as 'arc 5', thought to be specific for diagnosis of *E. granulosus* infection. Additional work has clearly demonstrated the usefulness of this test and, in particular, the diagnostic arc 5 (Coltorti & Varela-Díaz 1975a, Guisantes *et al.* 1975, López-Lemes & Varela-Díaz 1975a, Varela-Díaz *et al.* 1975a,c, Yarzábal *et al.* 1975). Recently arc 5 has been demonstrated with the sera of patients infected with *E. multilocularis* (Varela-Díaz *et al.* 1977b, Yarzábal *et al.* 1977a), *E. vogeli* (Varela-Díaz *et al.* 1978) and *T. solium* cysticercosis (Varela-Díaz *et al.* 1978, Schantz *et al.* 1980). Despite these reports, demonstration of the arc 5 still remains the most specific test for infection with *Echinococcus* spp., especially where cysticercosis is not prevalent. The IEP test is less capable of detecting low levels of specific antibody than the agglutination tests and the indirect antibody assays. The arc 5 can be detected with the serum of only 60–90 per cent of preoperative serum samples (Capron *et al.* 1967, 1970, Yarzábal *et al.* 1974, Schantz *et al.* 1980, Varela-Díaz *et al.* 1975c, Picardo & Guisantes 1981, Rickard 1984). However, it has been shown that if the criterion for positivity of the IHA test (Varela-Díaz *et al.* 1975b) and the ELISA test (Rickard *et al.* 1984) were taken as the highest dilution giving cross-reactions with other parasites, then the IEP has comparable sensitivity. An additional criterion that has been used for a positive IEP test is the presence of three or more arcs in the absence of arc 5 (Yarzábal *et al.* 1975, Varela-Díaz & Coltorti 1976, Rickard 1984) and this has increased the sensitivity of this test without reducing specificity with the sera examined.

Recently Coltorti and Varela-Díaz (1978) have described an arc 5 double diffusion test (DD5). This test relies on the specific detection in double diffusion of antibodies to antigen 5 using a standard antiserum for positive identification. It is easier to perform than IEP, more sensitive and uses less antigen. Further evaluation of this method (Bout *et al.* 1979, Schantz *et al.* 1980) suggests that the DD5 is as useful as IEP in diagnosing those cases where the antibody to antigen 5 is present. Counter-immunoelectrophoresis (CIEP) or immunoelectrodiffusion (IED) has also been applied to the diagnosis of hydatid disease and can be carried out in gels or on cellulose acetate membranes (Gentelini & Pinon 1972, Sorice *et al.* 1975, López-Lemes & Varela-Díaz 1975b, Pinon & Dropsy 1976, Richard-Lenoble *et al.* 1978, Pinon *et al.* 1979, Mansueto *et al.* 1982). Where identification of antibody to antigen 5 has been the criterion for a positive reaction, this method has been accurate and sensitive, and is rapid to perform. A further modification of this method has used peroxidase-conjugated anti-immunoglobulins to localise precipitation lines (Pinon & Dropsy 1977, Pinon *et al.* 1979). This technique also allows qualitative determination of immunoglobulin classes.

Application of serological tests in human hydatid disease

There are many factors which must be taken into account when determining which test or tests are most useful in a particular situation. Practical considerations such as the availability of equipment for carrying out the tests or for purifying antigen, supplies of antigen, conditions under which tests are to be performed and skill of the operators may be overriding considerations in determining the test of choice.

PRETREATMENT DIAGNOSIS IN CLINICAL CASES

At the present time, those methods which can positively identify antibody to antigen 5 are the most specific tests currently available although cross-reactions which occur between the *Echinococcus* spp. and *T. solium* may present a problem in some areas. A significant number of patients do not have detectable antibody to antigen 5 and therefore other methods are also important. The more tests that can be carried out, the greater is the degree of certainty with which an accurate diagnosis can be reached. Most serum samples submitted for examination are already pre-selected on the basis of a clinical syndrome or past history consistent with a possible diagnosis of echinococcosis. In addition, physical aids to diagnosis which are presently available, especially CAT scanning, may have already been carried out so that there may be good presumptive evidence of infection. In such cases serological methods serve to confirm the diagnosis and provide a 'bench mark' for post-therapy surveillance of the patient. LA, IHA or ELISA in combination with either DD5 or IEP are satisfactory for such applications. If it is intended to follow the progress of a patient serologically, the IEP, CFT or RAST are most likely to be useful and this is discussed more fully in a subsequent section.

PRETREATMENT SCREENING OR EPIDEMIOLOGICAL STUDIES

Theoretically, the most specific test available should be used for this purpose. Any test which is not 100 per cent specific will have very limited value for use as an epidemiological tool with a low incidence disease such as echinococcosis. Practically, it is generally not possible to use the most specific tests (relying on identification of antibody to antigen 5) because of the technical difficulty in handling large numbers of samples and/or the lack of adequate quantities of purified antigen. The LA test, IHA test and ELISA test using crude antigens are useful as a primary screen for detecting asymptomatic infection, but positive samples must be further tested using more specific methods such as IEP, DD5 or ELISA with antigen 5.

PROBLEMS ENCOUNTERED IN PREOPERATIVE DIAGNOSIS

Variations in technical skill, antigen preparations, equipment, etc., can all have a substantial influence on the performance of a given test. This creates a problem in trying to compare results obtained with a particular test in different laboratories and, ideally, all tests should be compared in a single laboratory on the same sera. Each laboratory must standardise and if possible evaluate the tests being carried out.

'False positive' results occur with most serological tests, especially where other parasite infections are common; for example significant cross-reactions have been reported with sera from patients with schistosomiasis (Matossian *et al.* 1979, Sorice *et al.* 1977, Iacona *et al.* 1980), filariasis (Felgner 1978, Speiser 1980, Rickard *et al.* 1984), taeniasis (Todorov *et al.* 1979), fascioliasis (Ben-Ismail *et al.* 1980) and cysticercosis (Schantz *et al.* 1980). Crude hydatid cyst fluid contains a complex mixture of antigens and it is quite likely that some antigens may be shared in common with other parasites. In addition, hydatid cysts are known to contain P_1 blood group antigen (Russi *et al.* 1974, Ben-Ismail *et al.* 1980) in common with *Fasciola hepatica* (Ben-Ismail *et al.* 1980) and perhaps other parasites, and the presence of anti-P_1 antibody could be a significant source of misleading results. Cross-reactions that occur between the more closely related parasites *Echinococcus* spp. and *T. solium* pose more difficult problems because all of these parasites can stimulate antibodies to antigen 5. Recent experiments (Gottstein *et al.* 1983) have used antibody affinity chromatography purification methods for preparing antigens which can discriminate between patients infected with *E. granulosus* and *E. multilocularis*.

Some other pathological disorders, notably hepatic cirrhosis (Kagan *et al.* 1960b, Iacona *et al.* 1980), also produce false positive reactions, and this has been attributed to autoantibodies to host serum protein contaminants in the hydatid cyst fluid antigen.

Negative serological tests in known infected patients, i.e. 'false negative' reactions, also occur, although the use of multiple tests will reduce their frequency of occurrence. The location and nature of the hydatid cyst influences serological reactivity and false negatives are less likely to occur with cysts located in the liver, peritoneal cavity and bone, or where multiple organs are infected, than with cysts located in the brain, spleen and lung. Simple hyaline cysts stimulate less reaction than those which are damaged and perhaps 'leaking' antigen. Infertile, degenerated or calcified cysts also provoke less immunological response. Excessive release of antigen may result in the formation of immune complexes (Richard-Lenoble *et al.* 1978, Ibarrola *et al.* 1981) and interfere with the detection of free antibody in the serum. Children (Todorov *et al.* 1976, Pinon *et al.* 1979) and pregnant women (Pinon *et al.* 1979) have been shown to have poor serological response to infection.

Strain variations in the parasite, as well as differences in the host–parasite relationship may significantly affect the serological response. For example, there are reports from Kenya of many cases of hepatic hydatid infection where conventional serological tests have not been very useful in detecting antibodies (Anon. 1981, Chemtai *et al.* 1981).

SEROLOGICAL SURVEILLANCE OF PATIENTS AFTER TREATMENT

Cases of hydatid disease treated by surgery often require multiple operations either because of the growth of previously undetected cysts or development of secondary cysts resulting from leakage of cyst material or spillage during surgery. It is of great value to the surgeon to have a reliable means for determining whether patients remain free from infection after operation. The majority of serological tests such as IHA, ELISA, RIA, LA have little to offer in this regard because positive tests can persist for long periods after successful cure. However, Todorov *et al.* (1976, 1979) suggested some criteria that may be usefully applied to these tests. A favourable prognosis is anticipated if (a) the tests are negative before surgery and remain negative up to the end of the first year afterwards; (b) the titres are low prior to surgery, become negative afterwards and remain negative for 12–18 months; (c) the reduction in titres is small but the downward trend continues up to the end of the second year after operation. Recurrence of hydatid disease is likely if (a) the titres remain high or show only slight fluctuations for 2 years after operation, whether or not there was an increased titre after surgery; (b) the titres decline after surgery and then rise steadily.

The CFT measures predominantly IgM antibody and because the IgM antibody titre declines rapidly when antigenic stimulation is withdrawn (Matossian *et al.* 1972), this test has been advocated for postoperative surveillance of patients (Matossian & Araj 1975, Lass *et al.* 1973). However, others have found that positive CFT titres persist for a considerable period (Todorov & Stojanov 1979). Indirect antibody methods such as ELISA and RIA which can measure specific immunoglobulin classes in the serum may also be useful for postoperative surveillance, although Matossian and Araj (1975) found that the IFA test was not useful because of a high level of non-specific reaction. In cases where specific IgE levels are elevated prior to or immediately after surgery, a rapid decline in levels indicates a favourable prognosis (Dessaint *et al.* 1975).

The IEP test has been advocated for the post-surgical surveillance of hydatid disease (Capron *et al.* 1970, Varela-Díaz & Coltorti 1976, Rickard 1984) and is probably useful for this purpose by virtue of its poorer capacity for detecting low levels of specific antibody. It has been suggested that IEP tests should become negative within 12 months after successful cure by surgery (Capron *et al.* 1970; Varela-Díaz & Coltorti 1976), although Rickard (1984) found that a positive IEP test persisted for 2 years in several patients, and beyond this time in four other cases where cure was apparently successful.

Results described so far suggest that serological diagnosis is unlikely to be of value in the surveillance of patients having chemotherapy as their only form of treatment (Bekhti *et al.* 1977, Eckert & Wissler 1978, Braithwaite 1981).

IMMUNOLOGICAL DIAGNOSIS OF *ECHINOCOCCUS* INFECTION IN ANIMALS

Research on immunodiagnosis of *Echinococcus* spp. infection in domesticated animals has been restricted to analysis of immune responses to *E. granulosus*. Immune responses to both *E. granulosus* and *E. multilocularis* infections have been investigated in laboratory animals, but these will not be dealt with here. The Casoni intradermal test and a variety of serological tests have been used for diagnosis of hydatid infection in animals, including representative tests from each of the categories described for human diagnosis. Literature to 1966 on diagnosis in animals has been reviewed by Kagan (1968).

Diagnosis in sheep

Sheep are the principal intermediate hosts of *E. granulosus* in most endemic regions of the world and the majority of research efforts on immunodiagnosis in animals have been carried out in this species.

Using IHA titres of 1:400 or greater as the criterion for a positive reaction, Sweatman *et al.* (1963) were able to differentiate 18 out of 20 sheep experimentally infected with *E. granulosus* from either non-infected controls or sheep experimentally infected with *T. hydatigena, T. ovis, Multiceps multiceps* or *Linguatula serrata*. Conder *et al.* (1980) reduced non-specificity of IHA by recording only titres equal to or more than 1:1024 as being positive in experimentally infected sheep. Other workers have not been able to identify experimentally or naturally infected sheep on the basis of IHA titre (Blundell-Hasell 1969, Schantz 1973b). By comparing IHA titres obtained using hydatid antigen to titres obtained using antigens from heterologous cestodes, Yong *et al.* (1978) were able to distinguish sheep experimentally infected with *E. granulosus* from those infected with either *T. hydatigena* or *T. ovis*. Such differentiation was not possible with sera from animals infected with both *T. hydatigena* and *T. ovis*. Using the same criteria, naturally infected sheep with viable cysts were positive in 12 out of 13 cases. Despite this limited success, Yong *et al.* (1978) concluded that, using their criteria for positivity, IHA was not suitable for either serodiagnostic or epidemiological studies in areas where more than one larval cestode species was present.

Antibodies to *E. granulosus* in sera from both experimentally infected and naturally infected sheep have also been examined using gel diffusion and IEP techniques (Yong & Heath 1979, Conder *et al.* 1980, Hamel & Ris 1982). Antibodies to various antigens including antigen 5 were found in the sera of some, but not all, *E. granulosus* infected animals. There was no correlation between the number of precipitin bands in IEP or the presence of arc 5 and the numbers of cysts in each animal (Yong & Heath 1979). Based on the presence of arc 5 in IEP, Yong and Heath (1979) were able to differentiate between animals with naturally acquired viable hydatid infections and either non-infected sheep or sheep with non-viable cysts. However, animals infected with *T. hydatigena* or *T. ovis* were also positive in IEP with hydatid antigens. Furthermore, Hamel and Ris (1982) demonstrated the arc 5 with the sera of animals having no apparent taeniid cestode infection. The presence of antibodies to a 'cathodic antigen' in IEP has also been suggested to be useful for the diagnosis of hydatid infection in both experimentally infected and naturally infected sheep although both false positive and false negative reactions to this antigen occur (Hamel & Ris 1982).

Positive reactions in intradermal tests and homologous skin sensitising serum activity to hydatid antigens have been described in sheep with hydatid parasitism (Schantz 1973a,b). However, the occurrence of non-responders in infected animals, as well as problems with cross-reactivity with *T. hydatigena* and *T. ovis* infection, limit the usefulness of intradermal tests for hydatid diagnosis in sheep.

ELISA techniques using a variety of antigens have been applied to the immunodiagnosis of hydatid infection (Craig 1981, Craig & Rickard 1981b, Craig *et al.* 1980, 1981, Lightowlers *et al.* 1984, Yong *et al.* 1984). In experimentally infected sheep, antibodies to hydatid antigens can be detected as early as 4–6 weeks post-infection (Craig 1981) and persist for at least 4 years (Lightowlers *et al.* 1984). However, serologic cross-reactions between *E. granulosus* and other cestode infections prohibit the specific diagnosis of hydatid infection by ELISA using crude parasite antigens (Craig 1981, Lightowlers *et al.* 1984, Yong *et al.* 1984).

Yong *et al.* (1984) tested antigens from somatic tissue, cyst fluids or *in vitro* culture for the diagnosis of taeniid cestode infections in sheep. All antigens detected antibodies in infected sheep and culture antigens from *T. ovis* adult worms gave the least non-specific background activity and the highest antibody titres in the sera of cestode-infected sheep. However, none of the antigens was suitable for species-specific diagnosis in either experimentally infected or naturally infected sheep.

Attempts to develop competitive assays using monoclonal antibodies to hydatid antigens (Craig *et al.* 1980) have not been successful for the diagnosis of hydatid infection in sheep. Affinity purification of crude antigens with antibodies from animals immunised with homologous antigen (Craig & Rickard 1981b), or affinity depletion of cross-reactive antigens with monoclonal antibody (Craig *et al.* 1981, Lightowlers *et al.* 1984), has only been partly successful in reducing cross-reactions. Lightowlers *et al.* (1984) found that components of ovine hydatid cyst fluid bound to sheep immunoglobulin non-specifically and contributed to 'false positive' reactions, even with sera from cestode-free animals. After affinity depletion of crude antigen with both the monoclonal antibody developed by Craig *et al.* (1981), and sheep immunoglobulin from animals not infected with hydatids, 'background' reactions were greatly reduced. Using this affinity depleted antigen it was possible to differentiate serologically between a flock of sheep with hydatid infection and non-infected controls from the same locality (Tasmania), but specific diagnosis of infection in individual sheep was not achieved. In contrast, serological activity in heavily infected sheep from another locality (mainland Australia) was low and variation in antibody responses to different parasite 'strains' was suggested as a possible cause of these differences.

Although false positive reactions associated with parasitism by related cestodes are recognised as a major problem for specific immunodiagnosis of hydatid infection, the problems posed by the apparently poor antibody response of sheep to naturally acquired hydatid infection has claimed much less attention. False negative reactions in serological tests for hydatid disease in sheep occur commonly (Blundell-Hasell 1969, Yong & Heath 1979, Hamel & Ris 1982, Lightowlers *et al.* 1984).

M. W. Lightowlers, R. D. Honey and M. D. Rickard (unpublished observations) failed to detect free circulating parasite antigen in the sera of sheep with hydatid infection using a competitive ELISA with a sensitivity of approximately 0.1 μg of antigen protein (crude cyst fluid antigen) per millilitre of serum.

Diagnosis in other natural intermediate hosts

Diagnosis of hydatid infection has been investigated in pigs (Pauluzzi & Castagnari 1965, Hutchinson 1967, Alencar Filho 1978, Martinez Gómez *et al.* 1980), cattle (Lamy *et al.* 1959, Pauluzzi & Castagnari 1965, Alencar Filho *et al.* 1974, Alencar Filho 1978, Martinez Gómez *et al.* 1980), goats (Martinez Gómez *et al.* 1980), buffaloes (Rao & Mittal 1973) and camels (Dada *et al.* 1981). In no case has specific serodiagnosis been demonstrated. Some studies have presented data as the results of serological surveys of infected and uninfected animals collected from different groups of animals, at different times, and without reference to infection with other taeniid cestodes. False positive reactions occur in these intermediate hosts (Lamy *et al.* 1959, Rao & Mittal 1973, Hutchinson 1967, Martinez Gómez *et al.* 1980, Dada *et al.* 1981), and as for sheep the serological response to infection is typically weak.

Diagnosis of infection in definitive hosts

Little research has been carried out on immunodiagnosis of *Echinococcus* infection in definitive hosts. A reliable species-specific diagnostic test for *E. granulosus* infection in dogs would be particularly valuable now because the ready availability of the cestocidal drug praziquantel complicates attempts to assess infection by arecoline purge. Williams and Pérez Esandi (1971) demonstrated homocytotropic skin-sensitising antibody in the sera of some dogs 10 weeks after infection with 20 000 *E. granulosus* protoscoleces. All dogs were serologically negative when analysed by IHA and Ouchterlony using sheep hydatid cyst fluid antigen. However, there are reports of serum antibody responses other than IgE during *E. granulosus* infection in dogs (Chordi *et al.* 1962, Movsesijan & Mladenović 1971, Jenkins & Rickard 1985).

Movsesijan and Mladenović (1971) were unable to detect specific antibody to hydatid infection in five dogs at 53 d post-infection using protoscoleces, germinal layer or brood capsules as antigen in indirect fluorescent antibody tests. However, antibodies to adult tapeworms were detected, and specific fluorescence occurred between the rostellum and the suckers, on the scolex tegument, and in the genital organs in the sub-terminal segment. No fluorescence was observed on the gravid terminal segments. Using ELISA, antibodies to protoscolex antigens were found by Jenkins and Rickard (1985) in the sera of dogs 32 d after infection with 100 000 *E. granulosus* protoscoleces.

FUTURE PROSPECTS

Despite the success of methods for serological diagnosis of hydatid disease in man there are still several avenues open for investigation, and methods for immunodiagnosis of infection in animals are inadequate. Detection of antibody to antigen 5 is the most specific method available for diagnosis in man, but this does not allow discrimination between infection with the various *Echinococcus* spp. and *T. solium* cysticercosis. Further extension of the antibody affinity chromatography methods described by Gottstein *et al.* (1983) may overcome this problem in man, although success has not been achieved in applying similar techniques to diagnosis in animals. Another question worthy of investigation is whether or not the antigen 5 common to the various cestode species may have particular antigenic determinants specific for each of them. This approach has important potential application for diagnosis in animals and man. Purified antigen 5 from the various cestode species could be used to raise epitope-specific monoclonal antibodies which could be useful for species-specific serological diagnosis in competitive binding assays. Specific monoclonal antibodies could also be useful for detecting circulating antigen in the serum of humans and animals. A recent report described a method for detecting antigen in sera from patients infected with either *E. granulosus* or *E. multilocularis* (Leĭkina *et al.* 1982). Antigen was found only in those patients with cysts apparently 'leaking' antigen and this may limit the general usefulness of such methods for preoperative diagnosis. However, they may have a useful application for postoperative surveillance. Also, in cases where antibody responses are poor despite heavy infection, e.g. the Turkana people in Kenya and in animal infections, antigen detection may be feasible.

Recent reports (Craig & Rickard 1981a, 1982) have described the early appearance of anti-oncospheral antibodies in the serum of lambs infected with taeniid cestodes and these antibodies declined rapidly in the absence of continued challenge infection. The presence of anti-oncospheral antibodies during *Echinococcus* spp. infection may be useful in providing an indication of recent transmission of the parasite. Specific information concerning the antibody response during early infection with *E. granulosus* in man is lacking, and obviously very difficult to obtain. However, use of antigens prepared from different stages of the parasite may yield information which could be particularly useful in epidemiological and transmission studies. For example, on the Australian mainland there are apparently two strains of *E. granulosus*, a pastoral strain which uses dogs and sheep as hosts, and a sylvatic strain in dingoes and wild dogs, and large marsupials (Thompson & Kumratilake 1982). Dingo trappers rarely show serological reactivity to cyst fluid antigen (unpublished results) despite being in frequent contact with heavily infected definitive hosts (Coman 1972). The debate concerning the danger to man of this sylvatic strain of *E. granulosus* is unresolved, and it would be interesting to examine the serum from these people for anti-oncospheral antibodies.

Early results on the serodiagnosis of *E. granulosus* infection in dogs seem promising (Jenkins & Rickard 1985). However, the development of methods for demonstrating *Echinococcus* spp. antigen in dogs' faeces also has great potential for diagnosis. Babos (1962) and Babos and Németh (1962) were able to detect *E. granulosus* antigen in the faeces of 14 infected dogs prior to worm patency using precipitation reactions with hyperimmune rabbit serum. Monoclonal antibody methods may be useful in the development of specific immunological probes to detect adult worm or oncospheral antigens in dogs' faeces.

Much work remains to be done to develop satisfactory methods for immunodiagnosis of hydatid infection in domesticated animals. Cross-reactions with other parasites are an obvious problem, but the weak antibody response to natural infection in animals is also a major hindrance to further work on serodiagnosis. The apparent differences between the poor antibody responses to hydatid infection in natural intermediate hosts and the strong responses in an 'abnormal' host, man, warrants investigation. Analysis of the reasons for non-responsiveness in some animals may provide a clue to methods for modulating the immune response in infected animals in order to facilitate serodiagnosis.

ACKNOWLEDGEMENTS

We are grateful to Ms B. Chambers for her skilful typing of the manuscript, and to Ms R. Honey for her helpful criticism.

REFERENCES

Alencar Filho, R. A. de 1978. Diagnóstico immunológico da hidatidose animal – resultados preliminares. *Arquivos Inst. Biol.* **45**, 101–16; *Helminthol. Abstr. A* **48**, 496 (1979).

Alencar Filho, R. A. de, D. R. Moreira and A. R. de Oliveira 1974. Reação de Casoni no diagnóstico da hidatidose em bovinos. *Biológico Brazil* **40**, 357–8; *Helminthol. Abstr. A* **45**, 436 (1976).

Ali-Khan, Z. 1974. Host–parasite relationship in echinococcosis. I. Parasite biomass and antibody response in three strains of inbred mice against graded doses of *Echinococcus multilocularis* cysts. *J. Parasitol.* **60**, 231–5.

Ali-Khan, Z. and R. Siboo 1982. *Echinococcus multilocularis*: immunoglobulin and antibody response in C57BL/6J mice. *Exp. Parasitol.* **53**, 97–104.

Ambroise-Thomas, P., P. T. Desgeorges and D. Monget 1978. Diagnostic immuno-enzymologique (ELISA) des maladies parasitaires par une micro-méthode modifée. 2. Résultatis pour la toxoplasmose, l'amibiase, la trichinose, l'hydatidose et l'aspergillose. *Bull. Wld Hlth Org.* **56**, 797–804.

Anon. 1981. Immunodiagnosis of hydatid disease in man. In *FAO/UNEP/WHO guidelines for surveillance, prevention and control of echinococcosis/hydatidosis.* J. Eckert, M. A. Gemmell and E. J. L. Soulsby (eds), 46–65. Geneva: WHO.

Babos, S. 1962. Untersuchungen über die Serodiagnostik der Echinokokkose. *Agnew. Parasitol.* **3**, 2–4.

Babos, S. and I. Németh 1962. Az echinococcis szérodiagnosztikájának kérdéséhez. *Magyar Állatorvosok Lapja* **17**, 58–60; *Helminthol. Abstr.* **33**, 387 (1964).

Ballad, N. E., M. Aminzhanov and Sh. A. Razzakov 1977. [Analysis of the immunogenic components of lydatid cyst fluid from sheep.] *Veterinariya, Moscow* **2**, 54–7 (in Russian); *Helminthol. Abstr. A* **46**, 686 (1977).

Bekhti, A., J. P. Schaaps, M. Capron, J. P. Dessaint, F. Santoro and A. Capron 1977. Treatment of hepatic hydatid disease with mebendazole: preliminary results in four cases. *Br. Med. J.* 1047–1051.

Ben-Ismail, R., B. Carme, G. Niel and M. Gentelini 1980. Non-specific serological reactions with *Echinococcus granulosus* antigens: role of anti-P_1 antibodies. *Am. J. Trop. Med. Hyg.* **29**, 239–45.

Bensted, H. J. and J. D. Atkinson 1953. Hydatid disease. Serologic reactions with standardized reagents. *Lancet i*, 265–8.

Biguet, J., A. Capron, P. Tran Van Ky and R. d'Haussy 1962. Étude immunoélectrophorétique comparée des antigènes de divers helminthes. *C. R. Acad. Sci., Paris* **254**, 3600–2.

Blundell-Hasell, S. K. 1969. Serological diagnosis of larval cestodes in sheep. *Aust. Vet. J.* **45**, 334–6.

Bombardieri, S., F. Giordano, F. Ingrao, S. Ioppolo, A. Siracusano and G. Vicari 1974. An evaluation of an agar gel diffusion test with crude and purified antigens in the diagnosis of hydatid disease. *Bull. Wld Hlth Org.* **51**, 525–30.

Bout, D., Y. Carlier and A. Capron 1979. Immunodiagnosis of hydatidosis using monospecific immune serum anti-Ag_5. *Biomedicine* **31**, 214–5.

Bout, D., J. Fruit and A. Capron 1974. Purification d'un antigène spécifique de liquide hydatique. *Annls Immunol. Inst. Pasteur* **125C**, 775–88.

Bout, D., J. -P. Dessaint, H. Dupas, L. Yarzabal and A. Capron 1977. Characterization of allergens in *Schistosoma mansoni, Fasciola hepatica* and *Echinococcus granulosus*. *Annls Immunol. Inst. Pasteur* **128C**, 687–98.

Bradstreet, C. M. P. 1969. A study of two immunological tests in the diagnosis and prognosis of hydatid disease. *J. Med. Microbiol.* **2**, 419–33.

Braithwaite, P. A. 1981. Long-term high-dose mebendazole for cystic hydatid disease of liver: failure in two cases. *Aust. N.Z. J. Surg.* **51**, 23–7.

Cameron, G. C. and J. M. Staveley 1957. Blood group P substance in hydatid cyst fluids. *Nature, Lond.* **179**, 147–8.

Capron, A., A. Vernes and J. Biguet 1967. Le diagnostic immuno-électrophorétique de l'hydatidose. In *Le Kystehydatique du foie*, 27–40 Lyon: SIMEP.

Capron, A., J. Biguet, A. Vernes and D. Afchain 1968. Structure antigénique des helminthes. Aspects immunologiques des relations hote-parasite. *Path. Biol., Paris* **16**, 121–38.

Capron, A., L. Yarzabal, A. Vernes and J. Fruit 1970. Le diagnostique immunologique de l'echinococcose humaine. *Path. Biol., Paris* **18**, 357–65.

Castagnari, L., S. Della and R. Pozzuoli 1968. Sulla distribuzione immuno-globilinica degli anticorpi sierici antiidatidei. *Boll. Ist. Sieroter. Milan* **47**, 63–9.

Chemtai, A. K., G. B. A. Okelo and J. Kyobe 1981. Application of immunoelectrophoresis (IEP 5) test in the diagnosis of human hydatid disease in Kenya. *E. Afr. Med. J.* **58**, 583–6.

Chordi, A. and I. G. Kagan 1965. Identification and characterization of antigenic components of sheep hydatid fluid by immunoelectrophoresis. *J. Parasitol.* **51**, 63–71.

Chordi, A., J. Gonzáles-Castro and Y. Tormo 1962. Aportacion al estudio de las helminthiasis intestinales en los perros. II. Resultados de la prueba de floculación con Ben-thid y de la de fijación de complemento en perros con *Echinococcus granulosus*. *Revta Ibér. Parasitol.* **22**, 285–90.

Coltorti, E. A. and V. M. Varela-Díaz 1972. IgG levels and host specificity in hydatid cyst fluid. *J. Parasitol.* **58**, 753–6.

Coltorti, E. A. and V. M. Varela-Díaz 1974. *Echinococcus granulosus*: penetration of macromolecules and their localization on the parasite membranes of cysts. *Exp. Parasitol.* **35**, 225–31.

Coltorti, E. A. and V. M. Varela-Díaz 1975a. Modification of the immuno-electrophoresis test for the immunodiagnosis of hydatidosis. *J. Parasitol.* **61**, 155–6.

Coltorti, E. A. and V. M. Varela-Díaz 1975b. Penetration of host IgG molecules into hydatid cysts. *Z. ParasitKde* **48**, 47–51.

Coltorti, E. A. and V. M. Varela-Díaz 1978. Detection of antibodies against *Echinococcus granulosus* arc 5 antigens by double diffusion test. *Trans. R. Soc. Trop. Med. Hyg.* **72**, 226–9.

Coman, B. J. 1972. Helminth parasites of the dingo and feral dog in Victoria with some notes on the diet of the host. *Aust. Vet. J.* **48**, 456–61.

Conder, G. A., F. L. Andersen and P. M. Schantz 1980. Immunodiagnostic tests for hydatidosis in sheep: an evaluation of double diffusion, immunoelectrophoresis, indirect hemagglutination and intradermal tests. *J. Parasitol.* **66**, 577–84.

Craig, P. S. 1981. *Studies on the immunodiagnosis of larval cestode infections in sheep and cattle*. PhD thesis, University of Melbourne.

Craig, P. S. and M. D. Rickard 1981a. Anti-oncospheral antibodies in the serum of lambs experimentally infected with either *Taenia ovis* or *Taenia hydatigena*. *Z. ParasitKde* **64**, 169–77.

Craig, P. S. and M. D. Rickard 1981b. Studies on the specific immunodiagnosis of larval cestode infections of cattle and sheep using antigens purified by affinity chromatography in an enzyme-linked immunosorbent assay (ELISA). *Int. J. Parasitol.* **11**, 441–9.

Craig, P. S. and M. D. Rickard 1982. Antibody responses of experimentally infected lambs to antigens collected during *in vitro* maintenance of the adult, metacestode or oncosphere stages of *Taenia hydatigena* and *Taenia ovis* with further observations on anti-oncospheral antibodies. *Z. ParasitKde* **67**, 197–209.

Craig, P. S., R. E. Hocking, G. F. Mitchell and M. D. Rickard 1981. Murine hybridoma-derived antibodies in the processing of antigens for the immunodiagnosis of hydatid (*Echinococcus granulosus*) infection in sheep. *Parasitology* **83**, 303–17.

Craig, P. S., G. F., Mitchell, K. M. Cruise and M. D. Rickard 1980. Hybridoma antibody immunoassays for the detection of parasitic infection: attempts to produce an immunodiagnostic reagent for a larval taeniid cestode infection. *Aust. J. Exp. Biol. Med. Sci.* **58**, 339–50.

Dada, B. J. O., D. S. Adegboye and A. N. Mohammed 1981. Experience in Northern Nigeria with countercurrent immunoelectrophoresis, double diffusion and indirect haemagglutination tests for diagnosis of hydatid cyst in camels. *J. Helminthol.* **55**, 197–202.

Davies, C., M. D. Rickard, D. T. Bout and J. D. Smyth 1978. Ultrastructural immunocytochemical localization of two hydatid fluid antigens (antigen 5 and antigen B) in the brood capsules and protoscoleces of ovine and equine *Echinococcus granulosus* and *E. multilocularis*. *Parasitology* **77**, 143–52.

Dessaint, J. P., D. Bout, P. Wattre and A. Capron 1975. Quantitative determination of specific IgE antibodies to *Echinococcus granulosus* and IgE levels in sera from patients with hydatid disease. *Immunology* **29**, 813–23.

Dighero, M. W. and C. M. P. Bradstreet 1979. The serodiagnosis of human hydatid disease: 1. The routine use of latex-agglutination and complement-fixation in diagnosis. *J. Helminthol.* **53**, 283–6.

Dottorini, S. and C. Tassi 1977. *Echinococcus granulosus*: characterization of the main antigenic component (Arc 5) of hydatid fluid. *Exp. Parasitol.* **43**, 307–14.

Dottorini, S. and C. Tassi 1978. *Echinococcus granulosus*: comparison between antigens in scolices and hydatid fluid. *Int. J. Parasitol.* **8**, 259–65.

Eckert, J. and K. Wissler 1978. Immunodiagnose und Therapie der Echinokokkose. *Ther. Umschau* **35**, 766–76.

Farag, H., D. Bout and A. Capron 1975. Specific immunodiagnosis of human hydatidosis by the enzyme linked immunosorbent assay (ELISA). *Biomedicine* **23**, 276–8.

Felgner, P. 1978. Antibody activity in stick-ELISA as compared to other quantitative immunological tests in sera of echinococcosis cases. *Tropenmed. Parasitol.* **29**, 417–22.

Fischman, A. 1960. Flocculation tests in hydatid disease. *J. Clin. Path.* **13**, 72–5.

Fischman, A. 1968. A new whole-scolex complement-fixation test for hydatid disease. *Bull. Wld Hlth Org.* **39**, 39–43.

Fraga de Azevado, J. and P. C. Rombert 1965. L'application de l'immuno-fluorescence au diagnostic de l'echinococcose. *Annls Parasitol. Hum. Comp.* **40**, 529–42.

Garabedian, G. A. 1971. Evaluation of the reactivity of hydatid whole-scolex antigen in hydatid disease serology. *Ann. Trop. Med. Parasitol.* **65**, 385–91.

Garabedian, G. A., R. M. Matossian and A. Y. Djanian 1957. An indirect haemagglutination test for hydatid disease. *J. Immunol.* **78**, 269–72.

Gentelini, M. and J. M. Pinon 1972. Intérêt de l'électrosynérèse sur membrane d'acétate de cellulose dans le diagnostic de l'hydatidose. *Annls Méd Interne* **123**, 883–6.

Gomez Garcia, V., M. Campos Bueno, J. Lozano Maldonado, M. Rodriguez Osorio and I. Mañas Almendros 1980. Antigenos comunes al hospedador y otras especies animales en extractos antigencos de cestodes. II. Ensayos realizados con sueros anti-gamma globulinas. *Revta Ibér. Parasitol.* **40**, 375–84.

Gore, R. W., E. H. Sadun and R. Haff 1970. *Echinococcus granulosus* and *E. multilocularis*: soluble antigen fluorescent antibody test. *Exp. Parasitol.* **28**, 272–9.

Gottstein, B., J. Eckert and H. Fey 1983. Serological differentiation between *Echinococcus granulosus* and *E. multilocularis* infections in man. *Z. ParasitKde* **69**, 347–56.

Guisantes, J. A., M. F. Rubio and R. Díaz 1981. Application of an enzyme-linked immunosorbent assay (ELISA) method to the diagnosis of human hydatidosis. *Bull. Pan Am. Hlth Org.* **15**, 260–6.

Guisantes, J. A., L. A. Yarzabal, V. M. Varela-Díaz, M. I. Ricardes and E. A. Coltorti 1975. Standardization of the immunoelectrophoresis test with whole and purified hydatid cyst fluid antigens for the diagnosis of human hydatidosis. *Revta Inst. Med. Trop. Sao Paulo* **17**, 69–74.

Hamel, K. L. and D. R. Ris 1982. The use of a cathodic antigen in the immunoelectrophoretic serodiagnosis of *Echinococcus granulosus* in sheep. *Vet. Immunol. Immunopath.* **3**, 419–25.

Hammerberg, B., A. J. Musoke and J. F. Williams 1977. Activation of complement by hydatid cyst fluid of *Echinococcus granulosus*. *J. Parasitol.* **63**, 327–31.

Hariri, M. N., C. W. Schwabe and M. Koussa 1965. Host–parasite relationships in echinococcosis. XI. The antigens of the indirect hemagglutination test for hydatid disease. *Am. J. Trop. Med. Hyg.* **14**, 592–604.

Hoghooghi, N., H. Sabbaghlan, E. Ghadirian, I. G. Kagan and E. L. Schiller 1976. Evaluation of the slide-latex agglutination and intradermal (Casoni) tests for echinococcosis. *Am. J. Trop. Med. Hyg.* **25**, 660–1.

Hrženjak, T., V. Muić and I. Ehrlich 1979. A comparative study of the polyhexosamine ceramide complex isolated from *Echinococcus granulosus* larv. and *Fasciola hepatica*. *Vet. Archiv* **49**, 21–32.

Hrženjak, T., I. Ehrlich, V. Muić and Z. Debogovic 1977. Immunochemical and serological properties of the polyhexosamine ceramide complex (PHC) isolated from the hydatidic fluid of *Echinococcus granulosus* larv. *Vet. Archiv* **47**, 317–22.

Huldt, G., G. O. Johansson and S. Lantto 1973. Echinococcosis in Northern Scandinavia. Immune reactions to *Echinococcus granulosus* in Kautokeino Lapps. *Arch. Environ. Hlth* **26**, 36–40.

Hustead, S. T. and J. F. Williams 1977. Permeability studies on taeniid metacestodes. I. Uptake of proteins by larval stages of *Taenia taeniaeformis, T. crassiceps*, and *Echinococcus granulosus*. *J. Parasitol.* **63**, 314–21.

Hutchison, W. F. 1967. Studies on *Echinococcus granulosus*. IV. Detection of *Echinococcus* antibodies in naturally infected Mississippi swine. *J. Parasitol.* **53**, 1241–4.

Iacona, A., C. Pini and G. Vicari 1980. Enzyme-linked immunosorbent assay (ELISA) in the serodiagnosis of hydatid disease. *Am. J. Trop. Med. Hyg.* **29**, 95–102.

Ibarrola, A. S., B. Sobrini, J. Guisantes, J. Pardo, J. Diez, J. M. Monfá and A. Purroy 1981. Membranous glomerulonephritis secondary to hydatid disease. *Am. J. Med.* **70**, 311–5.

Ito, K., Y. Horiuchi, M. Kumagai, M. Ueda, R. Nakamura, N. Kawanishi and Y. Kasai 1977. Evaluation of RAST as an immunological method for diagnosis of multilocular echinococcosis. *Clin. Exp. Immunol.* **28**, 407–12.

Jenkins, D. J. and M. D. Rickard 1985. Specific antibody responses to *Taenia hydatigena, T. pisiformis* and *Echinococcus granulosus* in dogs. *Aust. Vet. J.* **62**, 72–8.

Kagan, I. G. 1968. A review of serological tests for the diagnosis of hydatid disease. *Bull. Wld Hlth Org.* **39**, 25–37.

Kagan, I. G. 1978. Recent advances in the diagnosis of hydatidosis (1970-76). *Parasitologia Hung.* **11**, 31–50.

Kagan, I. G. and M. Agosin 1968. *Echinococcus* antigens. *Bull. Wld Hlth Org.* **39**, 13–24.

Kagan I. G. and L. Norman 1961. Antigenic analysis of *Echinococcus* antigens by agar diffusion techniques. *Am. J. Trop. Med. Hyg.* **10**, 727–34.

Kagan, I. G. and L. Norman 1963. Analysis of helminth antigens (*Echinococcus granulosus* and *Schistosoma mansoni*) by agar gel methods. *Ann. N.Y. Acad. Sci.* **113**, 130–53.

Kagan, I. G., L. Norman and D. S. Allain 1960a. Studies on echinococcosis: serology of crude and fractionated antigens prepared from *Echinococcus granulosus* and *Echinococcus multilocularis*. *Am. J. Trop. Med. Hyg.* **9**, 248–61.

Kagan, I. G., L. Norman, D. S. Allain and G. C. Goodchild 1960b. Studies on echinococcosis: nonspecific serologic reactions of hydatid fluid antigen with serum of patients ill with diseases other than echinococcosis. *J. Immunol.* **84**, 635–40.

Kagan, I. G., J. J. Osimani, J. C. Varela and D. S. Allain 1966. Evaluation of intradermal and serologic test for the diagnosis of hydatid disease. *Am. J. Trop. Med. Hyg.* **5**, 172–9.

Kent, N. H. 1963. Fractionation, isolation and definition of antigens from parasitic helminths. *Am. J. Hyg. Monogr. Ser.* **22**, 30–45.

Kertesz, V., P. W. Roberts and P. Sharp 1979. Evaluation of three serological tests for the diagnosis of hydatid disease. *Med. J. Aust.* **2**, 678–80.

Kilejian, A., L. A. Schinazi and C. W. Schwabe 1961. Host–parasite relationships in echinococcosis. V. Histochemical observations on *Echinococcus granulosus*. *J. Parasitol.* **47**, 181–8.

Lamy, L., J. Bénex and J. Gledel 1959. Étude de la réaction de fixation du complément a divers antigènes de cestodes chez le mouton. Deuxième note. *Bull. Soc. Path. Exp.* **2**, 193–8.

Lass, N., A. Laver and J. Lengy 1973. The immunodiagnosis of hydatid disease: Post-operative evaluation of the skin test and four serological tests. *Ann. Allergy* **31**, 430–6.

Lauriola, L., M. Piantelli, R. Pozzuoli, E. Arru and P. Musiani 1978. *Echinococcus granulosus*: preparation of monospecific antisera against antigens in sheep hydatid fluid. *Zbl. Bakt. ParasitKde Abt I, Abt. Orig. A* **240**, 251–7.

Leĭkina, E. S., E. A. Kovrova and N. N. Krasovskaya 1982. [Detection of circulating antigens in the sera of patients with unilocular or multilocular hydatidosis or with trichinelliasis.] *Med. Parazitol. Parazitarnye Bolezni* **51**, 7–15 (in Russian); *Helminthol. Abstr. A* **52**, 118 (1983).

Leykina, E. S., M. V. Dalin, N. E. Ballad, N. V. Tchebyshev, V. I. Zorikhina and O. G. Poletaeva 1981. Isolation of diagnostical helminth antigens and their use in serodiagnosis. *Helminthologia* **18**, 273–80.

Lightowlers, M. W., M. D. Rickard, R. D. Honey, D. L. Obendorf and G. F. Mitchell 1984. Serological diagnosis of *Echinococcus granulosus* infection in sheep using cyst fluid antigen processed by antibody affinity chromatography. *Aust. Vet. J.* **61**, 101–8.

López-Lemes, M. H. and V. M Varela-Díaz 1975a. Application of the immunoelectrophoresis test for hydatidosis in patients with a presumptive diagnosis of the disease. *Trop. Geog. Med.* **17**, 301–4.

López-Lemes, M. H. and V. M. Varela-Díaz 1975b. Evaluation of crossed-over electrophoresis test for the immunodiagnosis of human hydatid disease. *Trop. Geog. Med.* **27**, 295–300.

Mahajan, R. C., N. K. Ganguly and N. L. Chitkara 1976. Evaluation of immunodiagnostic techniques for hydatid disease. *Indian J. Med. Res.* **64**, 405–9.

Mansueto, S., M. D. Miceli, D. M. Picone and S. Tripi 1982. Ulteriori osservazioni su un test rapido di controimmunoelettroforesi (CIEP) su membrana di acetato di cellulose (cellogel) nella diagnostica della idatidosi. *Giom. Mal. Infett. Parassitol.* **34**, 453–6.

Martinez Gomez, F., S. Hernandez Rodriguez, I. Navarrete López-Cózar and R. Calero Carretero 1980. Serological tests in relation to the viability, fertility and localization of hydatid cysts in cattle, sheep, goats and swine. *Vet. Parasitol.* **7**, 33–8.

Matossian R. M. 1977. The immunological diagnosis of human hydatid disease. *Trans. R. Soc. Trop. Med. Hyg.* **71**, 101–4.

Matossian, R. M. 1981. A simplified radioimmunoassay technique for hydatid disease and human trichinosis. *J. Helminthol.* **55**, 49–57.

Matossian, R. M. and G. F. Araj 1975. Serologic evidence of postoperative persistence of hydatid cysts in man. *J. Hyg., Camb.* **75**, 333–40.

Matossian, R. M., S. Y. Alami, I. Salti and G. F. Araj 1976. Serum immunoglobulin levels in human hydatidosis. *Int. J. Parasitol.* **6**, 367–71.

Matossian, R. M., G. J. Kane, S. M. Chantler, I. Batty and H. Sarhadian 1972. The specific immunoglobulin in hydatid disease. *Immunology* **22**, 423.

Matossian, R. M., M. L. McLaren, C. C. Draper, C. M. P. Bradstreet, M. W. Dighero, G. J. Kane, L. M. Mackinlay and M. D. Rickard 1979. The serodiagnosis of human hydatid disease. 2. Additional studies on selected sera using indirect haemagglutination (IHA), enzyme linked immunosorbent assay (ELISA) and defined antigen substrate spheres (DASS). *J. Helminthol.* **53**, 287–91.

Merritt, M. and J. Hardy 1955. Notes on a serum containing anti-P in high titre. *J. Clin. Path.* **8**, 329–30.

Miggiano, V. C., S. Ferrari and F. Ingrao 1966. *Echinococcus granulosus* and lymphocyte stimulation. *Lancet ii*, 1244.

Movsesijan, M. and Ž. Mladenović 1971. Ispitivanje mogućnosti korišćenja raznih razvojnih oblika *E. granulosus* u detekciji specifičnih antitela prema istom parazitu. *Vet. Glasnik* **25**, 159–63.

Muntyan, N. A. 1971. [Antigenic composition of hydatid fluid, extracts of scoleces and germinal membranes of hydatid cysts.] *Medskaya Parazit.* **40**, 528–32 (in Russian); *Helminthol. Abstr. A* **41**, 275 (1972).

Musiani, P., M. Piantelli, E. Arru and R. Pozzuoli 1974. A solid phase radioimmunoassay for the diagnosis of human hydatidosis. *J. Immunol.* **112**, 1674–9.

Musiani, P., M. Piantelli, L. Lauriola, E. Arru and R. Pozzuoli 1978. *Echinococcus granulosus*: specific quantification of the two most immunoreactive antigens in hydatid fluids. *J. Clin. Path.* **31**, 475–8.

Norman, L., I. G. Kagan and A. Chordi 1964. Further studies on the analysis of sheep hydatid fluid by agar gel methods. *Am. J. Trop. Med. Hyg.* **13**, 816–21.

Oriol, C. and R. Oriol 1975. Physicochemical properties of a lipoprotein antigen of *Echinococcus granulosus*. *Am. J. Trop. Med. Hyg.* **24**, 96–100.

Oriol, R., J. F. Williams, M. V. Pérez Esandi and C. Oriol 1971. Purification of lipoprotein antigens of *Echinococcus granulosus* from sheep hydatid fluid. *Am. J. Trop. Med. Hyg.* **20**, 569–74.

Pauluzzi, S. and L. Castagnari 1965. La fissazione del complemento per l'idatidosi V. Risultati della reazione di fissazione del complemento e confronto con la reazione di emoagglutinazione indiretta nell'idatidosi animale. *Ann. Sclavo* **7**, 93–103.

Pauluzzi, S. and S. Dottorini 1972. Gli antigeni idatidei. I. Analisi chemico-fisica delle frazioni chromatogratiche del liquido cistico. *Boll. Ist. Sieroter. Milan.* **51**, 130–5; *Helminthol. Abstr. A* **43**, 278 (1974).

Pauluzzi, S., S. Dottorini and R. F. Frongillo 1972a. Gli antigeni idatidei. II. Analisi antigenica delle frazioni cromatografiche del liquido cistico. *Boll. Ist. Sieroter. Milan.* **51**, 136–44; *Helminthol. Abstr. A* **43**, 278 (1974).

Pauluzzi, S., S. Dottorini and A. Piras 1972b. Gli antigeni idatidei. III. Ultracentrifugazione su gradienti di densità della frazione globulinica del liquido cistico. *Ann. Sclavo* **14**, 191–6; *Helminthol Abst. A* **43**, 33 (1974).

Piantelli, M., R. Pozzuoli, E. Arru and P. Musiani 1977. *Echinococcus granulosus*: identification of subunits of the major antigens. *J. Immunol.* **119**, 1382–6.

Picardo, N. G. A. and J. A. Guisantes 1981. Comparison of three immunological tests for seroepidemiological purposes in human echinococcosis. *Parasite Immunol.* **3**, 191–9.

Pinon, J. M. and G. Dropsy 1976. Immunological study of hydatidosis. I. Evaluation of the test of immunoelectrodiffusion in the humoral study of human hydatidosis. *Biomedicine* **25**, 341–4.

Pinon, J. M. and G. Dropsy 1977. ELIEDA (enzyme-linked immunoelectro-diffusion assay): application of a combined immunoelectro-diffusion and immunoenzyme method to the study of immune response in parasitic infections. *J. Immunol. Meth.* **16**, 15–22.

Pinon, J. M., A. Sulahian, G. Remy and G. Dropsy 1979. Immunological study of hydatidosis. I. Evaluation of immunoelectrodiffusion tests and enzyme-linked immunoelectrodiffusion assay (ELIEDA) in human hydatidosis. *Am. J. Trop. Med. Hyg.* **28**, 318–24.

Pozzuoli, R., P. Musiani, E. Arru, C. Patrono and M. Piantelli 1974. *Echinococcus granulosus*: evaluation of purified antigens' immunoreactivity. *Exp. Parasitol.* **35**, 52–60.

Pozzuoli, R., P. Musiani, E. Arru, M. Piantelli and R. Mazzarella 1972. *Echinococcus granulosus*: isolation and characterization of sheep hydatid fluid antigens. *Exp. Parasitol.* **32**, 45–55.

Pozzuoli, R., M. Piantelli, C. Perucci, E. Arru and P. Musiani 1975. Isolation of the most immunoreactive antigens of *Echinococcus granulosus* from sheep hydatid fluid. *J. Immunol.* **115**, 1459–63.

Rao, B. V. and K. R. Mittal 1973. Studies on hydatidosis in Indian buffaloes (*Bubalus bubalis*). 1. Some serological observations in natural infections of hydatids in buffaloes. *Z. Tropenmed. Parasitol.* **24**, 476–80.

Richard-Lenoble, D., M. D. Smith and M. Loisy 1978. Human hydatidosis: evaluation of three serodiagnostic methods, the principal subclass of specific immunoglobulin and the detection of circulating immune complexes. *Ann. Trop. Med. Parasit.* **72**, 553–60.

Rickard, M. D. 1979. The immunological diagnosis of hydatid disease. *Aust. Vet. J.* **55**, 99–104.

Rickard, M. D. 1984. Serological diagnosis and post-operative surveillance of human hydatid disease. I. Latex agglutination and immunoelectrophoresis using crude cyst fluid antigen. *Pathology* **16**, 207–10.

Rickard, M. D. and J. F. Williams 1982. Hydatidosis/cysticercosis: immune mechanisms and immunization against infection. *Adv. Parasitol.* **21**, 229–96.

Rickard, M. D., C. Davies, D. T. Bout and J. D. Smyth 1977. Immuno-histological localisation of two hydatid antigens (antigen 5 and antigen B) in the cyst wall, brood capsules and protoscoleces of *Echinococcus granulosus* (ovine and equine) and *E. multilocularis* using immunoperoxidase methods. *J. Helminthol.* **51**, 359–64.

Rickard, M. D., R. D. Honey, J. L. Brumley and G. F. Mitchell 1984. Serological diagnosis and post-operative surveillance of human hydatid disease. II. The enzyme-linked immunosorbent assay (ELISA) using various antigens. *Pathology* **16**, 211–6.

Russi, S., A. Siracusano and G. Vicari 1974. Isolation and characterization of a blood P_1 active carbohydrate antigen of *Echinococcus granulosus* cyst membrane. *J. Immunol.* **112**, 1061–9.

Schantz, P. M. 1973a. Homocytotropic antibody to *Echinococcus* antigen in sheep with homologous and heterologous larval cestode infection. *Am. J. Vet. Res.* **34**, 1179–81.

Schantz, P. M. 1973b. Immunodiagnostic tests with *Echinococcus* antigens in sheep with homologous and heterologous larval cestode infections. *Rev. Inst. Med. Trop. São Paulo* **15**, 179–94.

Schantz, P. M. and B. Gottstein 1985. Echinococcosis (hydatidosis). In *Immunoserology of parasitic diseases*, K. F. Walls and P. M. Schantz (eds.), in press. New York: Academic Press.

Schantz, P. M. and I. G. Kagan 1980. Echinococcosis (hydatidosis). In *Immunologic investigation of tropical parasitic diseases*, V. Houba (ed.), 104–29. New York: Churchill Livingstone.

Schantz, P. M., R. E. Ortiz-Valqui and H. Lumbreras 1975. Nonspecific reactions with the intradermal test for hydatidosis in persons with other helminth infections. *Am. J. Trop. Med. Hyg.* **24**, 849–52.

Schantz, P. M., D. Shanks and M. Wilson 1980. Serologic cross-reactions with sera from patients with echinococcosis and cysticercosis. *Am. J. Trop. Med. Hyg.* **29**, 609–12.

Smyth, J. D. 1968. *In vitro* studies and host-specificity in *Echinococcus*. *Bull. Wld Hlth Org.* **39**, 5–12.

Sorice, F., S. Delia and L. Castagnari 1975. Counterimmunoelectrophoresis in diagnosis of hydatid disease. *Lancet ii*, 617.

Sorice, F., S. Delia and L. Castagnari 1977. Il test ELISA nella immunodiagnosi dell'idatidosi umana. Osservazioni preliminari. *Boll. Inst. Sieroter. Milan* **56**, 152–6.

Sorice, F., S. Delia, V. Vullo, A. Aceti and U. Ferone 1979. Sensitivity and specificity of the RAST (radioallergosorbent test) in biological diagnosis of hydatidosis. *Ann. Sclavo* **21**, 800–15.

Speiser, F. 1980. Application of the enzyme-linked immunosorbent assay (ELISA) for the diagnosis of filariasis and echinococcosis. *Tropenmed. Parasit.* **31**, 459–66.

Sweatman, G. K., R. J. Williams, K. M. Moriarty and T. C. Henshall 1963. On acquired immunity to *Echinococcus granulosus* in sheep. *Res. Vet. Sci.* **4**, 187–98.

Szyfres, B. and I. G. Kagan 1963. A modified slide latex screening test for hydatid disease. *J. Parasitol.* **49**, 69–72.

Tassi, C., S. Dottorini and F. Baldelli 1982. Confronto tra la reazione di Emoagglutinazione Indiretta ed ELISA per la diagnosi della idatidosi umana. *Giorn. Mal. Infett. Parasit.* **34**, 493–4.

Tassi, C., S. Dottorini, G. Scalise and N. Geranio 1981. *Echinococcus granulosus*: diagnosis of human hydatid disease by the indirect haemagglutination reaction with antigens from hydatid fluid and scoleces. *Int. J. Parasitol.* **11**, 85–8.

Tassi, C., S. Dottorini, A. G. Tolu and F. De Rosa 1980. Diagnosis of hydatid disease in sheep by indirect hemagglutination test. *Rev. Parasitol.* **41**, 61–6.

Thompson, R. C. A. and L. M. Kumratilake 1982. Intraspecific variation in *Echinococcus granulosus*: the Australian situation and perspectives for the future. *Trans. R. Soc. Trop. Med. Hyg.* **76**, 13–6.

Todorov, T. and G. Stojanov 1979. Circulating antibodies in human echinococcosis before and after surgical treatment. *Bull. Wld Hlth Org.* **57**, 751–8.

Todorov, T., I. Dakov, M. Kosturkova, S. Tenev and A. Dimitrov 1979. Immunoreactivity in pulmonary echinococcosis. I. A comparative study of immunodiagnostic tests. *Bull. Wld Hlth Org.* **57**, 735–40.

Todorov, T., G. Stojanov, L. Rohov, R. Rasev and N. Alova 1976. Antibody persistence after surgical treatment of echinococcosis. *Bull. Wld Hlth Org.* **53**, 407–15.

Varela-Díaz, V. M. and E. A. Coltorti 1972. Further evidence of the passage of host immunoglobulins into hydatid cysts. *J. Parasitol.* **58**, 1015–6.

Varela-Díaz, V. M. and E. A. Coltorti 1973. The presence of host immunoglobulins in hydatid cyst membranes. *J. Parasitol.* **59**, 484–8.

Varela-Díaz, V. M. and E. A. Coltorti 1976. *Techniques for the immunodiagnosis of human hydatid disease.* Buenos Aires: Pan American Zoonosis Center.

Varela-Díaz, V. M., E. A. Coltorti and A. D'Alessandro 1978. Immunoelectrophoresis tests showing *Echinococcus granulosus* arc 5 in human cases of *Echinococcus vogeli* and cysticercosis-multiple myeloma. *Am. J. Trop. Med. Hyg.* **27**, 554–7.

Varela-Díaz, V. M., E. A. Coltorti, M. D. Rickard and J. M. Torres 1977a. Comparative antigenic characterisation of *Echinococcus granulosus* and *Taenia hydatigena* cyst fluids by immunoelectrophoresis. *Res. Vet. Sci.* **23**, 213–6.

Varela-Díaz, V. M., E. A. Coltorti, M. I. Ricardes, J. A. Guisantes and L. A. Yarzábal 1974. The immunoelectrophoretic characterization of sheep hydatid cyst fluid antigens. *Am. J. Trop. Med. Hyg.* **23**, 1092–6.

Varela-Díaz, V. M., J. Eckert, R. L. Rausch, E. A. Coltorti and U. Hess 1977b. Detection of *Echinococcus granulosus* diagnostic arc 5 in sera from patients with surgically-confirmed *E. multilocularis* infection. *Z. ParasitKde* **53**, 183–8.

Varela-Díaz, V. M., J. A. Guisantes, M. I. Ricardes, L. A. Yarzábal and E. A.

Coltorti 1975a. Evaluation of whole and purified hydatid fluid antigens in the diagnosis of human hydatidosis by the immunoelectrophoresis test. *Am. J. Trop. Med. Hyg.* **24**, 298–303.

Varela-Díaz, V. M., M. H. López-Lemes, U. Prezioso, E. A. Coltorti and L. A. Yarzábal 1975b. Evaluation of four variants of the indirect hemagglutination test for human hydatidosis. *Am. J. Trop. Med. Hyg.* **24**, 304–11.

Varela-Díaz, V. M., E. A. Coltorti, U. Prezioso, M. H. López-Lemes, J. A. Guisantes and L. A. Yarzábal 1975c. Evaluation of three immunodiagnostic tests for human hydatid disease. *Am. J. Trop. Med. Hyg.* **24**, 312–9.

Williams, J. F. 1972. An evaluation of the Casoni test in human hydatidosis using an antigen solution of low nitrogen concentration. *Trans. R. Soc. Trop. Med. Hyg.* **66**, 160–4.

Williams, J. F. and M. V. Pérez Esandi 1971. Reaginic antibodies in dogs infected with *Echinococcus granulosus*. *Immunology* **20**, 451–5.

Williams, J. F. and U. Prezioso 1970. Latex agglutination test for hydatid disease using Boerner slides. *J. Parasitol.* **56**, 1253–4.

Williams, J. F., M. V. Pérez Esandi and R. Oriol 1971. Evaluation of purified lipoprotein antigens of *Echinococcus granulosus* in the immunodiagnosis of human infection. *Am. J. Trop. Med. Hyg.* **20**, 575–9.

Yarzábal, L. A., J. Leiton and M. H. López-Lemes 1974. The diagnosis of human pulmonary hydatidosis by the immunoelectrophoresis test. *Am. J. Trop. Med. Hyg.* **23**, 662–6.

Yarzábal, L. A., P. M. Schantz and M. H. López-Lemes 1975. Comparative sensitivity and specificity of the Casoni intradermal and the immunoelectrophoresis tests for the diagnosis of hydatid disease. *Am. J. Trop. Med. Hyg.* **24**, 843–8.

Yarzabál, L. A., D. T. Bout, F. R. Naquira and A. R. Capron 1977a. Further observations on the specificity of antigen 5 of *Echinococcus granulosus*. *J. Parasitol.* **63**, 495–9.

Yarzabál, L., H. Dupas, D. Bout and A. Capron 1976. *Echinococcus granulosus*: distribution of hydatid fluid antigens in tissues of the larval stage 1. Localization of the specific antigen of hydatid fluid (antigen 5). *Exp. Parasitol.* **40**, 391–6.

Yarzabál, L. A., H. Dupas, D. Bout, F. Naquira and A. Capron 1977b. *Echinococcus granulosus*: the distribution of hydatid fluid antigens in the tissues of the larval stage II. Localization of the thermostable lipoprotein of parasitic origin (antigen B). *Exp. Parasitol.* **42**, 115–20.

Yong, W. K. and D. D. Heath 1979. 'Arc 5' antibodies in sera of sheep infected with *Echinococcus granulosus, Taenia hydatigena* and *Taenia ovis*. *Parasite Immunol.* **1**, 27–38.

Yong, W. K., D. D. Heath and S. N. Parmeter 1978. *Echinococcus granulosus, Taenia hydatigena, T. ovis*: evaluation of cyst fluids as antigen for serodiagnosis of larval cestodes in sheep. *N.Z. Vet. J.* **26**, 231–4.

Yong, W. K., D. D. Heath and F. van Knapen 1984. Comparison of cestode antigens in an enzyme-linked immunosorbent assay for the diagnosis of *Echinococcus granulosus, Taenia hydatigena* and *T. ovis* infections in sheep. *Res. Vet. Sci.* **36**, 24–31.

Yusuf, J. N., G. J. Frayha and A. H. Malakian 1975. *Echinococcus granulosus*: host lymphocyte transformation by parasite antigens. *Exp. Parasitol.* **38**, 30–7.

9 Prospects for treatment of the metacestode stage of *Echinococcus*

J. ECKERT

INTRODUCTION

Surgical intervention is the basic form of treatment of many cases of cystic (unilocular) and alveolar echinococcosis in man, caused by the metacestode stages of *Echinococcus granulosus* and *E. multilocularis*, respectively (Posselt 1928, Schicker 1976, Akovbiantz *et al.* 1978, Kasai *et al.* 1980, Mosimann 1980, Bähr 1982, Schantz 1982).

In cystic echinococcosis, surgery provides cure in about 50–60 per cent (French 1981) to over 90 per cent of cases (Schantz *et al.* 1982), depending on the number and localisation of cysts, severity and selection of cases, quality of medical facilities, operative technique and other factors. Among such cases the frequency of recurring (secondary) echinococcosis after an operation for primary hydatid disease is generally in the order of 2–11 per cent (for a review see Schantz *et al.* 1982) but may be as high as 30 per cent (Schicker 1976, French 1981). Lethality associated with a first, second and third operation has been reported as 2.5, 6.0 and 20.0 per cent, respectively (Amir-Jahed *et al.* 1975).

Alveolar echinococcosis is a fatal disease in a large percentage of cases (Drolshammer *et al.* 1973, Schicker 1976, Mosimann, 1980, Wilson & Rausch 1980). According to Schicker (1976) 93 per cent of 66 patients died within 10 years after the diagnosis of the disease and lethality rates in different groups of patients were not significantly influenced by palliative treatment or radical operation (Schicker 1976). The percentages of surgically resectable cases vary from 26 to 58 per cent (for a review see Schantz *et al.* 1982).

In both forms of echinococcosis, surgical intervention and postoperative treatment are expensive, and this may lead to considerable socio-economic problems. In Argentina the average number of days of hospitalisation per patient with cystic echinococcosis was 31.6 in 1979 (Varela-Díaz *et al.* 1983, see Ch. 3 for details). There is, therefore, an urgent need for effective chemotherapy against human echinococcosis (WHO 1981a,b). Moreover, anthelmintics against larval *Echinococcus* could be of future importance in the control of the infection in intermediate hosts of *E. granulosus*, such as cattle, sheep and camels (WHO 1981a).

In the past, attempts to develop a chemotherapy against the metacestode stage of *Echinococcus* were unsuccessful (for a review see Barandun 1978). With the discovery of the efficacy of benzimidazole derivatives against larval cestodes, including metacestodes of *Echinococcus* (Heath & Chevis 1974, Krotov *et al.* 1974, Thienpont *et al.* 1974a,b), a potential chemotherapy for human echinococcosis became feasible. This event was followed by intensive research, the main results of which are summarised below.

GENERAL CONSIDERATIONS: FACTORS INVOLVED IN CHEMOTHERAPY OF LARVAL ECHINOCOCCOSIS

Chemotherapy of naturally acquired larval echinococcosis requires the diagnosis of the infection and includes drug treatment, management of the disease and follow-up examinations.

Diagnosis of the infection

For the diagnosis of larval echinococcosis in humans, highly effective techniques for the detection of *Echinococcus* metacestodes or related lesions are available, such as radiology, radioisotope scanning, ultrasonography, intravenous viscerography and computer-assisted tomography (CAT), (Haertel *et al.* 1980, Morris 1981, Hübener & Metzger 1982, Otto *et al.* 1982, Pirschel 1982, Walther 1982). The latter method is suited to measure the density of cyst fluid or other contents and to determine the volume of a metacestode with high precision (Robotti 1983). At present CAT is the technique of choice but it is only available in clinical centres.

For primary detection of human echinococcosis and for confirmation of the clinical diagnosis based on CAT and other investigations immunodiagnostic methods play an important role (Schantz & Kagan 1980, Gottstein *et al.* 1983, for details see Ch. 8).

Drug treatment and management of the disease

A large number of factors are involved in drug treatment of larval echinococcosis (Fig. 9.1). Some of the current problems related to chemotherapy are discussed here, more information may be obtained from other sources (WHO 1981a,b). The management of the disease includes a variety of clinical procedures and measures of symptomatic treatment. To discuss these aspects would be beyond the scope of this article.

DRUG EFFICACY AND ABSORPTION

According to recent studies, albendazole, fenbendazole, flubendazole,

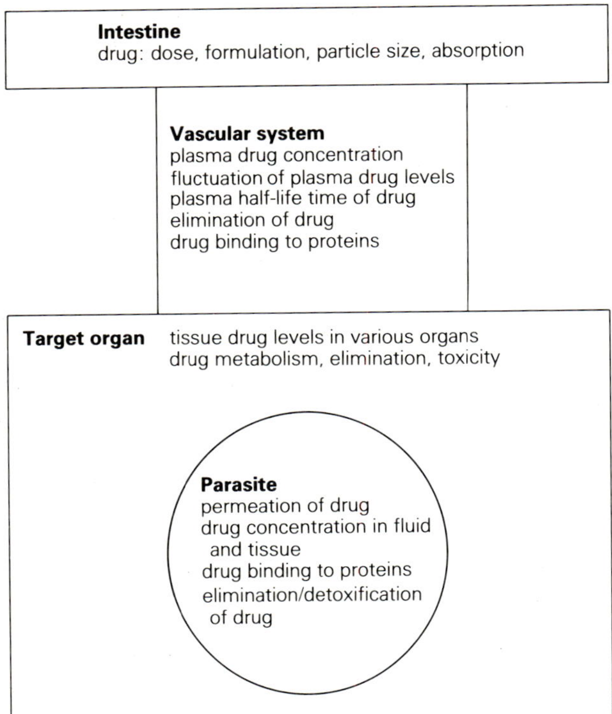

Possible drug effects against parasite
protoscolicidal
damage/destruction of cyst wall (especially of germinal layer)
suppression of proliferation
prevention of secondary echinococcosis and metastases formation
antigen release
release of cytotoxic substances

Possible host reactions
side effects of drug
parasite elimination/encapsulation
formation of antigen–antibody complexes
immunologic glomerulonephritis
allergic reactions

Figure 9.1 Factors involved in the chemotherapy of larval echinococcosis.

mebendazole★ and some other benzimidazole derivatives have certain anthelmintic effects against metacestode stages of *E. granulosus* and *E. multilocularis* in the animal model (see below).

Some of these drugs, albendazole, flubendazole and mebendazole, are used in trials for the treatment of human echinococcosis (see below). Since

★albendazole: methyl-5(6)-propylthiobenzimidazole-2-carbamate; fenbendazole: methyl-5(6)-phenylthiobenzimidazole-2-carbamate; flubendazole: methyl-5(6)-(*p*-fluorobenzoyl)benzimidazole-2-carbamate; mebendazole: methyl-5(6)-benzoylbenzimidazole-2-carbamate.

most studies were done with mebendazole, this drug can be used as an example to demonstrate some relevant pharmacological aspects.

Mebendazole was developed as an anthelmintic against gastrointestinal nematodes. To avoid side effects a substance with a low solubility in water was synthesised. Consequently most species, including humans, absorb less than 10 per cent of an orally administered dose (Brugmans *et al.* 1971, van Wijngaarden 1971). Absorption of poorly soluble chemicals is dependent on surface area (particle size) (Prichard 1978), and it has been suggested that a small particle size of mebendazole may be important in achieving a high efficacy against both larval and adult tapeworms (Gemmell & Johnstone 1981). In studies with dogs it was shown that micronised mebendazole powder was more efficient against intestinal *E. granulosus* as compared with a tablet preparation at equal oral doses (M. A. Gemmell pers. comm. 1984). This phenomenon may be due to changes in physical properties when powders are compressed into tablets. According to Wang *et al.* (1981) efficacy of mebendazole against porcine cysticercosis (caused by metacestodes of *Taenia solium*) was negligible when particle size exceeded 5 μm.

There is evidence that host factors influence intestinal absorption and may cause inter- and intraspecific variation of drug activity. For example, plasma mebendazole concentrations in rodents (*Meriones unguiculatus*) are approximately 10 times higher than in humans at comparable oral doses (Witassek *et al.* 1981). Such species-specific differences in absorption rates may play a role among other factors such as diet. In humans the systemic availability of mebendazole (Münst *et al.* 1979, 1980) and of flubendazole (Heykants *et al.* 1979) was enhanced by concomitant food ingestion.

PLASMA DRUG CONCENTRATIONS

After absorption mebendazole is distributed in the blood with 63 per cent in plasma and 37 per cent in the cellular fraction; in plasma 95 per cent is protein-bound (Braithwaite *et al.* 1982).

Several studies have shown that mebendazole plasma concentrations differ considerably between individual animals (Burkhardt 1981, Witassek *et al.* 1981) and patients (Wilson *et al.* 1978, Münst *et al.* 1980, Witassek *et al.* 1981, Braithwaite *et al.* 1982, Bryceson *et al.* 1982a,b) (Table 9.1). In one study the mean plasma concentration of mebendazole after a single dose was lower than during chronic therapy of patients (Braithwaite *et al.* 1982). In patients with normal liver function, mebendazole is rapidly metabolised in the liver and excreted via urine (1 per cent in dogs, 50 per cent in pigs) (Brugmans *et al.* 1971) and bile (up to 1.0 per cent in man) (Witassek *et al.* 1983). The elimination half-life times for mebendazole are short and were found to range between 1.5 and 9.0 h in several groups of patients (Münst *et al.* 1980, Witassek *et al.* 1981, Braithwaite *et al.* 1982). The anthelmintic effect against nematodes of the identified metabolites was lower than that of the parent compound (van den Bossche 1980).

There is evidence that several factors induce variability of mebendazole plasma concentrations, including irregular absorption (Münst *et al.* 1980,

Table 9.1 Range of plasma drug concentrations in patients with echinococcosis under oral treatment with benzimidazole compounds.

Drug	Dose ($mg\ kg^{-1}\ d^{-1}$)	Duration of treatment*	Number of patients	Plasma drug concentration ($ng\ ml^{-1}$)	Determination†		Authors
					Time (h)	Method	
mebendazole	16–63	5–36 m	27	15–295	4	HPLC	Witassek *et al.* (1981)
	40–60	3–11 m	7	7–90	1–3	RIA	Bryceson *et al.* (1982b)
	100–150	3–11 m	3	18–112	1–3	RIA	Bryceson *et al.* (1982b)
	200	3–11 m	6	14–297	1–3	RIA	Bryceson *et al.* (1982b)
albendazole	10–14	2–39 d	11	66–2000	—	HPLC	Saimot *et al.* (1983)
	10	5–8 d	4	420–1820	4–5	HPLC	Morris *et al.* (1983)
flubendazole	50	1 w–24 m	6	1–103	1–3	RIA	Roche *et al.* (1982a)

* d, days; w, weeks; m, months.

† Time is given in hours after the morning dose; methods are high performance liquid chromatography (HPLC) and radioimmunoassay (RIA).

Braithwaite *et al.* 1982, Witassek & Bircher 1983). Other factors are the impaired drug metabolising capacity of the liver (microsomal function) and/or reduced biliary elimination due to cholestasis which can account for prolonged plasma half-life times and for higher plasma mebendazole concentrations in patients with liver damage (Witassek *et al.* 1981, Witassek & Bircher 1983, Witassek *et al.* 1983). To avoid toxic side effects during mebendazole treatment, early and frequent monitoring of plasma drug levels is regarded as necessary in patients with cholestasis and liver diseases which drastically reduce microsomal function such as cirrhosis, hepatitis, alcoholic liver damage and advanced parasitic disease (Witassek & Bircher 1983).

Chemotherapy of human echinococcosis with constant doses of mebendazole, for example with 40 mg per kilogram of body weight per day, results in a wide variability of plasma drug levels. Therefore, it has been proposed to monitor plasma drug levels and adjust the daily drug dose to the individual patient's capacity to produce sufficiently high plasma levels (flexible dose schedule) (WHO 1981b, Witassek *et al.* 1981). However, in some patients increasing the daily mebendazole dose to 80 – 100 mg/kg^{-1} did not lead to 'effective' plasma drug concentrations (Witassek & Bircher 1983).

The 'effective' or 'therapeutic' plasma drug concentrations for treatment of echinococcosis are not well defined. In rodents (*Meriones*) experimentally infected with metacestodes of *E. multilocularis*, mebendazole concentrations above 74 ng/ml^{-1} were associated with a highly significant inhibition of parasite proliferation and with a 90–99 per cent reduction of metacestode weight as compared with untreated controls (Burkhardt 1981, Witassek *et al.* 1981). These data and results from human trials suggest that mebendazole plasma concentrations in excess of 80–100 ng/ml^{-1} maintained for long periods (several months to years) may be necessary to achieve an anthelmintic effect (Witassek *et al.* 1981, Bryceson *et al.* 1982a). Witassek *et al.* (1981) observed in patients on long-term therapy with 16–48 mg kg^{-1} mebendazole per day that plasma drug concentrations 4 h after the morning dose exceeded 74 ng ml^{-1} only in 52 per cent of the cases. Similar observations were described by other authors (Braithwaite *et al.* 1982, Bryceson *et al.* 1982a,b, Morris & Gould 1982).

Toxic mebendazole plasma concentrations for humans are not well defined, but levels higher than 590 ng ml^{-1} should be avoided, since above that value toxicity has been observed in rodents (Witassek *et al.* 1981).

Some examples for plasma concentrations of mebendazole and other drugs are given in Table 9.1. It appears that albendazole treatment is followed by relatively high and more constant plasma drug concentrations by comparison with mebendazole and flubendazole.

TISSUE DRUG CONCENTRATIONS

Tissue drug concentrations have been determined by various authors (Table 9.2). According to Braithwaite *et al.* (1982, 1983) mebendazole is

Table 9.2 Examples of drug concentrations in host tissues and cysts of *Echinococcus granulosus* from humans.

Drug	Dose (mg kg^{-1} d^{-1})	Number of patients	Drug concentration in							Authors
			Plasma (ng ml^{-1})	Liver (ng g^{-1})	Fat (ng g^{-1})	Cyst fluid (ng g^{-1})		Daughter cyst fluid (ng g^{-1})		
						Viable	Dead	Viable	Dead	
mebendazole	40	1–4	116–200*	157–404	86–270	46	84–154	6–23	60–89	Braithwaite *et al.* (1983)
mebendazole	50	5–7	10–84	—	—	0.4–14.5	—	—	—	Morris and Gould (1982)
flubendazole	50	7	0.5–10	88–142	—	0.05	—	—	—	Saimot *et al.* (1981)
albendazole	10–14	8–11	66–2000	272–8239	—	94–4365	—	—	—	Saimot *et al.* (1983)

* Maximum concentrations.
Abbreviations: g, wet weight; d, day.

concentrated in the liver tissue, in which drug levels are significantly higher than maximum concentrations found in plasma. In fatty tissues and the hydatid cyst wall, mebendazole equilibrated at 68–75 per cent of the maximum plasma drug concentration.

DRUG UPTAKE BY THE METACESTODE

The efficacy of chemotherapy will depend on the influx of a certain quantity of drug into the metacestode from the host organ. As mebendazole levels vary in host tissues (see above) parasites located in the liver, lung, kidneys and other organs are likely to be exposed to different external drug concentrations.

Echinococcus granulosus In cases of *E. granulosus* infection the drug has first to pass the adventitious capsule formed around the metacestode cyst by the host (Fig. 9.2). Thickness, structure and chemical composition of this layer can vary considerably depending on several factors. For example, in man host capsules of 0.5–1.0 cm in thickness have been reported, but mostly they are thinner (Lehmann 1928). It is further known that cysts located in the liver and kidney may have much stronger capsules than those found in the lung or in the peritoneal cavity (Lehmann 1928). Cellular composition, calcareous deposits and degree of degenerative changes are also variables which may influence drug distribution and its local concentration. The metacestode wall is composed of an outer acellular 'laminated layer' and an inner cellular syncytial 'germinal layer' (see Ch. 1). The latter is regarded as an absorptive tegument, similar to that of adult cestodes, with microtriches projecting into the laminated layer (Morseth 1967, Bortoletti & Ferretti 1973, Richards *et al.* 1983).

Significant differences of these two layers were observed in *E. granulosus* cysts isolated from different hosts in Sardinia (Bortoletti & Ferretti 1978). In cysts from humans, the laminated layer was thicker (360–2750 μm) and the germinal layer more proliferating (9.0–75.0 μm) than in cysts from cattle (8.0–50.0 and 0.1–3.5 μm, respectively). Cysts from pigs and sheep ranged between these extremes. Such structural differences may be related to host influences, to the age of the infection, the parasite strain and possibly other factors. Furthermore, daughter cysts may be enclosed in a mother cyst so that the drug would have to pass a double barrier of laminated and germinal layers.

In relation to chemotherapy, the question of permeability of the parasite wall to chemicals is very important. Using *E. granulosus* cysts obtained from secondarily infected mice, Rotunno *et al.* (1974) demonstrated *in vitro* under steady state conditions that water diffused through cyst walls rapidly (diffusional permeability 1.88×10^{-4} cm s^{-1}), whereas permeability to Na^+ and Cl^- was relatively low (0.13 and 0.35 μmol h^{-1} cm^{-2}, respectively). The cyst wall is also permeable to larger molecules, such as host cholesterol (Frayha 1968), albumin and immunoglobulins (Chordi & Kagan 1965, Coltorti & Varela-Díaz 1972, 1974, 1975, Hustead & Williams 1977).

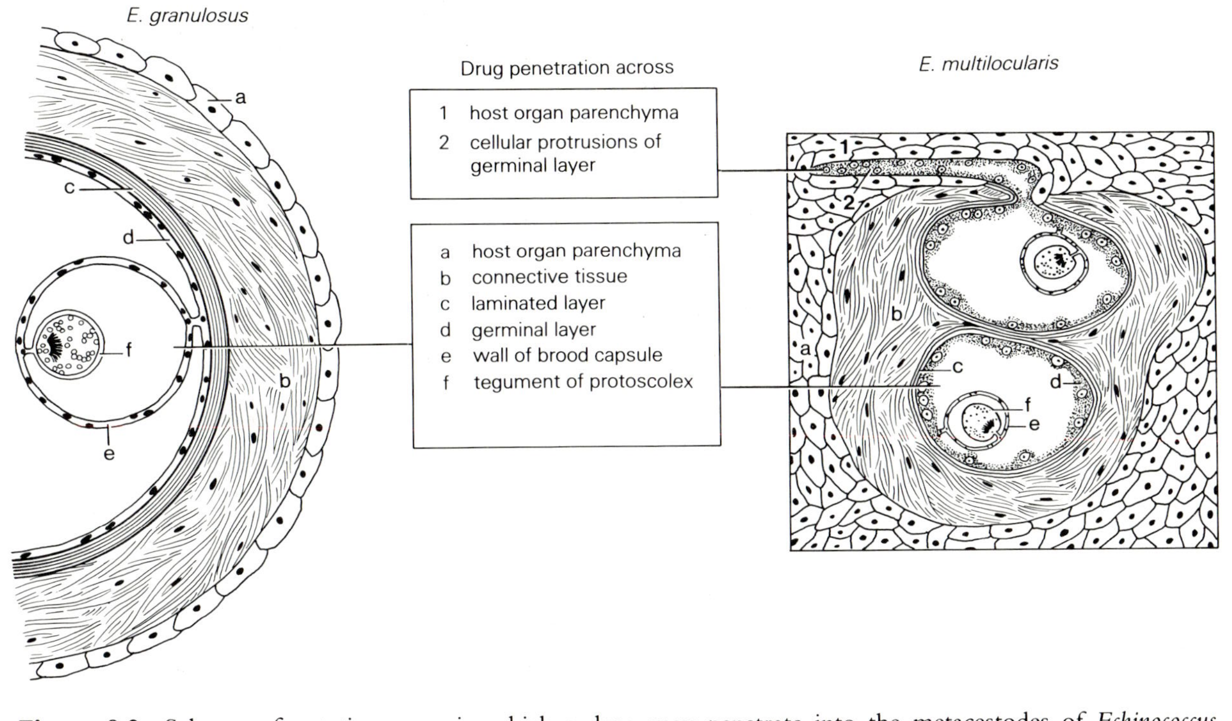

Figure 9.2 Scheme of putative ways in which a drug may penetrate into the metacestodes of *Echinococcus granulosus* and *E. multilocularis*.

Sheep hydatid cyst fluid was found to contain between 1.3–13.0 and 3.0–34.0 μg ml^{-1} host IgG and albumin, respectively (Coltorti & Varela-Díaz 1972). The differences in albumin concentrations between serum and the cyst fluids were in the order of 1000–10 000 (Coltorti & Varela-Díaz 1972). That these molecules had entered the cysts from the host tissues was proven by finding recipient IgG in fluid of cysts transplanted previously into heterologous host species (Varela-Díaz & Coltorti 1972). Further evidence was obtained by the demonstration of host IgG in the hydatid cyst wall (Varela-Díaz & Coltorti 1973) and by results which supported the ability of IgG to penetrate into the laminated layer and to reach the germinal layer of cysts (Coltorti & Varela-Díaz 1974).

The degree of host protein penetration into the cysts is variable. In a study by Coltorti and Varela-Díaz (1972) host IgG was detected in 15 of 18 (83 per cent) peritoneal cysts obtained from experimentally infected gerbils and in 18 of 61 (29 per cent) mouse hydatid cysts which had been transplanted into the peritoneal cavity of gerbils for periods ranging from 1 d to 2 years. Host IgG concentrations in the fluids of different cysts varied between 0.007 and 3.7 μg ml^{-1}, but no association could be detected between these concentrations and the time period after cyst implantation. Hustead and Williams (1977) found that only 20 per cent of intact cysts took up ^{125}I-labelled bovine serum albumin *in vitro*. The same authors concluded from incorporation studies with ^{125}I-labelled rat IgG_2 that uptake of external proteins can occur but that they may be rapidly degraded in hydatid cyst fluid by proteases.

The mechanisms by which host macromolecules penetrate into hydatid cysts are not known. Available data suggest that they readily penetrate the laminated layer but the germinal layer may form an obstacle for further permeation. Coltorti and Varela-Díaz (1975) suggested that the irregular finding of host IgG in hydatid cyst fluid may be a result of 'random events like the occasional fissuring of the cyst tegument'. This irregularity of protein uptake may also influence drug transport across the cyst wall if drugs are bound to proteins. As mentioned above, the plasma fraction of mebendazole is 95 per cent protein-bound (Braithwaite *et al.* 1982).

At present it is unknown whether free or protein-bound mebendazole, or both forms, penetrate the cyst wall in the living organism. *In vitro* studies with incubation of cysts in Krebs–Ringer solution have shown that the permeability of the cyst wall to mebendazole (solubilised in dimethylsulphoxide) is very similar to water but 500–2000 times higher than to Na^+ and Cl^- (see above), and that drug concentration in cyst fluid can rapidly reach values similar to those of the incubation fluid (Reisin *et al.* 1977).

The fact that metacestodes of *E. granulosus* and *E. multilocularis* in animals (see below) are affected by treatment with mebendazole and some other compounds indirectly indicates that drugs can penetrate the parasites *in vivo*. This is confirmed by the detection of drugs in metacestodes of *E. granulosus* isolated from mice (Kammerer & Miller 1981) or humans under chemotherapy (Table 9.2).

Data obtained from cases with *E. granulosus* infection show that *total* mebendazole concentrations in hydatid fluid of cysts from different patients vary greatly (Table 9.2). According to Luder *et al.* (1985) mebendazole drug levels in cyst fluid are significantly correlated with plasma drug concentrations (4 h after the morning dose) which themselves vary widely from patient to patient (see above). There is evidence that mebendazole in humans can penetrate into viable and dead cysts of *E. granulosus*, the latter having up to six times higher concentrations, whereas daughter cysts were found to have lower drug levels than the corresponding mother cysts (Braithwaite *et al.* 1983, Luder *et al.* 1985).

It has been suggested that viable cysts may have active mechanisms for prevention or reduction of drug penetration and/or of excretion and detoxification of chemicals (Braithwaite *et al.* 1983). The suggestion of a regulatory mechanism of drug uptake is supported by recent data of Luder *et al.* (1985). These authors found that *total* mebendazole concentrations (free and protein-bound fractions) in hydatid cysts were on average less than one-third of corresponding plasma levels. Since albumin uptake by cysts is fluctuating (see above) the lower concentrations of total mebendazole in cyst fluid in comparison to plasma may be in part explained by an irregular transport across the cyst wall of the albumin-bound drug fraction. Most interestingly, in the study of Luder *et al.* (1985) the concentrations of *free* mebendazole in plasma and hydatid fluid were very similar. Thus it may be that free mebendazole readily diffuses across the cyst wall *in vivo* as *in vitro* (Reisin *et al.* 1977) whereas the transport of protein-bound mebendazole fluctuates depending on the ability of cysts to incorporate proteins from the environment. If this ability depends on fissuring of the cyst wall (Coltorti & Varela-Díaz 1975), albumin concentrations in cyst fluid could indicate the degree of cyst wall damage. However, protein binding of mebendazole may also occur in the cyst fluid. The free mebendazole fraction in cyst fluid accounts for 5–100 per cent of the total mebendazole concentration (Luder *et al.* 1985) and may be of special importance for drug action.

With regard to drug concentrations and their stability in hydatid cysts, it has to be considered that the parasite may metabolise or detoxify the drug. Repetto and Morello (1981) detected glutathione-*S*-transferase in protoscoleces of *E. granulosus*. This enzyme catalyses the conjugation of 'substances' with glutathione as a first step of detoxification. Nothing is known of the capacity of *Echinococcus* metacestodes to metabolise mebendazole or other drugs.

Echinococcus multilocularis According to new knowledge (Vogel 1978, Eckert *et al.* 1983, Mehlhorn *et al.* 1983) the metacestode stage of *E. multilocularis* in rodents consists of a network of solid cellular protrusions of the germinal layer, tube-like structures and cystic expansions (Fig. 9.2). There is evidence that cellular protrusions also occur in metacestodes of *E. multilocularis* located in the human liver (Eckert *et al.* 1983). It is suggested that detached parts of the cellular protrusions (Ali-Khan *et al.* 1983, Eckert *et al.* 1983, Mehlhorn *et al.* 1983) may be involved in the spread of the parasite via the vascular system and in resultant metastases formation in various organs. The latter is a complication of human alveolar echinococcosis.

In *Meriones*, cellular protrusions and tube-like structures, devoid of a laminated layer, have been found infiltrating host organs in intimate contact with surrounding host cells and not being separated by a fibrous capsule from the host organ parenchyma (Mehlhorn *et al.* 1983). It can be speculated that drug penetration from host tissues into these structures may differ from that into cystic structures which are surrounded by a laminated layer and an adventitious host reaction. In human cases of alveolar liver echinococcosis, the metacestode is mostly embedded within a strong layer of connective tissue and parts of the living parasite may be engulfed by necrotic areas (Posselt 1928). However, in these cases, cellular protrusions infiltrating the host organ may be more intensively exposed to drug action than parts of the parasites within cysts surrounded by a laminated layer and/or by fibrous tissue and necrotic material.

There is ample indirect evidence from experiments with artificially infected rodents that mebendazole and other drugs penetrate into the metacestode stage of *E. multilocularis* (see below).

MODE OF DRUG ACTION

Ultrastructural examinations of metacestodes of *Taenia taeniaeformis* indicate that mebendazole disrupts the microtubular system, induces destruction of microtriches and finally degeneration of the tegument (Borgers *et al.* 1975, Verheyen *et al.* 1978). Similar changes were observed in the germinal layer of metacestodes of *E. granulosus* (Gemmell *et al.* 1981, Verheyen 1982) and of *E. multilocularis* (Swiderski & Eckert 1978). In consequence, glucose uptake is blocked, the endogenous glycogen reserves are depleted and the parasites die. Binding of mebendazole to parasite tubulin is regarded as a primary mode of action of certain benzimidazole compounds against cestodes and nematodes. This is followed by structural and metabolic changes (for a review see Eckert & Köhler 1983). Moreover, mebendazole appears to render larval cestodes more vulnerable to attack by the immune reaction of the host, as increased numbers of host cells were attached to the tegument after chemotherapy (Borgers *et al.* 1975, Verheyen *et al.* 1978).

INDICATIONS OF DRUG ACTIVITY AGAINST THE METACESTODE AND CRITERIA FOR EVALUATION OF DRUG EFFICACY

Several drugs tested in animal experiments have certain anthelmintic effects against the metacestode stages of *E. granulosus* and *E. multilocularis* (see below). From studies with rodents and sheep it can be concluded that the main indicators of drug activity against metacestodes of *E. granulosus* are: loss of viability (motility, flame cell activity) and infectivity of protoscoleces, destruction of protoscoleces, damage or destruction of the germinal layer, loss of cyst fluid and collapse of the cyst wall. The

Figures 9.3 and 9.4 Cysts of *Echinococcus granulosus* from the peritoneal cavity of *Meriones unguiculatus* (467 days post infection).

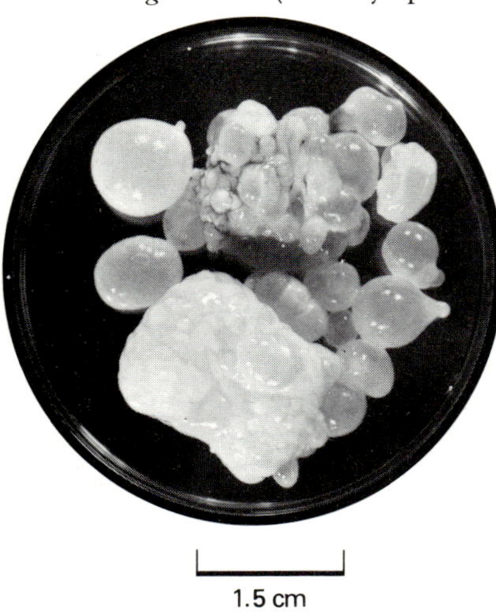

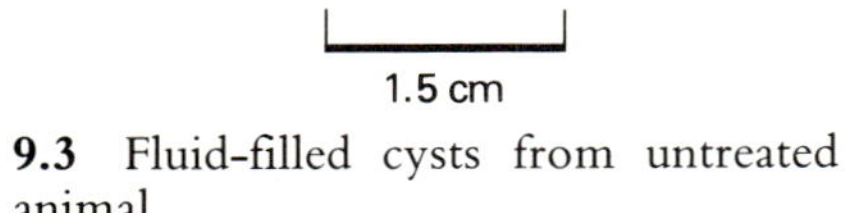

9.3 Fluid-filled cysts from untreated animal.

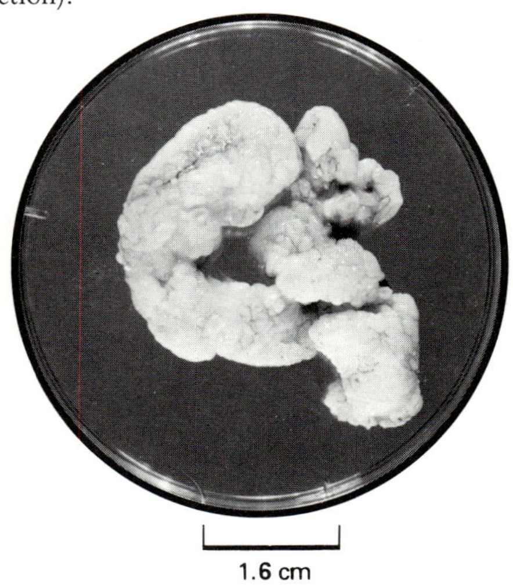

9.4 Collapsed and shrunken cysts from animal after 60 days of flubendazole treatment (500 ppm in food, about 30–50 mg/kg of body weight).

Figures 9.5 and 9.6 Historical section of a cyst wall of *Echinococcus granulosus* isolated from *Meriones*.

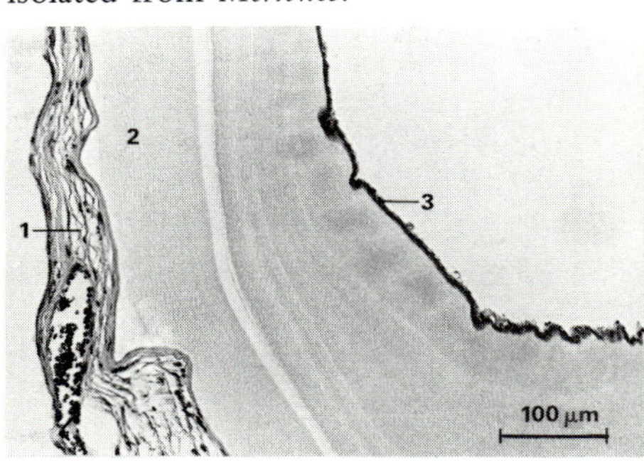

9.5 From untreated animal. 1, Adventitious layer; 2, laminated layer; 3, intact germinal layer.

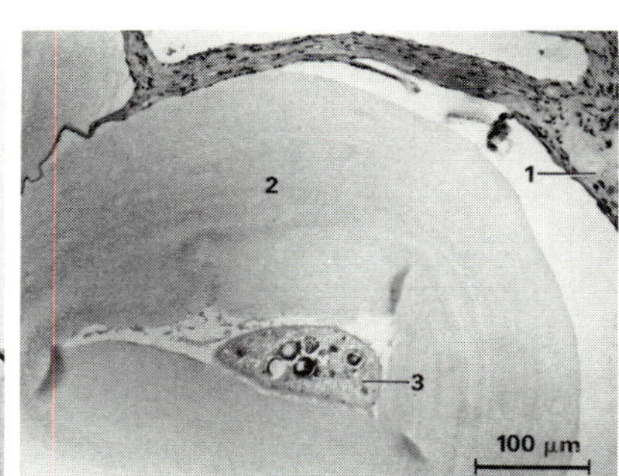

9.6 After 80 days of mebendazole treatment (500 ppm). 1, Adventitious layer; 2, unchanged laminated layer; 3, remnants of destroyed germinal layer (from Eckert *et al.* 1978).

laminated layer may show vacuolation or may remain unchanged for some time after drug treatment (see Figs 9.3–6).

Criteria of drug efficacy against the metacestode of *E. multilocularis* in rodents include: damage or destruction of protoscoleces, partial destruction of the histological structure of the metacestode, reduction of parasite weight in the order of more than 80 per cent, prevention of metastases formation and prolonged survival times of infected and treated animals as compared with untreated controls (see Figs 9.7–10).

Figures 9.7 and 9.8 *Meriones* (dorsal view) 134 (Fig. 9.7) and 230 (Fig. 9.8) days after subcutaneous transplantation of 0.1 g metacestode tissue of *Echinococcus multilocularis*.

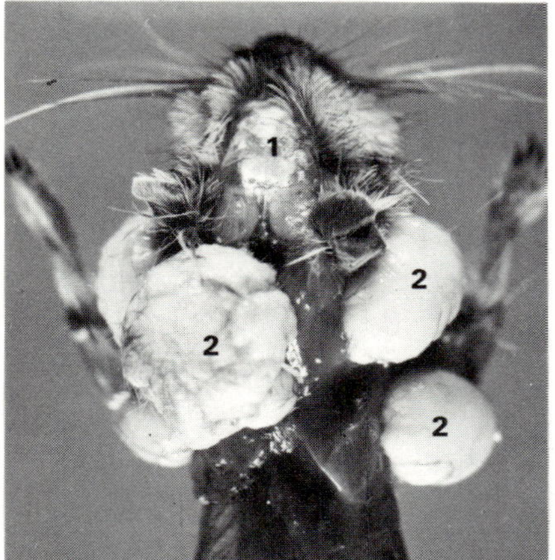

9.7 Significantly enlarged transplant (1) and metastases (2) in draining lymph nodes.

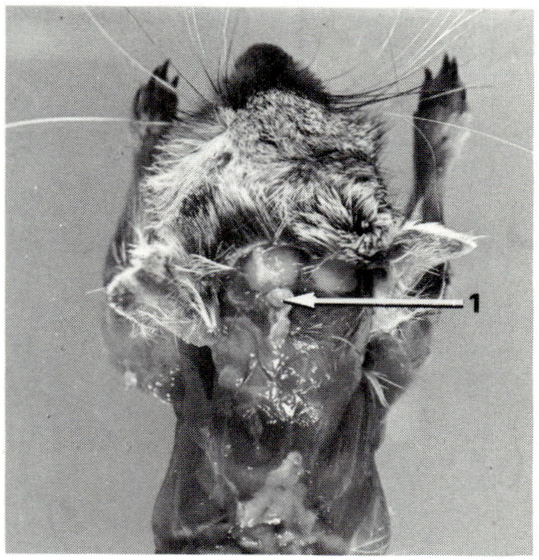

9.8 Remnants of parasite tissue at implantation site (arrow 1), no metastases, after 223 days of mebendazole treatment (500 ppm) (from Eckert & Burkhardt 1980).

Figures 9.9 and 9.10 Histological sections of metacestodes of *Echinococcus multilocularis* from *Meriones*.

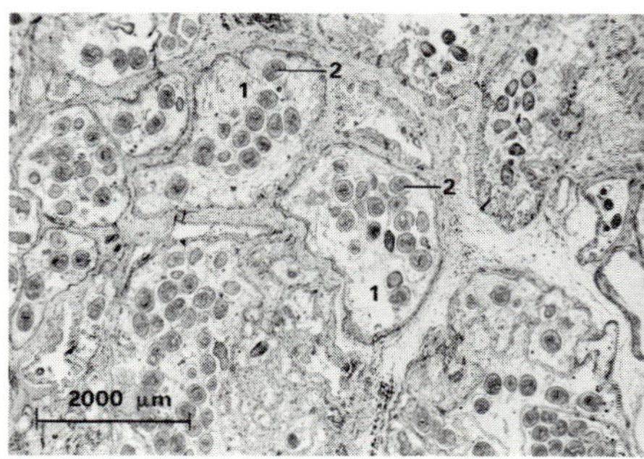

9.9 Untreated animal. 1, Cysts; 2, protoscoleces.

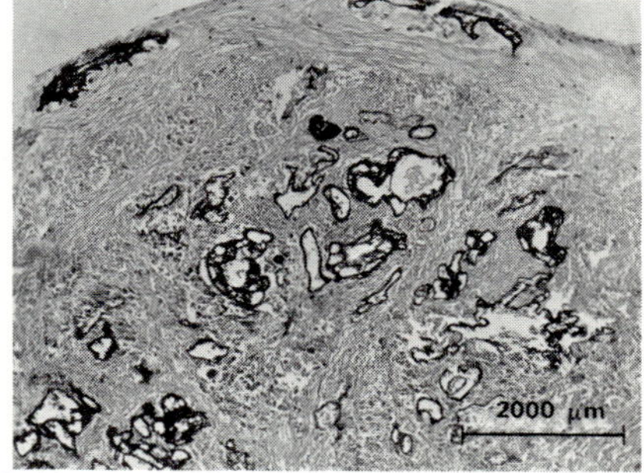

9.10 Animal treated for 60 days with mebendazole (500 ppm): normal cystic structure partially destroyed (from Eckert *et al.* 1978).

Table 9.3 Summary of main criteria used for evaluation of drug efficacy against echinococcosis in humans* (modified after WHO 1981b).

Echinococcus granulosus infection
- disappearance of cysts
- significant reduction of size and number of cysts, loss of fluid, collapse of cyst wall
- expectoration of cysts from lungs
- no dissemination of parasites after cyst rupture
- clinical improvement (decrease of liver size, pain and tenderness etc.)
- presumably therapeutic plasma drug levels (see earlier text)
- loss of parasite viability.

Echinococcus multilocularis infection
- parasite-induced lesions unchanged or reduced
- no metastases formation
- no progression of disease
- clinical improvement (weight, working capacity, hepatomegalia, signs of portal hypertension, liver function)
- prolongation of survival time
- presumed therapeutic plasma drug levels (see earlier text)

* Criteria based on findings in animals that cysts of *E. granulosus* may be severely damaged or killed by chemotherapy with certain drugs, whereas only the proliferation of *E. multilocularis* metacestodes is inhibited.

Detailed technical instructions for the determination of drug efficacy against metacestodes of *Echinococcus* species have been published by WHO (1981a). It is evident that only a combination of criteria allows definite conclusions regarding drug efficacy against the metacestodes in animals.

Essentially the same techniques used for the examination of metacestodes from animals can be employed for parasite material isolated from humans by biopsy, operation or autopsy.

Evaluation of drug efficacy against *Echinococcus* metacestodes in humans and follow-up examinations

The main problem in the evaluation of chemotherapy in echinococcosis of humans is the lack of easy measurable parameters which would closely reflect the course of the disease, the effect of the drug against the parasite and parasite viability. Trials carried out during the last few years indicate that several parameters can provide direct or indirect information on drug efficacy. These are summarised in Table 9.3.

Practical difficulties in the assessment of these parameters include the non-uniformity in the status of the disease at the beginning of treatment, the lack of untreated control patients, limited knowledge of the natural history of the disease (for example, spontaneous cure), and the fluctuations of plasma drug levels. Several studies have shown (Kern *et al.* 1979, Müller *et al.* 1982, Bryceson *et al.* 1982a) that the course of *Echinococcus* antibody titres as determined by conventional techniques does not correlate with the clinical or parasitological status of the patient. For example, declining IFAT and IHAT titres during long-term chemotherapy were observed both in patients with progressive *E. multilocularis* infection and with clinical improvement (Müller *et al.* 1982). In a study of 17 patients with alveolar echinococcosis, Schantz *et al.* (1983) observed a marked decline of hemagglutinating antibody titres during the first year following radical surgical resection of the lesions; in three cases clinical evidence of recurrence was preceded by rising serologic titres. In contrast, antibody had persisted at high levels in non-resected patients treated continuously with high doses of mebendazole. This finding is in agreement with the fact that the larval parasite is only inhibited in proliferation but not killed in laboratory animals (see below). The significance of other immunological tests, such as the determination of parasite-specific immunoglobulin classes (Gottstein *et al.* 1984) or circulating antigens and immune complexes is still under investigation.

It has to be concluded that evaluation of drug efficacy in echinococcosis of humans is at present based on prolonged observation of patients which includes follow-up examinations of certain main parameters (Table 9.3). Guidelines for clinical trials have been worked out by WHO (1981b). They should be consulted for detailed information.

CHEMOTHERAPY OF EXPERIMENTAL LARVAL ECHINOCOCCOSIS

Models for drug evaluation

In chemotherapeutic studies for the evaluation of drug efficacy the potential of the metacestodes of *Echinococcus* spp. to proliferate asexually has to be considered. Besides the metacestodes of *E. granulosus* and *E. multilocularis* in rodents (*Meriones*, cotton rats, mice) some other larval cestodes with this potential may be used as models in drug screening programmes. It has been shown that tetrathyridia of *Mesocestoides corti* and cysticerci of *Taenia crassiceps* inhabiting the peritoneal cavity of mice are highly sensitive to drugs that also show activity against metacestodes of *E. granulosus* and *E. multilocularis* in laboratory rodents (WHO 1981a). As these metacestodes can be maintained easily, at low costs and without danger for man they provide useful primary screening models (WHO 1981a).

Guidelines for drug screening with metacestodes of *Echinococcus* spp. and of other cestode species in the rodent model and with metacestodes of *E. granulosus* in farm animals have been published by WHO (1981a). It has to be considered that these models only partially reflect the disease condition in man. Therefore, research to develop more adequate model systems is required.

Trials in laboratory animals

For many years the search for drugs active against larval cestodes was unsuccessful. Various groups of drugs, including cytostatics, antibiotics,

Table 9.4 Selected data on the efficacy of drugs against metacestodes of *Echinococcus granulosus* in rodents.

Drug	Animals*	Dose (oral)†	Time and (duration) of treatment (days p.i.‡)	Metacestode		Germinal layer	Viability¶	Authors
				Controls, average weight (g)	Treated (% reduction) §			
fenbendazole	*Meriones* ($n = 6$)	500 ppm	195–275 (= 80)	20.5	91	destroyed	dead	Eckert *et al.* (1978)
flubendazole	mouse ($n = 6$)	500 ppm	300–321 (= 21)	—	—	only few collapsed	n.d.	Thienpont *et al.* (1976)
	mouse ($n = 6$)	1000 ppm	300–321 (= 21)	—	—	cysts present	n.d.	Thienpont *et al.* (1976)
	Meriones ($n = 19$)	500 ppm	383–443 (= 60)	12.9	68	destroyed	n.d.	J. Eckert (unpublished)
mebendazole	mouse ($n = 24$)	1000 ppm	(= 21)	—	—	damaged	n.d.	Heath *et al.* (1975)
	mouse ($n = 5$)	50 mg kg^{-1} d^{-1}	300–310 (= 10)	100‖	15‖	damaged	n.d.	Kammerer and Judge (1976)
	Meriones ($n = 6$)	500 ppm	195–275 (= 80)	20.5	84	destroyed	dead	Eckert *et al.* (1978)

* *n*, number of treated animals, controls not included.
† 500 ppm in the food corresponding to about 30–50 mg per kilogram of body weight per day in *Meriones* and to 60–70 mg kg^{-1} in mice.
‡ p.i., post infection.
§ In comparison to untreated controls.
¶ Viability test (see earlier text).
‖ Mean number of total cysts.
Abbreviations: n.d., not done; —, no information; d, day.

sulphonamides, antiprotozoic compounds and several anthelmintics, have been tested with generally poor results (for a review see Barandun 1978). In 1974 Thienpont *et al.* (1974a,b) detected a high anthelmintic effect of mebendazole, a benzimidazole derivative, against metacestodes of *T. taeniaeformis* in mice. In the same year this drug and some other benzimidazole compounds were shown to have certain anthelmintic effects against the metacestode stages of *M. corti, T. pisiformis, E. granulosus* and *E. multilocularis* (Campbell & Blair 1974a,b, Heath & Chevis 1974, Krotov *et al.* 1974; for further literature see Eckert & Pohlenz 1976, Eckert *et al.* 1981, Gemmell & Johnstone 1981, WHO 1981a, Schantz *et al.* 1982).

CHEMOTHERAPY AGAINST LARVAL *ECHINOCOCCUS GRANULOSUS*

Efficacy of benzimidazole derivatives According to recent studies (Table 9.4) cysts of *E. granulosus* in the peritoneal cavity of rodents (*Meriones unguiculatus*) can be severely damaged or killed by long-term treatment for 60–80 d with mebendazole, fenbendazole or flubendazole applied in the food at dose rates of 500 ppm (corresponding to about 30–50 mg per kilogram of body weight per day) (Eckert *et al.* 1978, J. Eckert *et al.* unpublished). This treatment caused a reduction of cyst weight, mainly due to loss of hydatid fluid, morphological changes of the cyst wall with complete destruction of the germinal layer and partial vacuolation of the laminated layer, and the loss of parasite viability as demonstrated by transplantation experiments. An anthelmintic effect of these drugs was also observed after shorter periods of treatment and/or with other doses but parasite viability was not evaluated in these tests (Table 9.4).

Efficacy of other drugs Several other drugs, such as thymol (Kammerer & Perez-Esandi 1975), bithionol (Kammerer & Judge 1976) and levamisole (Kovalenko *et al.* 1976) did not exhibit significant efficacy against cysts of *E. granulosus* in rodents (for further literature see Barandun 1978).

Praziquantel applied at doses of 30 mg per mouse as a subcutaneously implanted rubber silicone disc 3 d before or on the day of infection with protoscoleces of *E. granulosus* reduced the development of secondary cysts by 91–97 per cent but was less effective (75–78 per cent) when treatment was started 3 d after infection (Marshall & Edwards 1982).

CHEMOTHERAPY AGAINST LARVAL *ECHINOCOCCUS MULTILOCULARIS*

Efficacy of benzimidazole derivatives Extensive chemotherapeutical trials have been performed with *E. multilocularis* in rodents (*Meriones unguiculatus* and mice) (for reviews see Barandun 1978, Eckert *et al.* 1978, Eckert 1980, Eckert & Burkhardt 1980, Burkhardt 1981, Eckert *et al.* 1981, WHO 1981a, Schantz *et al.* 1982). Recent results (Table 9.5) indicate that long-term treatment of experimentally infected *Meriones* during 60–300 d with 500 ppm mebendazole in the food (about 30–50 mg per kilogram of

Table 9.5 Selected data on the efficacy of drugs at doses of 500 ppm* applied in the food against metacestodes of *Echinococcus multilocularis* in *Meriones unguiculatus*.

Drug	Animal numbers†	Time and (duration) of treatment (days p.i.‡)	Metacestode		Structure¶	Viability‖	Authors
			Controls, average weight (g)	Treated (% reduction)§			
albendazole	10	7–67 (= 60)	13.2	99	damaged	living	Burkhardt (1981)
	10	40–100 (= 60)	8.4	93	damaged	living	Burkhardt (1981)
fenbendazole	7	7–67 (= 60)	10.7	99	damaged	living	Barandun (1978)
	15	40–207 (= 167)	9.1	95	damaged	living	Burkhardt (1981)
	14	7–207 (= 200)	9.1	97	damaged	living	Burkhardt (1981)
flubendazole	6	7–67 (= 60)	10.2	98	damaged	living	Barandun (1978)
	10	40–207 (= 167)	9.1	83	damaged	living	Burkhardt (1981)
	7	7–207 (= 200)	9.1	97	damaged	living	Burkhardt (1981)
mebendazole	17	7–67 (= 60)	10.4	99	damaged	living	Eckert *et al.* (1978)
	6	40–100 (= 60)	9.9	95	damaged	living	Eckert *et al.* (1978)
	10	40–160 (= 120)	16.1	97	damaged	living	Eckert *et al.* (1978)
	28	7–307 (= 300)	7.8	99	damaged	living	Eckert and Burkhardt (1980)
praziquantel	6	7–67 (= 60)	10.7	21	PS mostly damaged	living	Barandun (1978)

* Corresponding to about 30–50 mg per kilogram of body weight per day.
† Only treated animals, controls not included.
‡ p.i., post-infection.
§ In comparison to untreated controls.
¶ PS, protoscoleces.
‖ Transplantation tests (see earlier text).

body weight per day) resulted in average reductions of metacestode weights of 95–99 per cent as compared with untreated controls. Treatment starting 40 d post-infection was equally effective as therapy beginning as early as 7 d after infection. Similar effects were obtained with 500 ppm fenbendazole and flubendazole for 60–200 d and with albendazole for 60 d (Table 9.5).

In several experiments it was demonstrated that infected *Meriones* under long-term treatment had significantly longer survival times than untreated controls (Barandun 1978, Eckert *et al.* 1978, Burkhardt 1981). Moreover, such treatment completely prevented the formation of 'metastases' in lymph nodes and lungs of *Meriones* subcutaneously infected with metacestode tissue of *E. multilocularis* whereas 70 per cent untreated control animals developed metastases (Eckert & Burkhardt 1980, Burkhardt 1981).

Histological examinations of metacestodes of treated animals revealed a relatively high drug sensitivity of protoscoleces which were destroyed within 30–60 d of continuous treatment with various benzimidazole drugs (Eckert *et al.* 1978, Burkhardt 1981). In contrast, the germinal cells of *E. multilocularis* are less sensitive to drug action. Although severe alterations of the normal metacestode structure were observed in histological sections after long-term treatment of up to 300 d, most of the larval parasites resumed growth after transplantation into naive homologous recipient hosts (see Table 9.5). This indicates that the parasites were only suppressed and did not proliferate during chemotherapy.

The parasite weights were negatively correlated with mebendazole plasma concentrations and with the duration of therapy but not with the mebendazole content of the food (oral mebendazole dose). In man, the mebendazole plasma concentrations are considerably lower than in *Meriones* after comparable oral doses of the drug (Witassek *et al.* 1981). This fact indicates that in chemotherapeutic studies the rodent model of experimental echinococcosis is only partially comparable to the disease in humans.

Efficacy of other drugs Among the many other drugs used unsuccessfully against larval *E. multilocularis* in rodents (for reviews see Barandun 1978, Burkhardt 1981) some deserve brief comments.

Thymol (2-isopropyl-5-methylphenol) (e.g. Thymoloverm®: palmintine acid-thymol ester) has been used for the treatment of *E. granulosus* and *E. multilocularis* infections in man and *E. multilocularis* in rodents with little or no success (lit. Burkhardt 1981).

Praziquantel, which has a high efficacy against metacestodes of *Taenia saginata* and *T. solium* (Andrews *et al.* 1983), had a damaging effect against protoscoleces of *E. multilocularis* in rodents. However, it was not parasiticidal against the metacestode, even after application for 60 d at a daily dose of about 30–50 mg kg^{-1} (500 ppm in the food) (Eckert *et al.* 1977, Sakamoto 1977, Barandun 1978, Thomas & Gönnert 1978; Table 9.5).

Levamisole partially inhibited the proliferation of larval *E. multilocularis*, damaged protoscoleces but did not affect the cyst wall structure (Kovalenko *et al.* 1976, Krotov *et al.* 1976).

Trials in domestic animals

Only a few trials have been carried out on the efficacy of mebendazole against porcine and ovine *E. granulosus* infections (Pawlowski *et al.* 1976, Tinar 1979, Gemmel *et al.* 1981). Results in sheep indicate (Gemmel *et al.* 1981) that long-term treatment for up to 3 months with high daily doses (50 mg kg^{-1}) may be required to achieve strong efficacy against protoscoleces and germinal tissue of the cysts. Three studies with praziquantel treatment (one using 50 mg kg^{-1} subcutaneously and two using 100 mg kg^{-1} *per os*, respectively) of sheep have failed to demonstrate an effect against cysts of *E. granulosus* (Heath & Lawrence 1978, Tinar 1979, Gemmell & Parmeter, cit. Andrews *et al.* 1983).

Conclusions from animal experiments

Based on present knowledge of research on treatment of experimental echinococcosis the following conclusions can be drawn:

(a) In both laboratory rodents and farm animals, cysts of *E. granulosus* are sensitive to treatment with benzimidazole drugs if applied in high doses over prolonged periods of time. Minimum doses and treatment schedules to achieve maximum efficacy have not yet been defined.
(b) The proliferation of metacestodes of *E. multilocularis* may be suppressed by chemotherapy with benzimidazoles but generally the parasites are not killed.
(c) As plasma levels of mebendazole in man are lower than in rodents, the antiparasitic effect may be less distinct in humans as compared with rodents.

CHEMOTHERAPY OF HUMAN ECHINOCOCCOSIS

Background and general observations

A few years after the publication of reports on the efficacy of mebendazole against metacestodes of *Echinococcus* in animals, the drug was used to treat humans with inoperable echinococcosis caused by *E. granulosus* (Goodman 1976, Bekhti *et al.* 1977, Danis *et al.* 1977) or *E. multilocularis* (Akovbiantz *et al.* 1977, Wilson *et al.* 1978). Until 1980, mebendazole, and to a lesser extent flubendazole, had been used in treating at least 303 published cases of cystic and 17 of alveolar echinococcosis (for a review see Schantz *et al.* 1982). At a workshop held in November 1980, further information on 243 and 31 treated patients suffering from these forms of the disease was reported; some of the cases had been already described in previous publications (for a review see Schantz *et al.* 1982). The treatment schedules were inconsistent and varied widely. Daily mebendazole doses of 16–200 mg kg^{-1} were given for 3 weeks up to 1 year against cystic echinococcosis, and of 40–50 mg kg^{-1} d^{-1} for 1 month up to 6 years in cases of alveolar echinococcosis. The data available at this time were critically reviewed by Schantz *et al.* (1982). They concluded that mebendazole or flubendazole treatment of humans infected with *E. granulosus* was followed by subjective improvement in most cases, evidence of regression of cysts in some patients and progression of the disease in others. In several patients cysts continued to grow and were proven viable even after several months of high-dose mebendazole therapy. In patients with *E. multilocularis* infection, the progressive course of the disease appeared to be arrested, but treatment apparently did not kill the parasite. Chemotherapy was well tolerated in the majority of patients; side effects in some cases have included allergic reactions, alopecia, and reversible neutropenia (see Schantz *et al.* 1982).

Since 1980 many further reports have been published, some of which are summarised in Tables 9.6 and 9.7.

Based on recent experience a fixed and a flexible dose schedule for mebendazole treatment have been proposed (WHO 1981b).

In the *fixed dose schedule* standard doses of mebendazole should be taken three times a day with meals. Starting with 500 mg per adult person twice a day, doses of 4.5 g d^{-1} (64 mg kg^{-1} for 70 kg body weight; three tablets at 500 mg three times a day) should be reached within 2 weeks. In several studies (see Ammann *et al.* 1979 and below) similar schedules have been applied, mostly with a maintenance dosage around 30–50 mg kg^{-1} d^{-1}. The duration of treatment in several studies varied between 1 month and 6 years (Tables 9.6 & 9.7).

In the *flexible dose schedule* mebendazole is given three times a day in gradually increasing doses while monitoring plasma drug concentrations until presumed therapeutic levels above 80 ng ml^{-1} are reached (WHO 1981b). This dose schedule has the purpose of achieving similar plasma drug levels in all patients.

Continuous mebendazole treatment is regarded as necessary in inoperable or non-radically operated cases of *E. multilocularis*, whereas other cases are treated for shorter periods of several months (Tables 9.6 & 9.7). Some examples for the dosage of albendazole and flubendazole are given in Tables 9.6 and 9.7.

Chemotherapy of cystic (*E. granulosus*) echinococcosis

Recent data (Table 9.6) support former observations that only a small percentage of patients with cystic echinococcosis favourably responds to high-dose and long-term oral mebendazole treatment. For example, chemotherapy with daily mebendazole doses of 30–200 mg kg^{-1} during 4–12 months was reported to be ‘at least partially successful’ in only four

Table 9.6 Summary of selected recent data on chemotherapy of cystic echinococcosis in humans.

Treatment	No. patients	Site of cysts	Results	Reference
albendazole				
10 mg kg^{-1} d^{-1} for 1–2 months	4	liver (two), abdominal (one), thoracic (one)	significant reduction of cyst size in three patients and no recurrence in 3–6 months; one anaphylactic, others feverish with nausea within 48 h of treatment; high plasma drug levels	Morris *et al.* (1983)
10–14 mg kg^{-1} d^{-1} for 30 d; repeated courses (up to six) at intervals of 2 weeks	10	liver (three), abdominal (two), bone (five)	three liver cysts cured; no recurrence in two abdominal cysts after cyst rupture and treatment; no improvement in bone cysts in spite of high drug levels (1000 ng per gram wet weight); all patients had high plasma drug levels and drug was well tolerated	Saimot *et al.* (1983)
mebendazole				
40 mg kg^{-1} d^{-1} for 1 month	16	liver and abdominal	in all patients there was no reduction in size or number of cysts, no side effects; anti-body persistence	Okello and Chemati (1981)
30–200 mg kg^{-1} d^{-1} for 4–12 months	11	liver (five), lung (one), bone (four), other (one)	four patients showed a reduction in cyst size; cysts were unchanged or progressed in other patients; in several patients there were viable cysts even after 24 months of treatment; the successes and failures of this treatment were presumably correlated with plasma drug levels	Bryceson *et al.* (1982a)

(36 per cent) of 11 cases, as indicated by significant reduction in cyst size (Bryceson *et al.* 1982a). However, complete cure could not be demonstrated, and some patients contained viable cysts even after 24 months of intensive treatment (Bryceson *et al.* 1982a).

In a few cases, cure of pulmonary or mediastinal infections have been reported (for example, Oppermann *et al.* 1982, Shivashankar *et al.* 1982, van den Brink *et al.* 1983), sometimes with unchanged liver cysts in the same patient. Recent observations suggest that single pulmonary and liver cysts may be more sensitive to chemotherapy than multiple cysts and those in other locations. It has to be considered, however, that about

Table 9.6 – *continued*

Treatment	No. patients	Site of cysts	Results	Reference
30–40 mg kg^{-1} d^{-1} for 2–14 months	4		clinical improvement in three patients; initial decrease of lung lesions in one patient, later no change; no serious adverse reactions	Müller *et al.* (1982)
50 mg kg^{-1} d^{-1} for 1 month; repeated courses; cumulated doses of 114–892 g per patient	15	liver (11), lung (six)	of the 11 liver cyst patients, three showed clinical improvement and two a reduction of cyst size; of the six lung cyst patients, one showed clinical improvement and five a reduction of cyst size; allergic reactions occurred in four patients with lung cysts and there was a decrease in antibody titres in a few patients	Kern (1983)
35–50 mg kg^{-1} d^{-1} for 94 d	1	liver	plasma drug concentrations 39–274 ng ml^{-1}, after operation cyst viable (mouse inoculation test)	Petersen *et al.* (1983)
50, 200 and 50 mg kg^{-1} d^{-1} for each of 2 weeks; two times 100 mg d^{-1} for 3 months	15	liver, lung, other	follow-up carried on for 3–7 years; 10 of 15 patients showed objective and clinical improvement; two of these relapsed 1–6 years after completing therapy; single liver and lung cysts showed best response; others showed little or no change	Kammerer and Schantz (1984)

Further publications: Lorenzo Garcia *et al.* (1980), Loughran and McCarey (1980), Mulhall (1980), Alvarez *et al.* (1981), Garcia Merida *et al.* (1981), Scholz and Michael (1981), Ammann *et al.* (1982), Fiennes and Thomas (1982), Kern and Dietrich (1982), Kern and Volkmer (1982), Shivashankar *et al.* (1982), van den Brink *et al.* (1983).

30–50 per cent of the patients may spontaneously eliminate their lung cysts (Pinch & Wilson 1973, Zhongxi *et al.* 1980).

Thus, it has to be concluded that the effect of the drug against cystic echinococcosis in humans is variable and insufficient to achieve cure in the majority of patients. This failure of success seems to be related to inadequate drug concentrations in the patients' plasma and secondarily in the parasite cysts (see above).

According to recent reports albendazole has better absorption properties than mebendazole, leading to more stable plasma drug levels after 2–4 d of treatment (Morris *et al.* 1983, Saimot *et al.* 1983). Treatment at daily doses

Table 9.7 Summary of selected recent data on chemotherapy of hepatic alveolar echinococcosis in humans.

Treatment	No. of patients	Results	Reference
flubendazole			
2–6 g per patient per day for 10–24 months	10	inconclusive	Mistilopoulos (1982)
50 mg kg^{-1} d^{-1} for 7–21 months	6	subjective improvement in all patients during first months of therapy; in three cases relapse of disease after interruption of chemotherapy, in two cases after re-treatment	Roche *et al.* (1982b)
mebendazole			
40 mg kg^{-1} d^{-1} for 1–30 months	12	clinical improvement in 11 patients after 3 months of therapy; one patient died after 6 months of therapy; liver lesions unchanged	Junge and Friedl (1982)
30–40 mg kg^{-1} d^{-1} for 5–34 months	24	clinical improvement in 11 of 15 symptomatic cases, one patient died after 8 months of therapy; in 10 monitored cases no definite signs of increase or decrease of lesions; in six radically operated cases no remission under treatment	Müller *et al.* (1982)
40 mg kg^{-1} d^{-1} for 6.4 years	5	no progression of the disease; no metastases formation; regression of lesions in one case; all patients well, survival 100 per cent after 9.5 years post-diagnosis as compared to 30 per cent of 13 untreated patients; one other patient with severe alcoholic liver disease and echinococcosis died 17 days after initiation of chemotherapy	Wilson and Rausch (1982)
50 mg kg^{-1} d^{-1} for continuous or intermittent	8	of seven patients, four showed clinical improvement and two showed reduction in size of lesions; no decline of antibody titres	Kern (1983)

Further publications: Ammann *et al.* (1982), Biedermann (1982), Härlin *et al.* (1982), Kern and Dietrich (1982), Klemm (1982), Lindboe *et al.* (1983).

of 10–14 mg kg^{-1} in single or repeated courses of 30 d resulted in a cure for three patients with hepatic cysts (Saimot *et al.* 1983) and in significant regression of cyst size in three or four other patients with involvement of liver, lungs and other organs (Morris *et al.* 1983). However, there was no evidence of improvement in five patients with bone hydatid disease although very high levels of the active metabolite, albendazole sulphoxide, were found in the bone (Saimot *et al.* 1983). In the study by Morris *et al.* (1983), one patient did not respond to a 2 month course of albendazole treatment.

Experiences with flubendazole treatment are limited (see Schantz *et al.* 1982); drug concentrations achieved in plasma and cysts are low and do not encourage further studies (Saimot *et al.* 1981, Morris & Gould 1982).

Chemotherapy of alveolar (*E. multilocularis*) echinococcosis

Oral mebendazole treatment at daily doses of 30–50 mg kg^{-1}, mainly applied continuously for periods of several months up to more than 6 years, has induced in the majority of the patients (Table 9.7) transient or usually long-lasting improvement of clinical parameters, including general condition, weight, pain, pruritus and serum concentrations of bilirubin, alkaline phosphatase and transaminases (see Table 9.7). Some of these patients had far advanced hepatic alveolar echinococcosis with metastatic lung lesions. In one study (Wilson & Rausch 1982), survival times of treated patients were significantly prolonged by comparison with untreated cases (Table 9.7). In the majority of patients the progressive course of the disease appeared to be arrested and metastases' formation prevented. On the other hand hepatic lesions extended into contiguous structures in five (16 per cent) of 32 untreated patients and distant metastases (brain, lung, mediastinum) were found in six (19 per cent) (Wilson & Rausch 1980). However, in treated patients regression of organ lesions was only rarely observed.

Parasite material removed by biopsy after 5, 16 and 30 months of continuous mebendazole treatment, respectively, resumed growth after transplantation to animals (Schantz *et al.* 1983). This finding together with persistence of high *Echinococcus* antibody levels may indicate that mebendazole treatment does not kill the parasite but prevents proliferation and metastases formation in humans as in laboratory animals (see above and Schantz *et al.* 1983).

Side effects of treatment

High doses of albendazole, flubendazole and mebendazole were generally well tolerated by patients with cystic and alveolar echinococcosis in previous and recent clinical trials (see Schantz *et al.* 1982, Tables 9.6 & 9.7). Apparent side effects observed in some of the patients include pain at the site of the cyst, allergic reactions, fevers, alopecia and reversible neutropenia (see Schantz *et al.* 1982, Kern 1983). Glomerulonephritis, probably due to immune complex or antigen trapping in glomerula of the kidney has been observed in a few cases of untreated (Sanchez Ibarrola *et al.* 1981) and mebendazole treated patients with cystic echinococcosis (Kern 1983). A previous report of severe progressive glomerulonephritis in African pastoralists after mebendazole treatment (French 1980) was recently supported by histological findings that five treated patients had variable degrees of diffuse proliferative changes whereas the kidneys of two untreated patients were normal (Kung'u 1982). It seems possible that both the primary disease and mebendazole treatment (the latter inducing intensive antigen release), are perhaps causally related to kidney lesions, especially in patients with heavy infections. Generalised amyloidosis, including the kidneys, has been observed in rodents infected with *E. multilocularis* (Ali-Khan *et al.* 1982, Mettler *et al.* 1982).

According to recent observations, reversible neutropenia apparently due to bone marrow suppression under high-dose mebendazole therapy, may occur in about 5 per cent of patients (Levin *et al.* 1983, Braithwaite *et al.* 1985). Evidence suggests that this toxic side effect is related to high plasma drug levels (Levin *et al.* 1983). Therefore, careful monitoring of plasma drug levels is recommended (Witassek *et al.* 1983).

The embryotoxic and teratogenic effects of several benzimidazole compounds observed in some animal species are reasons of concern for the use of these drugs for long-term treatment of human patients. Therefore, the WHO code of ethics and the recommended exclusion criteria for therapy have to be closely followed in clinical trials (WHO 1981b).

GENERAL CONCLUSIONS AND PROSPECTS

Since 1974 considerable progress has been achieved in chemotherapy of the metacestode stage of *Echinococcus*. In animals, cysts of *E. granulosus* can be killed and metacestodes of *E. multilocularis* inhibited in proliferation by chemotherapy with benzimidazole drugs. Adequate models and techniques for drug testing in animals are now available and considerable clinical, pharmacological and parasitological knowledge has accumulated. Treatment of human cases of cystic (*E. granulosus*) and alveolar (*E. multilocularis*) echinococcosis with albendazole, flubendazole and mebendazole has so far only been partially effective. However, experiences from animal experiments and human trials represent a basis for future studies, including new drugs with a better potential of efficacy against the metacestode stage of *Echinococcus*. As there is evidence that an effective chemotherapy of human echinococcosis may become feasible, intensive research should be continued and supported.

REFERENCES

Akovbiantz, A., R. Ammann and J. Eckert 1978. Gibt es eine Chemotherapie der Echinokokkose des Menschen? *Schweiz. Med. Wschr.* **108**, 1101–3.

Akovbiantz, A., J. Eckert, U. Hess and M. Schmid 1977. Clinical experience with mebendazole treatment of human echinococcosis. *XIth Int. Congr. Hydatidosis, Athens* 5.

Ali-Khan, Z., S. Jothy and R. Siboo 1982. Amyloidosis in experimental murine alveolar hydatidosis. *Trans. R. Soc. Trop. Med. Hyg.* **76**, 169–71.

Ali-Khan, Z., R. Siboo, M. Gomersall and M. Faucher 1983. Cystolytic events and the possible role of germinal cells in metastasis in chronic alveolar hydatidosis. *Ann. Trop. Med. Parasitol.* **77**, 497–512.

Alvarez, J. L. R., M. Carazo Carazo, L. R. Gonzales and D. D. Lopez 1981. Hidatidosis peritoneal secundaria masiva y mebendazol. *Revta Esp. Enf. Ap. Digest.* **59**, 255–66.

Amir-Jahed, A. K., R. Fardin, A. Farzad and K. Bakshandeh 1975. Clinical echinococcosis. *Ann. Surg.* **182**, 541–6.

Ammann, R., A. Akovbiantz, J. Eckert and F. Largiadèr 1979. Therapie der Echinokokkose. *Dt. Med. Wschr.* **104**, 1429–31.

Ammann, R., E. Müller, A. Akovbiantz, J. Bircher, J. Eckert, K. Wissler, F. Witassek, B. Wüthrich and W. Woodtli 1982. Medikamentöse Behandlung der Echinokokkose mit Mebendazol. In *Probleme der Echinokokkose unter Berücksichtigung parasitologischer und klinischer Aspekte*, R. Bähr (ed.), 92–5. Bern: Huber.

Andrews, P., H. Thomas, R. Pohlke and J. Seubert 1983. Praziquantel. *Med. Res. Rev.* **3**, 147–200.

Bähr, R. (ed.) 1982. *Probleme der Echinokokkose unter Berücksichtigung parasitologischer und klinischer Aspekte.* Bern: Huber.

Barandun, G. 1978. *Untersuchungen zur Chemotherapie der alveolären Echinokokkose und der* Mesocestoides corti-*Infektion bei Labortieren.* Veterinary dissertation, Zürich.

Bekhti, A., J. -P. Schaaps, M. Capron, J. -P. Dessaint, F. Santoro and A. Capron 1977. Treatment of hepatic hydatid disease with mebendazole: preliminary results in four cases. *Br. Med. J.* **2**, 1047–51.

Biedermann, H. 1982. Vier Jahre klinische Erfahrung mit der Mebendazol-Behandlung des inoperablen *Echinococcus multilocularis* bzw. des Rezidivs. In *Probleme der Echinokokkose unter Berücksichtigung parasitologischer und klinischer Aspekte*, R. Bähr (ed.), 98–9. Bern: Huber.

Borgers, M., S. De Nollin, A. Verheyen, O. Vanparijs and D. Thienpont 1975. Morphological changes in cysticerci of *Taenia taeniaeformis* after mebendazole treatment. *J. Parasitol.* **61**, 830–43.

Bortoletti, G. and G. Ferretti 1973. Investigation on larval forms of *Echinococcus granulosus* with electron microscope. *Riv. Parassitol.* **34**, 89–110.

Bortoletti, G. and G. Ferretti 1978. Ultrastructural aspects of fertile and sterile cysts of *Echinococcus granulosus* developed in hosts of different species. *Int. J. Parasitol.* **8**, 421–31.

Braithwaite, P. A., M. S. Roberts, R. J. Allan and T. R. Watson 1982. Clinical pharmacokinetics of high dose mebendazole in patients treated for cystic hydatid disease. *Eur. J. Clin. Pharmacol.* **22**, 161–9.

Braithwaite, P. A., R. J. Allan, M. Dawson, M. S. Roberts and T. R. Watson 1983. Cyst and host tissue concentrations of mebendazole in patients undergoing surgery for hydatid disease. *Med. J. Aust.* **2**, 383–4.

Braithwaite, P. A., R. J. S. Thomas and R. C. A. Thompson 1985. Hydatid disease: the alveolar variety in Australia. A case report with comment on the toxicity of mebendazole. *Aust. N.Z. J. Surg.*(in press).

Brugmans, J. P., D. C. Thienpont, I. van Wijngaarden, O. F. Vanparijs, V. L. Schuermans and H. L. Lauwers 1971. Mebendazole in enterobiasis: radiochemical and pilot clinical study in 1278 subjects. *J. Am. Med. Ass.* **217**, 313–6.

Bryceson, A. D. M., A. G. A. Cowie, C. MacLeod, S. White, D. Edwards, J. D. Smyth and D. P. McManus 1982a. Experience with mebendazole in the treatment of inoperable hydatid disease in England. *Trans. R. Soc. Trop. Med. Hyg.* **76**, 510–8.

Bryceson, A. D. M., R. Woestenborghs, M. Michiels and H. van den Bossche 1982b. Bioavailability and tolerability of mebendazole in patients with inoperable hydatid disease. *Trans. R. Soc. Trop. Med. Hyg.* **76**, 563–4.

Burkhardt, B. 1981. *Beiträge zur experimentellen Chemotherapie der larvalen Echinokokkose mit Untersuchungen zur biologischen Verfügbarkeit von Mebendazol bei Nagetieren.* Veterinary dissertation, Zürich.

Campbell, W. C. and L. S. Blair 1974a. Prevention and cure of hepatic cysticercosis in mice. *J. Parasitol.* **60**, 1049–52.

Campbell, W. C. and L. S. Blair 1974b. Treatment of the cystic stage of *Taenia crassiceps* and *Echinococcus multilocularis* in laboratory animals. *J. Parasitol.* **60**, 1053–4.

Chordi, A. and I. G. Kagan 1965. Identification and characterization of antigenic components of sheep hydatid fluid by immunoelectrophoresis. *J. Parasitol.* **51**, 63–71.

Coltorti, E. A. and V. M. Varela-Díaz 1972. IgG levels and host specificity in hydatid cyst fluid. *J. Parasitol.* **58**, 753–6.

Coltorti, E. A. and V. M. Varela-Díaz 1974. *Echinococcus granulosus*: Penetration of macromolecules and their localization on the parasite membranes of cysts. *Exp. Parasitol.* **35**, 225–31.

Coltorti, E. A. and V. M. Varela-Díaz 1975. Penetration of host IgG molecules into hydatid cysts. *Z. ParasitKde* **48**, 47–51.

Danis, M., G. Brücker, M. Gentilini, D. Richard-Lenoble and M. Smith 1977. Treatment of hepatic hydatid disease. *Br. Med. J.* **2**, 1356.

Drolshammer, I., E. Wiesmann and J. Eckert 1973. Echinokokkose beim Menschen in der Schweiz 1956–1969. *Schweiz. Med. Wschr.* **103**, 1337–41; 1386–92.

Eckert, J. 1980. Neue Medikamente gegen Echinokokkose. In *Importierte Infektionskrankheiten. Epidemiologie und Therapie*, O. Gsell (ed.), 136–40. Stuttgart: Thieme.

Eckert, J. and B. Burkhardt 1980. Chemotherapy of experimental echinococcosis. *Acta Tropica* **37**, 297–300.

Eckert, J. and P. Köhler 1983. Anthelmintics. In *Facts and reflections. IV. Resistance of parasites to anthelmintics*, F. H. M. Borgsteede, Sv. Aa. Henriksen and H. J. Over (eds), 61–78. Lelystad (Netherlands): Central Veterinary Institute.

Eckert, J. and J. Pohlenz 1976. Zur Wirkung von Mebendazol auf Metazestoden von *Mesocestoides corti* und *Echinococcus multilocularis. Tropenmed. Parasitol.* **27**, 247–62.

Eckert, J., J. Annen and G. Barandun 1977. Untersuchungen zur Chemotherapie der Echinokokkose. *Tropenmed. Parasitol.* **28**, 274–5.

Eckert, J., G. Barandun and J. Pohlenz 1978. Chemotherapie der larvalen Echinokokkose bei Labortieren. *Schweiz. Med. Wschr.* **108**, 1104–12.

Eckert, J., M. A. Gemmell and T. Wikerhauser 1981. Echinococcosis and other larval cestode infections. In *Review of advances in parasitology*, W. Slusarski (ed.), 365–92. Warszawa: PWN.

Eckert, J., R. C. A. Thompson and H. Mehlhorn 1983. Proliferation and metastases formation of larval *Echinococcus multilocularis*. 1. Animal model, macroscopical and histological findings. *Z. ParasitKde* **69**, 737–48.

Fiennes, A. G. T. W. and D. G. T. Thomas 1982. Combined medical and surgical treatment of spinal hydatid disease: a case report. *J. Neurol. Neurosurg. Psych.* **45**, 927–31.

Frayha, G. J. 1968. A study on the synthesis and absorption of cholesterol in hydatid cysts (*Echinococcus granulosus*). *Comp. Biochem. Physiol.* **27**, 875–8.

French, C. M. 1980. Experience with mebendazole therapy of hydatid disease in the Turkana District, Kenya. Workshop paper, 24–25 Nov. 1980, Janssen, Beerse (Belgium).

French, M. 1981. The treatment of *Echinococcus granulosus* infection in man in the Turkana district, north-western Kenya, from 1 January 1976 to June 1981. Paper presented at the WHO Parasite Discussion Programme, 29 June to 1 July 1981, Geneva.

Garcia Merida, M., P. Iglesia, J. A. Esteban and J. Alba 1981. Tratamiento de la siembra hidatidica peritoneal con mebendazol. Estudio preliminar. *An. Esp. Pediatr.* **14**, 160–7.

Gemmell, M. A. and P. D. Johnstone 1981. Cestodes. *Antibiot. Chemother.* **30**, 54–114.

Gemmell, M. A., S. N. Parmeter, R. J. Sutton and N. Khan 1981. Effect of mebendazole against *Echinococcus granulosus* and *Taenia hydatigena* cysts in naturally infected sheep and relevance to larval tapeworm infections in man. *Z. ParasitKde* **64**, 135–47.

Goodman, H. 1976. Mebendazole. *Med. J. Aust.* **2**, 662.

Gottstein, B., J. Eckert and H. Fey 1983. Serological differentiation between *Echinococcus granulosus* and *Echinococcus multilocularis* infections in man. *Z. ParasitKde* **69**, 347–56.

Gottstein, B., J. Eckert and W. Woodtli 1984. Determination of parasite-specific immunoglobulins using the ELISA in patients with echinococcosis treated with mebendazole. *Z. ParasitKde* **70**, 385–9.

Härlin, M., M. Weinzierl, U. Scherer and E. Egarter 1982. Abfall von indirektem Hämagglutinationstiter (IHA), indirektem Immunfluoreszenztiter (IFA) und Immunglobulin (IgE) unter zweijähriger Therapie mit Mebendazol bei *Echinococcus multilocularis* der Leber. In: *Probleme der Echinokokkose unter Berücksichtigung parasitologischer und klinischer Aspekte*, R. Bähr (ed.), 108–10. Bern: Huber.

Haertel, M., Ch. Fretz and W. A. Fuchs 1980. Zur computertomographischen Diagnose der Echinokokkose. *Fortschr. Röntgenstr.* **133**, 164–70.

Heath, D. D. and R. A. F. Chevis 1974. Mebendazole and hydatid cysts. *Lancet ii*, 218–9.

Heath, D. D. and S. B. Lawrence 1978. The effect of mebendazole and praziquantel on the cysts of *Echinococcus granulosus, Taenia hydatigena* and *T. ovis*. *N.Z. Vet. J.* **26**, 11–5.

Heath, D. D., M. J. Christie and R. A. F. Chevis 1975. The lethal effect of mebendazole on secondary *Echinococcus granulosus*, cysticerci of *Taenia pisiformis* and tetrathyridia of *Mesocestoides corti*. *Parasitology* **70**, 273–85.

Heykants, I., J. Geuens, H. Scheyground and H. van den Bossche 1979. Dose-dependence and influence of a meal on the absorption and plasma levels of flubendazole in volunteers. *Janssen Pharmaceutica Clin. Res. Rep.* R. 17889/18, June, Beerse, Belgium.

Hübener, K. H. and H. O. F. Metzger 1982. Computertomographische Diagnostik der Echinokokkose. In *Probleme der Echinokokkose unter Berücksichtigung parasitologischer und klinischer Aspekte*, R. Bähr (ed.), 75–9. Bern: Huber.

Hustead, S. T. and J. F. Williams 1977. Permeability studies on taeniid metacestodes. I. Uptake of proteins by larval stages of *Taenia taeniaeformis, T. crassiceps*, and *Echinococcus granulosus*. *J. Parasitol.* **63**, 314–21.

Junge, U. and P. Friedl 1982. Die medikamentöse Therapie des inoperablen *Echinococcus multilocularis* mit Mebendazol. In *Probleme der Echinokokkose unter Berücksichtigung parasitologischer und klinischer Aspekte*, R. Bähr (ed.), 100–3. Bern: Huber.

Kammerer, W. S. and D. M. Judge 1976. Chemotherapy of hydatid disease (*Echinococcus granulosus*) in mice with mebendazole and bithionol. *Am. J. Trop. Med. Hyg.* **25**, 714–7.

Kammerer, W. S. and K. L. Miller 1981. *Echinococcus granulosus*: permeability of hydatid cysts to mebendazole in mice. *Int. J. Parasitol.* **11**, 183–5.

Kammerer, W. S. and M. V. Perez-Esandi 1975. Chemotherapy of experimental *Echinococcus granulosus* infection. Trials in CF_1 mice and jirds (*Meriones unguiculatus*). *Am. J. Trop. Med. Hyg.* **24**, 90–5.

Kammerer, W. S. and P. M. Schantz 1984. Long term follow-up of human hydatid disease (*Echinococcus granulosus*) treated with a high-dose mebendazole regimen. *Am. J. Trop. Hyg.* **33**, 132–7.

Kasai, Y., S. Koshino, N. Kawanishi, H. Sakamoto, E. Sasaki and M. Kumagai 1980. Alveolar echinococcosis of the liver. Studies on 60 operated cases. *Ann. Surg.* **191**, 145–52.

Kern, P. 1983. Human echinococcosis: follow-up of 23 patients treated with mebendazole. *Infection* **11**, 17–24.

Kern, P. and M. Dietrich 1982. Wertigkeit der hochdosierten Mebendazol-Chemotherapie der Echinokokkose. In *Probleme der Echinokokkose unter Berücksichtigung parasitologischer und klinischer Aspekte.* R. Bähr (ed.), 104–5. Bern: Huber.

Kern, P. and K.-J. Volkmer 1982. Zystenruptur bei Patienten mit Lungenechinokokkose unter einer Chemotherapie mit Mebendazol. In *Probleme der Echinokokkose unter Berücksichtigung parasitologischer und klinischer Aspekte.* R. Bähr (ed.), 106–7. Bern: Huber.

Kern, P., M. Dietrich and K.-J. Volkmer 1979. Chemotherapy of echinococcosis with mebendazole: clinical observations of 7 patients. *Tropenmed. Parasitol.* **30**, 65–72.

Klemm, D. 1982. Erfolgreiche Mebendazol-Behandlung bei einem Fall von Leberechinokokkose mit Spontanperforation in den Magen. In *Probleme der Echinokokkose unter Berücksichtigung parasitologischer und klinischer Aspekte.* R. Bähr (ed.), 96–7. Bern: Huber.

Krotov, A. I., A. I. Chernyaeva and I. S. Budanova 1976. [Experimental therapy of alveococcosis. Part III. Influence of thiabendazole, sarcolysinacridine, levamisole and mebendazole on the development of *Alveococcus* larvocysts in albino mice.] *Med. Parazitol.* **45**, 164–8 (in Russian).

Krotov, A. I., A. I. Chernyaeva, F. P. Kovalenko, D. G. Bayandina, I. S. Budanova, O. E. Kuznetsova and L. V. Voskoboinik 1974. [Experimental therapy of alveococcosis. Part II. Effectiveness of some antinematode agents in the alveococcosis of laboratory animals.] *Med. Parazitol.* **43**, 314–9 (in Russian).

Kovalenko, F. P., A. I. Krotov, I. S. Budanova and Sh. A. Razakov 1976. [Experimental therapy of echinococcosis. Part I. Laboratory model of echinococcosis and influence exerted by sarcolysinacridine, levamisole and mebendazole on the development of *Echinococcus granulosus* larvocysts.] *Med. Parazitol.* **45**, 546–51 (in Russian).

Kungu'u, A. 1982. Glomerulonephritis following chemotherapy of hydatid disease with mebendazole. *E. Afr. Med. J.* **59**, 404–9.

Lehmann, J. C. 1928. Allgemeine Pathologie und Klinik der Echinokokkenkrankheit. In: *Die Echinokokkenkrankheit*, G. Hosemann, E. Schwarz, J. C. Lehmann and A. Posselt (eds), 115–304. Stuttgart: Enke.

Levin, M. H., R. A. Weinstein, J. L. Axelrod and P. M. Schantz 1983. Severe, reversible neutropenia during high-dose mebendazole therapy for echinococcosis. *J. Am. Med. Ass.* **249**, 2929–31.

Lindboe, C. F., J. A. Wilson and P. E. Hesla 1983. Echinokokkose. Et tilfelle av *Echinococcus multilocularis* cerebri behandlet med mebendazol. Tidsskr. Nor. Loegeforen **103**, 16–8.

Lorenzo Garcia, M. L., J. A. Rodriguez Montes, A. Tieso Herreros, J. Simal Fernandez, L. Asensio Prianes and S. Fernandez de Lis 1980. Posibilidades terapeuticas del mebendazol en la hidatidosis hepatica. *Revta Clin. Espanol.* **159**, 133–6.

Loughran, C. F. and A. G. McCarey 1980. Coincident pelvic and pulmonary hydatid disease in a young girl: the chest radiograph following treatment with mebendazole. *Br. J. Radiol.* **53**, 1020–51.

Luder, P. M., F. Witassek, K. Weigand, J. Eckert and J. Bircher 1985. Treatment of cystic echinococcosis (*Echinococcus granulosus*) with mebendazole: assessment of bound and free drug levels in cyst fluid and of parasite vitality in operative specimens. *Eur. J. Clin. Pharmacol.* **28**, 279–85.

Marshall, I. and G. T. Edwards 1982. The effects of sustained release praziquantel on the survival of protoscolices of *Echinococcus granulosus equinus* in laboratory mice. *Ann. Trop. Med. Parasitol.* **76**, 649–51.

Mehlhorn, H., J. Eckert and R. C. A. Thompson 1983. Proliferation and metastases formation of larval *Echinococcus multilocularis*. II. Ultrastructure. *Z. ParasitKde* **69**, 749–63.

Mettler, F., G. Barandun and B. Burkhardt 1982. Generalisierte Amyloidose bei der Wüstenrennmaus (*Meriones unguiculatus*) nach Infektion mit Finnen von *Echinococcus multilocularis*. *Zbl. Vet. Med. A* **29**, 704–9.

Mistilopoulos, S. 1982. *L'échinococcose alveolaire hepatique humaine.* Thèse, Université Besançon.

Morris, D. L. 1981. Management of hydatid disease. *Br. J. Hosp. Med.* June 1981, 586–90.

Morris, D. L. and S. E. Gould 1982. Serum and cyst concentrations of mebendazole and flubendazole in hydatid disease. *Br. Med. J.* **285**, 175.

Morris, D. L., P. W. Dykes, B. Dickson, S. E. Marriner, J. A. Bogan and F. G. O. Burrows 1983. Albendazole in hydatid disease. *Br. Med. J.* **286**, 103–4.

Morseth, D. J. 1967. Fine structure of the hydatid cyst and protoscolex of *Echinococcus granulosus*. *J. Parasitol.* **53**, 312–25.

Mosimann, F. 1980. Is alveolar hydatid disease of the liver incurable? *Ann. Surg.* **192**, 118–23.

Müller, E., A. Akovbiantz, R. W. Ammann, J. Bircher, J. Eckert, K. Wissler, F. Witassek and B. Wüthrich 1982. Treatment of human echinococcosis with mebendazole. Preliminary observations in 28 patients. *Hepato-gastroenterology* **29**, 236–9.

Münst, G. J., G. Karlaganis and J. Bircher 1979. Biologische Verfügbarkeit von Mebendazol als Voraussetzung einer wirksamen Pharmakotherapie der Echinokokkose. *Schweiz. Med. Wschr.* **109**, 627.

Münst, G. J., G. Karlaganis and J. Bircher 1980. Plasma concentrations of mebendazole during treatment of echinococcosis. Preliminary results. *Eur. J. Clin. Pharmacol.* **17**, 375–8.

Mulhall, P. P. 1980. Treatment of a ruptured hydatid cyst of lung with mebendazole. *Br. J. Dis. Chest* **74**, 306–8.

Okello, G. B. A. and A. K. Chemtai 1981. Treatment of hepatic hydatid disease with mebendazole: report of 16 cases. *E. Afr. Med. J.* **58**, 608–10.

Oppermann, H. C., R. G. Appell, F. Bostel, G. van Kaick and U. Wahn 1982. Mediastinal hydatid disease in childhood: CT documentation of response to treatment with mebendazole. *J. Comput. Assist. Tomogr.* **6**, 175–6.

Otto, R., W. Woodtli and R. Ammann 1982. Sonographie versus Computertomographie bei Lebermanifestationen der Echinokokkose. *Dt. Med. Wschr.* **107**, 1717–21.

Pawlowski, Z., B. Kozakiewicz and J. Zatonski 1976. Effect of mebendazole on hydatid cysts in pigs. *Vet. Parasitol.* **2**, 299–302.

Petersen, E., G. Thoren and R. Bergquist 1983. Mebendazole treatment of *Echinococcus granulosus* infection. Report of a case. *Am. J. Trop. Med. Hyg.* **32**, 1071–4.

Pinch, L. W. and J. F. Wilson 1973. Non-surgical management of cystic hydatid disease in Alaska: a review of 30 cases of *Echinococcus granulosus* infection treated without operation. *Ann. Surg.* **178**, 45–8.

Pirschel, J. 1982. Sonographie der Echinokokkose. In *Probleme der Echinokokkose unter Berücksichtigung parasitologischer und klinischer Aspekte*, R. Bähr (ed.), 69–74. Bern: Huber.

Posselt, A. 1928. Der Alveolarechinokokkus und seine Chirurgie. In *Die Echinokokkenkrankheit*, G. Hosemann, E. Schwarz, J. C. Lehmann and A. Posselt (eds), 303–418. Stuttgart: Enke.

Prichard, R. K. 1978. Sheep anthelmintics. In *The epidemiology and control of gastrointestinal parasites of sheep in Australia*. A. D. Donald, W. H. Southcott and J. K. Dineen (eds), 75–107. Sydney: Division of Animal Health, CSIRO.

Reisin, I. L., C. A. Rabito, C. A. Rotunno and M. Cereijido 1977. The permeability of the membranes of experimental secondary cysts of *Echinococcus granulosus* to [^{14}C]mebendazole. *Int. J. Parasitol.* **7**, 189–94.

Repetto, Y. and A. Morello 1981. Detoxification mechanisms in *Echinococcus granulosus*: glutathione-*S*-transferase. *IRCS Med. Sci.* **9**, 698.

Richards, K. S., C. Arme and J. F. Bridges 1983. *Echinococcus granulosus equinus*: an ultrastructural study of the laminated layer, including changes on incubating cysts in various media. *Parasitology* **86**, 399–405.

Robotti, G. 1983. Quantitative radiologische Verlaufskontrolle bei *Echinococcus multilocularis*-Befall. *Abstr. Symp. aktuelle Probleme Echinokokkose, Zürich.*

Roche, G., Ph. Canton, A. Gerard and J. B. Dureux 1982a. Traitement de l'échinococcose alvéolaire du foie par le flubendazole. Etude pharmacologique. *Path. Biol., Paris* **30**, 452–7.

Roche, G., Ph. Canton, A. Gerard, D. Colin, P. Boissel, C. Chaulieu and J. B. Dureux 1982b. Essai de traitement de l'échinococcose alvéolaire par le flubendazole. A propos de 7 observations. *Méd. Malad. Infect.* **12**, 218–30.

Rotunno, C. A., W. S. Kammerer, M. V. Pérez Esandi and M. Cereijido 1974. Studies on the permeability to water, sodium and chloride of the hydatid cyst of *Echinococcus granulosus*. *J. Parasitol.* **60**, 613–20.

Saimot, A. G., A. Meulemans, J. M. Hay, J. Mohler, C. Manuel and J. P.

Coulaud 1981. Etude pharmacocinétique du flubendazole au cours de l'hydatidose humaine à *E. granulosus*. *Nouv. Presse Méd.* **10**, 3121–4.

Saimot, A. G., A. C. Cremieux, J. M. Hay, A. Meulemans, M. D. Giovanangeli, B. Delaitre and J. P. Coulaud 1983. Albendazole as a potential treatment for human hydatidosis. *Lancet ii*, 652–6.

Sakamoto, T. 1977. Die cestozide Wirkung von Praziquantel auf die Larvenstadien von *Hydatigera taeniaeformis, Mesocestoides corti* und *Echinococcus multilocularis* bei Labortieren. *Vet. Med. Nachr., Marburg* **2**, 153–62.

Sanchez Ibarrola, A. S., B. Sobrini, J. Guisantes, J. Pardo, J. Diez, J. M. Monfa and A. Purroy 1981. Membranous glomerulonephritis secondary to hydatid disease. *Am. J. Med.* **70**, 311–5.

Schantz, P. M. 1982. Echinococcosis. In *CRC handbook series in zoonoses*, J. H. Steele (ed.), *Section C: Parasitic Zoonoses*, Vol. I, Parts 1/2, 231–77. Boca Raton, Fla: CRC Press.

Schantz, P. M. and I. G. Kagan 1980. Echinococcosis (hydatidosis). In *Immunological investigation of tropical diseases*. V. Houba (ed.), 104–29. Edinburgh: Churchill Livingstone.

Schantz, P. M., H. van den Bossche and J. Eckert 1982. Chemotherapy for larval echinococcosis in animals and humans: report of a workshop. *Z. ParasitKde* **67**, 5–26.

Schantz, P. M., J. F. Wilson, S. P. Wahlquist, L. P. Boss and R. L. Rausch 1983. Serological tests for diagnosis and post-treatment evaluation of patients with alveolar hydatid disease (*Echinococcus multilocularis*). *Am. J. Trop. Med. Hyg.* **32**, 1381–6.

Schicker, H. J. 1976. *Die Echinokokkose des Menschen. Stand von Diagnose, Therapie und Prognose bei Echinokokkenerkrankungen in Baden-Württemberg in den Jahren 1960 bis 1972*. Dissertation, Tübingen.

Scholz, A. and C. Michael 1981. Zur Therapie der *Echinococcus multilocularis*-Erkrankung mit Mebendazol. *Med. Welt* **32**, 1541–4.

Shivashankar, A., L. H. Lature and P. S. Shankar 1982. Treatment of pulmonary hydatid cyst with mebendazole. *J. Ass. Physns India* **30**, 317–8.

Swiderski, Z. and J. Eckert 1978. Ultrastructural changes of larval *Echinococcus multilocularis* tissue caused by mebendazole treatment. *Fourth Int. Congr. Parasitol. Warszawa*, Sect. C, II, 7, 130–1.

Thienpont, D., O. Vanparijs and L. Hermans 1974a. The anthelmintic action of mebendazole on *Cysticercus fasciolaris* in mice. *Proc. Third Int. Congr. Parasitol. München* **2**, 593.

Thienpont, D., O. Vanparijs and L. Hermans 1974b. Anthelmintic activity of mebendazole against *Cysticercus fasciolaris*. *J. Parasitol.* **60**, 1052–3.

Thienpont, D., O. Vanparijs and L. Hermans 1976. Anthelmintic activity of flubendazole on larval stages of *Echinococcus granulosus* in mice. Preclinical research report, Janssen Pharmaceutica, Beerse, Belgium.

Tinar, R. 1979. Contribution á l'étude d'efficacité de quelques anthelminthiques nouveaux sur les kystes hydatiques chez les agneaux infestés expérimentalement. *Veteriner Fakültesi Dergisi* **26**, 145–68.

Thomas, H. and R. Gönnert 1978. Zur Wirksamkeit von Praziquantel bei der experimentellen Cysticercose und Hydatidose. *Z. ParasitKde* **55**, 165–79.

Van den Bossche, H. 1980. Peculiar targets in anthelmintic chemotherapy. *Biochem. Pharmacol.* **29**, 1981–90.

Van den Brink, W. T. J., F. van Knapen and A. M. van der Elst 1983. [Treatment of echinococcosis with mebendazole (Vermox) in a patient with multiple cysts.]

Ned. Tijdschr. Geneeskd. **127**, 423–8 (in Dutch).

Van Wijngaarden, I. 1971. Excretion and metabolism of ^{14}C-labelled mebendazole in rats and men. Janssen Pharmaceutica Biological Research Report R 17635/2, Beerse (Belgium).

Varela-Díaz, V. M. and E. A. Coltorti 1972. Further evidence of the passage of host immunoglobulins into hydatid cysts. *J. Parasitol.* **58**, 1015–6.

Varela-Díaz, V. M. and E. A. Coltorti 1973. The presence of host immunoglobulins in hydatid cyst membranes. *J. Parasitol.* **59**, 484–8.

Varela-Díaz, V. M., E. A. Guarnera, N. Marchevsky, L. Rapoport, H. Conesa and S. Espinola 1983. Review of hospital cases in the assessment of hydatidosis as a health problem in the Argentine province of Chubut. *Z. ParasitKde* **69**, 507–15.

Verheyen, A. 1982. *Echinococcus granulosus*: the influence of mebendazole therapy on the ultrastructural morphology of the germinal layer of hydatid cysts in humans and mice. *Z. ParasitKde* **67**, 55–65.

Verheyen, A., O. Vanparijs, M. Borgers and D. Thienpont 1978. Scanning electron microscopic observations of *Cysticercus fasciolaris* (*Taenia taeniaeformis*) after treatment of mice with mebendazole. *J. Parasitol.* **64**, 411–25.

Vogel, H. 1978. Wie wächst der Alveolarechinokokkus? *Tropenmed. Parasitol.* **29**, 1–11.

Walther, E. 1982. Konventionelle Röntgendiagnostik der Echinokokkose. In *Probleme der Echinokokkose unter Berücksichtigung parasitologischer und klinischer Aspekte*, R. Bähr (ed.), 61–8. Bern: Huber.

Wang, J., B. Yifang, X. Guanghua, J. Changfa, G. Liren, Q. Jinggi, L. Ruilin, Z. Jiqun and J. Yulong 1981. [Effect of mebendazole in experimental treatment of cysticerciasis.] *Acta Acad. Med. Sin.* **3**, 63–5.

WHO 1981a. *FAO/UNEP/WHO Guidelines for surveillance, prevention and control of echinococcosis/hydatidosis*, J. Eckert, M. A. Gemmell and E. J. L. Soulsby (eds). Geneva: World Health Organisation.

WHO 1981b. *Treatment of human echinococcosis*, Report of an Informal WHO Meeting, 29 June–1 July, PDP/82.1. Geneva: World Health Organisation.

Wilson, J. F. and R. L. Rausch 1980. Alveolar hydatid disease. A review of clinical features of 33 indigenous cases of *Echinococcus multilocularis* infection in Alaskan Eskimos. *Am. J. Trop. Med. Hyg.* **29**, 1340–55.

Wilson, J. F. and R. L. Rausch 1982. Mebendazole and alveolar hydatid disease. *Ann. Trop. Med. Parasitol.* **76**, 165–73.

Wilson, J. F., M. Davidson and R. L. Rausch 1978. A clinical trial of mebendazole in the treatment of alveolar hydatid disease. *Am. Rev. Resp. Dis.* **118**, 747–57.

Witassek, F. and J. Bircher 1983. Chemotherapy of larval echinococcosis with mebendazole: microsomal liver function and cholestasis as determinants of plasma drug level. *Eur. J. Clin. Pharmacol.* **25**, 85–90.

Witassek, F., R. J. Allan, T. R. Watson, W. Woodtli, R. Ammann and J. Bircher 1983. Preliminary observations on the biliary elimination of mebendazole and its metabolites in patients with echinococcosis. *Eur. J. Clin. Pharmacol.* **25**, 81–4.

Witassek, F., B. Burkhardt, J. Eckert and J. Bircher 1981. Chemotherapy of alveolar echinococcosis. Comparison of plasma mebendazole concentrations in animals and man. *Eur. J. Clin. Pharmacol.* **20**, 427–33.

Zhongxi, Q., G. Shuiyuan, T. Guoxue, L. Ruilin, W. Mingbai, Q. Jun and Kurban 1980. Evaluation of Barrett's technique in 167 cases of pulmonary hydatid cyst. *Chinese Med. J.* **93**, 577–80.

Index

Readers should note that many major items such as 'antigens', 'biochemistry', 'chemotherapy', 'immunology', etc. are to be found under their own headings rather than as umbrella entries under '*Echinococcus*' or 'hydatid disease'. Numbers in italics refer to text illustrations.